Workbook and Competency Evaluation Review

Mosby's Essentials for Nursing Assistants

Sixth Edition

Kimberly Gibbs, BSN, RN
Director of Nursing
Kindred Healthcare
Louisville, Kentucky

ELSEVIER

ELSEVIER

3251 Riverport Lane
St. Louis, Missouri 63043

WORKBOOK AND COMPETENCY EVALUATION REVIEW FOR
MOSBY'S ESSENTIALS FOR NURSING ASSISTANTS, SIXTH EDITION

ISBN: 978-0-323-56968-2

Notices

Knowledge and best practice in this field are constantly changing. As new research and experience broaden our understanding, changes in research methods, professional practices, or medical treatment may become necessary.

Practitioners and researchers must always rely on their own experience and knowledge in evaluating and using any information, methods, compounds, or experiments described herein. In using such information or methods they should be mindful of their own safety and the safety of others, including parties for whom they have a professional responsibility.

With respect to any drug or pharmaceutical products identified, readers are advised to check the most current information provided (i) on procedures featured or (ii) by the manufacturer of each product to be administered, to verify the recommended dose or formula, the method and duration of administration, and contraindications. It is the responsibility of practitioners, relying on their own experience and knowledge of their patients, to make diagnoses, to determine dosages and the best treatment for each individual patient, and to take all appropriate safety precautions.

To the fullest extent of the law, neither the Publisher nor the authors, contributors, or editors, assume any liability for any injury and/or damage to persons or property as a matter of products liability, negligence or otherwise, or from any use or operation of any methods, products, instructions, or ideas contained in the material herein.

International Standard Book Number: 978-0-323-56968-2

Senior Content Strategist: Nancy O'Brien
Content Development Manager: Luke Held
Content Development Specialist: Kelly Skelton
Publishing Services Manager: Deepthi Unni
Senior Project Manager: G Janish Paul
Design Direction: Renee Duenow

Printed in United States

Last digit is the print number: 9 8 7 6 5 4 3

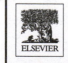

PREFACE

This workbook is written to be used with *Mosby's Essentials for Nursing Assistants*, sixth edition, by Sheila A. Sorrentino and Leighann N. Remmert. Any reference to the "textbook" in this workbook refers to *Mosby's Essentials for Nursing Assistants*, sixth edition.

This workbook is designed to help you apply what you have learned in each chapter. You are encouraged to use this workbook as a study guide. Various types of study questions (matching, fill in the blank, multiple choice, and labeling) and other learning activities are included to help you understand and apply the information in the textbook.

Case Studies are provided for each chapter. They will help you think about what you have learned and apply your knowledge in practical situations. The **Additional Learning Activities** encourage discussion and practical application of the information presented in each chapter. These activities are meant to challenge you and expand the learning experience.

Procedure Checklists are provided that correspond with the procedures in *Mosby's Essentials for Nursing Assistants*, sixth edition. NATCEP® skills are identified. These checklists are intended to help you become confident and skilled when performing procedures that affect the quality of care you provide.

The answers to the workbook questions are provided as part of the instructor resources. Your instructor will provide the answers as needed.

The **Competency Evaluation Review** includes a general review section and two practice exams with answers to help you prepare for the written certification exam. It also features a skills review guide that helps you practice procedures required for certification.

Nursing assistants are important members of the health team. Completing the exercises in this workbook will increase your knowledge, skills, and confidence. The goal is to prepare you to provide the best possible care and to help you develop pride in the important work you do.

1 INTRODUCTION TO HEALTH CARE

MATCHING

Match each term with the correct definition.

1. _____ A nurse who has completed a 1-year nursing program and has passed a licensing test
2. _____ Provides emergency care, surgery, nursing care, x-ray procedures and treatments, and laboratory testing
3. _____ The many health care workers whose skills and knowledge focus on the person's total care
4. _____ Provides a room, meals, laundry, and supervision
5. _____ A person who has passed a nursing assistant training and competency evaluation program; performs delegated nursing tasks under the supervision of a licensed nurse
6. _____ A governing body
7. _____ An agency or program for persons who are dying
8. _____ Those who provide nursing care; RNs, LPNs/LVNs, and nursing assistants
9. _____ A nurse who has completed a 2-, 3-, or 4-year nursing program and has passed a licensing test
10. _____ Provides housing, personal care, support services, health care, and social activities in a home-like setting to persons needing help with daily activities

A. Board and care home
B. Health care team (interdisciplinary health team)
C. Licensed practical nurse (LPN)
D. Registered nurse (RN)
E. Hospitals
F. Nursing team
G. Nursing assistant
H. Board of trustees or Board of directors
I. Assisted living residence (ALR)
J. Hospice

Match each description with the correct health team member.

11. _____ Diagnoses and treats diseases and injuries
12. _____ Assesses and plans for nutritional needs. Teaches about diet and healthy eating
13. _____ Prevents, diagnoses, and treats foot disorders
14. _____ Assists ill and injured persons with movement and pain management
15. _____ Diagnoses and treats communication and swallowing disorders
16. _____ Deals with social, emotional, and environmental issues affecting illness and recovery
17. _____ Assists nurses and gives care. Supervised by a licensed nurse
18. _____ Tests hearing; prescribes hearing aids; works with persons who are hard-of-hearing

A. Physical therapist
B. Podiatrist
C. Speech-language pathologists/speech therapist
D. Audiologist
E. Dietitian
F. Social worker
G. Physician
H. Nursing assistant

FILL IN THE BLANKS

19. Hospitals and long-term care centers provide _____ health care services. _____ is the focus of care.

20. Define the following terms.

   A. Acute illness _____

   _____

   _____

   B. Chronic illness _____

   _____

   _____

   C. Terminal illness _____

   _____

   _____

ADDITIONAL LEARNING ACTIVITIES

1. Search for the information online. List the hospitals, nursing centers, and assisted living residences (ALRs) in your community. If the services provided are identified, list them.

2. Collect brochures from the hospitals, nursing centers, and ALRs in your community. Compare the content.
   A. What services are provided?

   B. Are hospice services available?

   C. Is Alzheimer disease and dementia care available?

D. What other information about the hospital, nursing center, or ALR is provided?

3. Look at your health insurance policy.
   A. Do you know which services are covered and which are not?

   B. Does your policy limit where you can go for health care? Explain.

2 THE PERSON'S RIGHTS

MATCHING

Match each term with the correct definition.

1. _____ Someone who supports or promotes the needs and interests of another person
2. _____ The care provided to maintain or restore health, improve function, or relieve symptoms
3. _____ Separating a person from others against his or her will, keeping the person in a certain area, or keeping the person away from his or her room without consent
4. _____ A person with the legal right to act on the patient's or resident's behalf when he or she cannot do so for himself or herself
5. _____ A federal law requiring that nursing centers provide care in a manner and in a setting that maintains or improves each person's quality of life, health, and safety

A. Involuntary seclusion
B. Ombudsman
C. Representative
D. Treatment
E. Omnibus Budget Reconciliation Act of 1987 (OBRA)

Match the action to promote dignity and privacy with the example.

6. _____ You gain the person's attention before giving care.
7. _____ You close the door when the person asks for privacy.
8. _____ You take the resident to his or her weekly card game.
9. _____ You cover the resident with a blanket during a bath.
10. _____ You show interest when a resident tells stories about his or her past.
11. _____ You file fingernails and apply polish as the resident requests.
12. _____ You make sure the resident is wearing his or her dentures when he or she goes to the dining room.
13. _____ You allow the resident to smoke in a designated area.
14. _____ You open containers and arrange food at meal times to assist the resident.

A. Courteous and dignified interaction
B. Courteous and dignified care
C. Privacy and self-determination
D. Personal choice and independence

FILL IN THE BLANKS

15. _____

_____ explains the person's rights and expectations during hospital stays.

16. Nursing centers must inform residents of their rights.
    A. When are residents informed of their rights?

    _____

    _____

B. How are residents informed of their rights?

_____

_____

_____

17. An _____ is used to inform a person of his or her rights if the person speaks and understands a foreign language or communicates by sign language.

18. Residents have the right to be free from abuse. This includes _____
_____.

19. Involuntary seclusion involves:

   A. _____
   _____
   _____

   B. _____
   _____
   _____

   C. _____
   _____
   _____

20. A doctor's order is needed for restraint use. Restraints are not used:

   A. For _____

   B. To _____

21. Nursing center activity programs enhance each person's _____
_____

MULTIPLE CHOICE

*Circle the **BEST** answer.*

22. Nursing center residents have the right to information. This includes the following *except* the right to
   A. See all of his or her records
   B. Be fully informed of his or her total condition
   C. Information about his or her doctor
   D. Information about his or her roommate

23. If a person does not give consent or refuses treatment, treatment cannot be given.
   A. True
   B. False

24. A resident received a letter from her daughter. You know that the person cannot read. You can open the letter without the person's consent.
   A. True
   B. False

25. Which action promotes courteous and dignified care?
   A. Styling the person's hair the way you like it
   B. Rearranging pictures in the person's room
   C. Allowing the person to choose what clothing to wear
   D. Doing everything for the person

26. Which action does *not* promote the person's privacy?
   A. Draping the person properly during care procedures
   B. Knocking on the door before entering the person's room
   C. Closing the bathroom door when the person uses the bathroom
   D. Providing care with the room door open

27. Residents have the right to choose which activities they wish to attend.
   A. True
   B. False

28. When residents and their families plan activities together, this meets the resident's right to
   A. Privacy
   B. Freedom from restraint
   C. Freedom from mistreatment
   D. Participate in resident and family groups

29. The resident you are caring for has many old holiday decorations covering her nightstand. If you throw away these items without her permission, you are denying her right to
   A. Privacy
   B. Work
   C. Keep and use personal items
   D. Freedom from abuse

30. A staff member tells a resident he cannot leave his room because he talks too much. This action denies the resident
   A. Freedom from abuse, mistreatment, and neglect (involuntary seclusion)
   B. Freedom from restraint
   C. Care and security of personal possessions
   D. Personal choice

31. When a resident is given certain drugs that affect his mood, behavior, or mental function, it may deny his right to
   A. Privacy
   B. Personal choice
   C. Freedom from restraint
   D. Freedom from abuse, mistreatment, and neglect

32. Which statement about restraints is *correct?*
   A. Restraints are always used when patients and residents are confused.
   B. To keep them safe, all older patients and residents are restrained at night.
   C. Restraints are always used for persons at risk for falling.
   D. A doctor's order is needed for restraint use.

CASE STUDY

Mrs. Joan Jeffers is an 86-year-old woman who suffers from dementia. She has been a resident at your facility for 5 years. She does not have any family that visits her on a regular basis. She has recently become combative and refuses to take baths. She says that "people are spying on her." You have noticed other staff members keeping her in bed for long periods at a time, and when she refuses a bath, they move on to the next resident. Mrs. Jeffers is beginning to have an odor, and today is bath day.

Answer the following questions:
1. What is your next appropriate action?

2. Does Mrs. Jeffers have the right to refuse a bath? Explain.

3. What could you do to help Mrs. Jeffers feel more at ease about bathing?

ADDITIONAL LEARNING ACTIVITIES

1. Visit a nursing center and ask for a copy of the Residents' Rights. Compare it with the information in this chapter. Was it the same? Was it different?

2. When you visit the nursing center, ask if you could speak with the director of nursing. If available, ask the director of nursing how he or she ensures residents' rights are met on a daily basis. Describe his or her answer below.

MATCHING

Match each term with the correct definition.

1. _____ To authorize another person to perform a nursing task in a certain situation
2. _____ Having the necessary ability, knowledge, or skill to perform a task safely and successfully
3. _____ A document that describes what the agency expects you to do
4. _____ Official recognition by a state that standards or requirements have been met
5. _____ Nursing care or a nursing function, procedure, activity, or work that can be delegated to nursing assistants when it does not require a nurse's professional knowledge or judgment

A. Delegate
B. Certification
C. Job description
D. Nursing task
E. Competent

FILL IN THE BLANKS

6. The Omnibus Budget Reconciliation Act of 1987 (OBRA) requires each state to have a nursing assistant

_____

_____

It must be successfully completed by nursing assistants working in _____

_____

_____

_____.

7. The _____ is an official listing of persons who have successfully completed a nursing assistant training and competency evaluation program.

8. What information about each nursing assistant is contained in the nursing assistant registry?

A. _____

_____

B. _____

_____

C. _____

_____

D. _____

_____

E. _____

_____

F. _____

_____

G. _____

_____

9. Agencies must provide educational programs for nursing assistants. They must also evaluate their work. What is the purpose of these requirements?

_____

_____

_____

_____

10. To protect persons from harm, you must understand:

A. _____

B. _____

C. _____

11. Before you perform a nursing task, you must make sure that:

A. _____

_____

B. _____

_____

C. _____

_____

D. _____

_____

12. The _____

tells you what the agency expects you to do.

13. Do not take a job that requires you to:

A. _____

_____

B. _____

_____

C. _____

_____

14. List eight role limits for nursing assistants (things a nursing assistant should never do).

A. _____

_____

B. _____

_____

C. _____

_____

D. _____

_____

E. _____

_____

F. _____

_____

G. _____

_____

H. _____

_____

15. RNs can delegate nursing tasks to _____

_____

16. Delegation decisions must protect _____

_____

17. List the four steps of delegation described by the National Council of State Boards of Nursing (NCSBN).

A. _____

_____

B. _____

_____

C. _____

_____

D. _____

_____

18. During the communication step, the nurse must provide clear and complete directions about the following.

A. _____

_____

B. _____

_____

C. _____

_____

D. _____

_____

E. _____

_____

F. _____

_____

19. After completing a delegated task, you must ____

_____.

20. The *Five Rights of Delegation* for nursing assistants is another way to view the delegation process. List the *Five Rights of Delegation*.

A. _____

_____

B. _____

_____

C. _____

_____

D. _____

_____

E. _____

_____

21. Write the meanings of the following abbreviations.

A. OBRA _____

_____

B. NATCEP _____

_____

C. NCSBN _____

_____

MULTIPLE CHOICE

Circle the **BEST** *answer.*

22. OBRA requires each state to have a nursing assistant training program. How many hours of instruction does OBRA require?
    A. 16
    B. 40
    C. 50
    D. 75

23. To successfully complete the competency evaluation, how many attempts does OBRA allow you?
    A. Only one attempt
    B. At least two attempts
    C. At least three attempts
    D. At least four attempts

24. The nursing assistant registry is
    A. A skills evaluation
    B. A list of rules and responsibilities for nursing assistants
    C. An official listing of persons who have successfully completed a nursing assistant training and competency evaluation program
    D. A procedure book

25. Retraining and a new competency evaluation program are required
    A. For nursing assistants who have not worked for 24 months
    B. Whenever a nursing assistant changes jobs
    C. If a nursing assistant has a poor performance review
    D. Whenever a nursing assistant is accused of abuse

26. Nursing assistants
    A. Function under the supervision of licensed nurses
    B. Decide what should or should not be done for a person
    C. Supervise other nursing assistants
    D. Take telephone orders from the doctor

27. The nurse asks you to perform a task that is not in your job description. You should
    A. Perform the task after the nurse shows you how
    B. Refuse to perform the task and explain why
    C. Ask a co-worker to assist you with the task
    D. Report the nurse to the administrator

28. The nurse asks you to apply an ankle brace to a patient's right ankle. You do not understand the directions. What should you do?
    A. Ask the patient to tell you how to apply the brace.
    B. Ask the nursing assistant who cared for the patient yesterday to show you how to apply the brace.
    C. Ask another nursing assistant to apply the brace.
    D. Explain to the nurse that you do not understand the instructions.

29. You agree to perform a task. You must do the following *except*
    A. Complete the task safely
    B. Ask for help when you are unsure
    C. Report what you did and your observations to the nurse
    D. Delegate the task to another nursing assistant if you are busy

30. You can refuse to perform a delegated task for the following reasons *except*
    A. The task is not in your job description
    B. You do not know how to use the equipment
    C. You do not want to perform the task because it is unpleasant
    D. The nurse's directions are unclear

31. Nursing assistants *do not* delegate.
    A. True
    B. False

32. Which is *not* a standard for nursing assistants?
    A. Respecting the person's decision
    B. Carrying out the directions and instructions of the nurse if you have time
    C. Functioning as a member of the health team
    D. Keeping the person's information confidential

33. An RN asks you to perform a task beyond the legal limits of your role. You agree to perform the task. Harm is caused. Who is responsible?
    A. You and the RN
    B. Only the RN
    C. Only you
    D. The entire nursing team

34. Sometimes refusing to follow the nurse's directions is your right and duty.
    A. True
    B. False

CASE STUDY

You work in a busy nursing center. Today you are responsible for caring for 12 residents. You have been able to keep up with all of your duties; however, the nurse is running behind on her day's task. She has requested you to deliver Miss Jones's medications to her. Miss Jones is alert and oriented. She knows what medications she takes and is able to swallow them without difficulties.

1. Is this a task within your role? Explain.

2. How do you respond to the nurse delegating this task to you?

3. Do you need to report the nurse's request to anyone? Explain.

ADDITIONAL LEARNING ACTIVITIES

1. Read the nursing assistants standards.
    A. List ways you might apply these standards in a job setting.
    B. Discuss the importance of these standards with your classmates.

4 ETHICS AND LAW

MATCHING

Match each term with the correct definition.

1. _____ Laws dealing with relationships between people
2. _____ Laws concerned with offenses against the public and society in general
3. _____ Injuring a person's name and reputation by making false statements to a third person
4. _____ The willful infliction of injury, unreasonable confinement, intimidation, or punishment that results in physical harm, pain, or mental anguish
5. _____ Saying or doing something to trick, fool, or deceive a person
6. _____ Unlawful restraint or restriction of a person's freedom of movement
7. _____ Violating a person's right not to have his or her name, photo, or private affairs exposed or made public without giving consent
8. _____ An unintentional wrong in which a person did not act in a reasonable and careful manner and a person or the person's property was harmed
9. _____ An act, behavior, or comment that is sexual in nature
10. _____ A rule of conduct made by a government body
11. _____ A person's behaviors and way of living that threaten his or her health, safety, and well-being
12. _____ Any knowing, intentional, or negligent act by a caregiver or any other person to an older adult; the act causes harm or serious risk of harm

A. Negligence
B. Fraud
C. Civil law
D. Elder abuse
E. False imprisonment
F. Law
G. Abuse
H. Criminal law
I. Self-neglect
J. Invasion of privacy
K. Defamation
L. Professional sexual misconduct

FILL IN THE BLANKS

13. Ethical behavior involves not being _____

    or _____ .

14. You discuss with a patient the problems you are

    having disciplining your teenager. This is _____

    _____ .

15. False imprisonment involves:

    A. _____

    B. _____

    C. _____

16. The Health Insurance Portability and Accountability Act of 1996 (HIPAA) protects the privacy and security of a person's health information. Protected health information refers to:

    A. _____

    B. _____

    _____

17. Failure to comply with HIPAA rules can result in

    _____

    _____ .

18. You are admitting a person to the hospital. You tell the person that you are a nurse. This is _____.

19. Consent is informed when _____

_____

_____

20. A patient is unconscious. The doctor orders intravenous therapy and oxygen. How is legal consent for these treatments obtained?

_____

_____

_____.

21. List three ways in which a person may give consent.

    A. _____

    B. _____

    C. _____

22. Abuse is a crime. Abuse has one or more of the following elements.

    A. _____

    B. _____

    C. _____

    D. _____

    E. _____

23. A nursing center resident is allowed to lie in bed in the same position all day. The person's son finds her bed wet with urine when he visits. The person is crying. The staff is guilty of _____.

24. You see a resident's daughter slap him. This is

_____.

25. Involuntary seclusion is _____

_____

26. A person refuses to take needed drugs and does not keep doctors' appointments. The person has poor nutrition and poor hygiene and refuses help from others. This is _____.

27. Child abuse and neglect involves

    A. _____

    B. _____

    C. _____

28. If you suspect intimate partner violence, share your concerns with _____.

29. Write the meanings of the following abbreviations.

    A. HIPAA _____

    _____

    B. OBRA _____

    _____

    C. CDC _____

    _____

    D. IPV _____

    _____

MULTIPLE CHOICE

30. The Code of Conduct for nursing assistants states
    A. Take risk when completing a task
    B. Follow the lead nursing assistant's direction
    C. Take drugs that do not belong to you because you are in pain
    D. Keep the person's information confidential

31. Maintaining professional boundaries includes
    A. Kissing your resident on the cheek
    B. Balancing your resident's checkbook
    C. Taking a resident to your home for Christmas because they do not have any family
    D. Not using any offensive language

32. A tort is
    A. A pastry
    B. A wrong committed against a person
    C. A wrong committed against an animal
    D. A criminal offense

33. You tell a co-worker a false statement about your nurse. You have committed
    A. Slander
    B. Libel
    C. False imprisonment
    D. Abuse

34. You observe another nursing assistant taking a picture of a resident. You tell your supervisor because
    A. This is abuse
    B. This is a HIPAA violation
    C. This is fraud
    D. This is defamation

35. Informed consent is given by a
    A. Responsible party
    B. Sedated person
    C. Confused person
    D. Minor

36. Abuse is the unwillful infliction of injury, unreasonable confinement, intimidation, or punishment that results in physical harm, pain, or mental anguish.
    A. True
    B. False
37. You suspect a person you are caring for is being abused. You must
    A. Tell the nurse
    B. Call the police
    C. Tell a co-worker
    D. Tell the person's doctor
38. Examples of emotional or mental abuse include
    A. Humiliation
    B. Burning
    C. Abandonment
    D. Neglect
39. Signs of self-neglect include which of the following?
    A. Wearing hearing aids
    B. Weight gain
    C. Confusion
    D. Going to the doctor as scheduled
40. Which is *not* a sign of elder abuse?
    A. Complaints of stiff and painful joints
    B. Weight loss
    C. Bleeding and bruising in the genital area
    D. Frequent injuries
41. You suspect child abuse, so what do you do next?
    A. Call the police
    B. Tell the parents
    C. Tell the nurse
    D. Nothing, it is not your business

CASE STUDY

Miss Mary Adams is a 52-year-old woman. She was admitted to the hospital 2 days ago with nausea, vomiting, and complaints of abdominal pain. The nurse tells you in a report that Miss Adams is very anxious. She also has some demanding behaviors. Miss Adams has had her call light on three times in the past 30 minutes. While walking by her room, you overhear a co-worker talking to Miss Adams in a loud voice. The co-worker tells Miss Adams: "I can't keep coming in here to straighten your linens. I am very busy. If you keep using your call light, I will take it away. I need to spend my time with patients who really need me."

Answer the following questions.

1. Is your co-worker's behavior toward Miss Adams a form of abuse? Explain.

2. What is your responsibility in this situation?

3. Whom should you notify about what you heard?

ADDITIONAL LEARNING ACTIVITIES

1. Read the code of conduct for nursing assistants (Box 4-1 on p. 31 in the textbook).
   A. List ways you might apply this code in a job setting.

   B. Discuss the importance of this code with your classmates.

2. If you are asked to perform a task that you feel is unsafe, how might you handle the request?
   A. What could you say?

   B. To whom will you talk to about your concerns?

3. List any job functions that you are opposed to doing for moral or religious reasons. How will you advise your employer of your concerns?

CROSSWORD

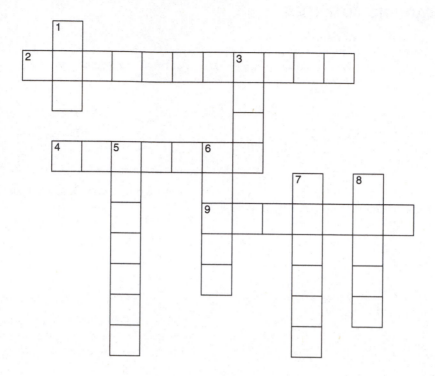

Across

2. Negligence by a professional person
4. Intentionally attempting or threatening to touch a person's body without his or her consent
9. Touching a person's body without his or her consent

Down

1. A rule of conduct made by a government body
3. A wrong committed against a person or the person's property
5. Making false statements orally
6. Making false statements in print, writing, or through pictures or drawings
7. Knowledge of what is right conduct and wrong conduct
8. An act that violates a criminal law

5 STUDENT AND WORK ETHICS

MATCHING

Match each term with the correct definition.

1. _____ Trusting others with personal and private information
2. _____ The most important thing at the time
3. _____ To spread rumors or talk about the private matters of others
4. _____ To trouble, torment, offend, or worry a person by one's behavior or comments
5. _____ Staff members work together as a group; each person does his or her part to provide safe and effective care
6. _____ Behavior in the workplace

A. Gossip
B. Harassment
C. Confidentiality
D. Teamwork
E. Work ethics
F. Priority

FILL IN THE BLANKS

7. Professionalism involves _____

_____

_____

8. Work ethics involves:

   A. _____

   B. _____

   C. _____

   D. _____

9. To give safe and effective care, you must be

   _____ and

   _____ healthy

10. Most adults need _____ hours of sleep daily.

11. Working under the influence of drugs affects the

    person's _____

    _____

    _____.

12. If you smoke, you must practice hand washing and good personal hygiene because _____

    _____

    _____

    _____.

13. You must never report to work under the influence of alcohol because _____

    _____

    _____

    _____

    _____.

14. Why should you keep your fingernails short and neatly shaped?

    _____

    _____

15. You should not wear perfume, cologne, or aftershave lotion to work because _____

    _____

    _____.

16. Explain why it is important for you to be at work on time and when scheduled.

    _____

    _____

    _____

17. Define the following qualities and traits for good work ethics.

    A. Caring _____

    _____

    _____

    B. Empathetic _____

    _____

    _____

    C. Honest _____

    _____

    _____

18. Teamwork involves

    A. _____

    B. _____

    C. _____

    D. _____

    E. _____

19. List 4 statements that signal a bad attitude.

    A. _____

    B. _____

    C. _____

    D. _____

20. You are scheduled to return from your meal break at noon. Explain why it is important to return

    from your meal break on time. _____

    _____

    _____

    _____

21. Setting priorities involves deciding

    A. _____

    B. _____

    C. _____

    D. _____

    E. _____

    F. _____

22. Priorities change as _____ change.

23. _____ is the response or change in the body caused by any emotional, physical, social, or economic factor.

24. Sexual harassment involves _____

    _____

25. You are resigning from a job. You should include the following in your notice.

    A. _____

    B. _____

    C. _____

MULTIPLE CHOICE

Circle the BEST answer.

26. To look professional, do the following *except*
    A. Wear a clean uniform daily
    B. Wear a lot of jewelry
    C. Wear your name badge or photo ID
    D. Wear a wristwatch with a second hand

27. You are always willing to help and work with others. You are being
    A. Cheerful
    B. Respectful
    C. Cooperative
    D. Enthusiastic

28. Knowing your own feelings, strengths, and weaknesses is the quality of
    A. Cooperation
    B. Self-awareness
    C. Caring
    D. Courtesy

29. Proper speech and language at work involves
    A. Speaking clearly
    B. Shouting to be heard
    C. Using abusive language when needed
    D. Arguing with the person when you know you are right

30. Which of these statements reflects a negative attitude?
    A. "Can I help you?"
    B. "Please show me how this works."
    C. "I can't; I'm too busy."
    D. "Thank you for your help."

31. You can share information about a resident with
    A. The resident's family
    B. The nurse supervising your work
    C. Your co-worker during lunch
    D. Your family and friends

32. Which action will keep personal matters out of the workplace?
    A. Letting family and friends visit you on the unit
    B. Using an agency copy machine to copy recipes for a co-worker
    C. Taking agency pens and pencils home
    D. Making personal phone calls during meals and breaks

33. Setting priorities involves the following *except* deciding
    A. Which person has the greatest needs
    B. What tasks need to be done at a set time
    C. What tasks you enjoy doing most
    D. How much help you need to complete a task

34. Stress in your personal life affects your work.
    A. True
    B. False

35. To reduce stress, do the following *except*
    A. Give yourself praise
    B. Get enough rest and sleep
    C. Spend time with unhappy people
    D. Laugh with others

36. Harassment is *not* legal in the workplace.
    A. True
    B. False

37. Harassment involves only sexual behavior.
    A. True
    B. False

38. Victims of sexual harassment are always women.
    A. True
    B. False

39. You feel that you are being harassed at work. Which is *correct?*
    A. Tell your co-workers.
    B. Ignore it. You do not want to cause trouble.
    C. Ask your family and friends for advice.
    D. Report it to your supervisor.

40. Common reasons for losing a job include the following *except*
    A. Poor attendance
    B. Falsifying a record
    C. Having, using, or distributing drugs in the work setting
    D. Politely refusing to perform a task you were not trained to do

41. You can lose your job for failing to maintain patient confidentiality.
    A. True
    B. False

CASE STUDY

Your co-worker, Linda Evans, is often 5 to 10 minutes late for work. She has difficulty completing her assignments. You see her walk by a patient's room when his call light is on. She tells you: "He is not my patient, and I am too busy to stop and answer the call light."

Answer the following questions:

1. How might Linda's actions affect the quality of care provided to the patient?

2. How might Linda's attitude affect the care of other patients?

3. Is Linda practicing good work ethics? Explain.

4. Can Linda's actions cause her to lose her job? Explain.

5. What are your responsibilities in this situation?

ADDITIONAL LEARNING ACTIVITIES

1. You have been having problems with one of the nurses at work; she ignores you and your requests. Discuss the following:

   A. How will you address this conflict with the nurse?

   B. What are the problem-solving steps you will use to resolve the issue?

6 HEALTH TEAM COMMUNICATIONS

MATCHING

Match each term with the correct definition.

1. _____ The exchange of information
2. _____ The method nurses use to plan and deliver nursing care; its five steps are assessment, nursing diagnosis, planning, implementation, and evaluation
3. _____ A report that the nurse gives at the end of the shift to the oncoming shift; change-of-shift report
4. _____ The legal account of a person's condition and response to treatment and care
5. _____ A written guide about the person's nursing care
6. _____ A health problem that can be treated by nursing measures
7. _____ The written account of care and observations; charting
8. _____ Things a person tells you about that you cannot observe through your senses; symptoms
9. _____ Setting priorities and goals
10. _____ The oral account of care and observations
11. _____ Using the senses of sight, hearing, touch, and smell to collect information
12. _____ An electronic version of a person's medical record

A. End-of-shift report
B. Recording
C. Medical record
D. Nursing process
E. Communication
F. Objective data
G. Nursing diagnosis
H. Subjective data
I. Reporting
J. Planning
K. Electronic health record
L. Nursing care plan

FILL IN THE BLANKS

13. Health team members share information about:

    A. _____

    B. _____

    C. _____

14. Agency policies about medical records address:

    A. _____

    B. _____

    C. _____

    D. _____

    E. _____

    F. _____

15. If you have access to charts, you have an _____

    _____

    _____.

16. Which medical record forms relate to your work?

    A. _____

    B. _____

    C. _____

    D. _____

    E. _____

17. The _____ is completed when the person is admitted to the agency. It has the person's identifying information.

18. The flow sheets and graphic sheets are used to record

    _____

    _____

    _____.

19. In long-term care, summaries of care describe

    _____

    _____.

20. List the five steps of the nursing process in the correct order.

    A. _____

    B. _____

    C. _____

    D. _____

    E. _____

21. You collect the following data about a patient. Identify the subjective data with an "S" and the objective data with an "O."

    A. _____ Pain

    B. _____ Nausea

    C. _____ Vomiting

    D. _____ Dizziness

    E. _____ Clear yellow urine

    F. _____ Warm moist skin

    G. _____ Numbness

    H. _____ Pulse rate of 80 beats per minute

22. _____ are what is most important for the person.

23. Goals are aimed at _____ _____ _____.

24. Describe the purpose of the nursing care plan.

    _____

    _____

    _____

    _____

    _____

25. The comprehensive care plan identifies:

    A. _____

    B. _____

    C. _____

    D. _____

26. The nurse uses an _____ to communicate delegated measures and tasks to you.

27. You do not understand a task on your assignment sheet. What should you do?

    _____

    _____

    _____

    _____

28. List when you report care and observations to the nurse.

    A. _____

    _____

    B. _____

    _____

    C. _____

    _____

    D. _____

    _____

29. Anyone who reads your charting should know:

    A. _____

    B. _____

    C. _____

30. Convert the following times from standard clock time to 24-hour clock time.

    A. 6:15 PM _____

    B. 8:00 AM _____

    C. 2:30 PM _____

    D. 5:02 PM _____

    E. 10:55 AM _____

    F. 1:29 PM _____

    G. 1:33 AM _____

    H. 9:00 PM _____

31. Convert the following times from 24-hour clock time to standard clock time.

    A. 1600 _____

    B. 0945 _____

    C. 1115 _____

    D. 2120 _____

    E. 1705 _____

32. List the word elements (parts of words).

    A. _____

    B. _____

    C. _____

33. Medical terms are formed by combining word elements. When translating medical terms, begin with the

    _____ .

34. Define the following directional terms.

    A. Anterior (ventral) _____

    B. Distal _____

    C. Lateral _____

    D. Medial _____

    E. Posterior (dorsal) _____

    F. Proximal _____

35. You are recording care given. You are unsure of an abbreviation. What should you do?

    _____

36. Computer systems _____ ,

    _____ ,

    _____ ,

    _____ ,

    and _____ information.

37. When speaking on the phone, you give much information by:

    A. _____

    B. _____

    C. _____

38. List the information you need to write when taking a phone message.

    A. _____

    B. _____

    C. _____

39. List the steps for transferring a phone call.

    A. _____

    _____

    B. _____

    _____

    C. _____

    _____

40. Write the meanings of the following abbreviations:

    A. ADL _____

    B. EHR _____

    B. ePHI _____

    C. MDS _____

MULTIPLE CHOICE

*Circle the **BEST** answer.*

41. For good communication, do the following *except*
    A. Use familiar words
    B. Be brief and concise
    C. Give unneeded information
    D. Give information in a logical, orderly manner

42. Which team members have access to a person's medical record?
    A. The person's family members
    B. Staff members involved in the person's care
    C. Laundry staff
    D. All dietary staff

43. All nursing interventions need a doctor's order.
    A. True
    B. False

44. Care is given during which step of the nursing process?
    A. Assessment
    B. Planning
    C. Implementation
    D. Evaluation

45. Nursing assistants have a key role in the nursing process.
    A. True
    B. False

46. Which statement about resident care conferences is *correct?*
    A. Family members are not allowed to attend.
    B. The resident is required to attend.
    C. Residents may refuse suggestions made by the health team.
    D. Residents attend only if invited by the doctor.

47. You are reporting resident care. Which is *incorrect?*
    A. Report your observations to the nurse.
    B. Report the care that was given by a co-worker.
    C. Reports must be prompt, thorough, and accurate.
    D. Report immediately any changes from normal.

48. When recording, do the following *except*
    A. Use ink
    B. Use only agency-approved abbreviations
    C. Use correct spelling and grammar
    D. Use correcting fluid if you make a mistake

49. When recording, do which of the following?
    A. Erase errors
    B. Skip lines
    C. Record your judgments
    D. Make sure writing is readable and neat

50. When using electronic charting, which action is *incorrect?*
    A. Using another person's username
    B. Checking the time your entry is made
    C. Checking for accuracy
    D. Saving your entry
51. Intake and output are recorded on the
    A. Graphic sheet
    B. Kardex
    C. Admission sheet
    D. Nursing care plan
52. Which is a nursing diagnosis?
    A. Breast cancer
    B. Pneumonia
    C. Bowel incontinence
    D. Diabetes
53. Priorities and goals are set. Which step in the nursing process is this?
    A. Assessment
    B. Planning
    C. Implementation
    D. Evaluation
54. Which prefix means "away from"?
    A. ab-
    B. anti-
    C. dis-
    D. epi-
55. Which root means "head"?
    A. broncho
    B. cephal(o)
    C. hema
    D. nephr(o)
56. The suffix "algia" means
    A. Cell
    B. Tumor
    C. Disease
    D. Pain
57. What does the medical term "gastritis" mean?
    A. Difficulty urinating
    B. Nerve pain
    C. Inflammation of the stomach
    D. Excision of the ovary
58. Which medical term means study of the skin?
    A. Glossitis
    B. Dermatology
    C. Neuralgia
    D. Bacteriogenic
59. You are using a computer to record care given. Which action will *not* protect the person's privacy?
    A. Preventing others from seeing what is on the screen
    B. Logging off after making an entry
    C. Not leaving printouts where others can read them
    D. Using personal e-mail to report confidential information
60. Which is *not* a guideline for answering phones?
    A. Give a courteous greeting.
    B. Cover the receiver with your hand when not speaking to the caller.
    C. Return to a caller on hold within 30 seconds.
    D. Do not give confidential information to any caller.

CASE STUDY

Mr. Juan Gomez is a 75-year-old resident of Valley View Nursing Center. You have been assigned his care this morning.

Mr. Gomez told you that he had a bowel movement at 0500 (5:00 AM).

You helped Mr. Gomez get ready for breakfast by assisting him with mouth care and with washing his face and hands. Mr. Gomez had breakfast sitting in the chair beside his bed. He ate everything on his breakfast tray. After breakfast, you took Mr. Gomez for a walk. He walked 20 feet and then complained of being tired. You assisted him back to his room and helped him into bed.

Answer the following questions.

1. What information would you report and record?

2. To whom should you report the information?

3. What form would you use to record each piece of information?

ADDITIONAL LEARNING ACTIVITIES

1. Practice answering the phone and taking a written message. Practice with a classmate or friend.
   A. How would you answer the phone in a professional, courteous manner?

   B. What information should you write down when taking a message?

   C. What steps would you take before putting a person on hold?

2. Practice your observation, recording, and reporting skills. Ask a classmate or member of your family to help. Use Box 6-2 on p. 55 in the textbook as a guide for recording your observations.
   A. Talk to the person for about 5 minutes. Use a note pad to write down your observations. Include the following.
      (1) Color and length of hair
      (2) Color of eyes
      (3) Description of any jewelry the person is wearing
      (4) Description of clothing the person is wearing
      (5) Any special features (birth marks, scars, and so on)
      (6) Any information the person gave you about himself or herself
   B. Use your notes to give a verbal report.
   C. Discuss the accuracy of your observations.

3. Read the following vignette involving conflict in the workplace. Then answer the questions at the end of the vignette.
   You are assigned to care for Mrs. Amy Martin. When you return from your lunch break, Mrs. Martin's call light is on. When you answer her call light, Mrs. Martin tells you that her light has been on for 25 minutes. Mrs. Martin also tells you that another nursing assistant walked into her room and told her that she would have to wait until her nursing assistant returned from lunch.
   A. How might you feel?

   B. What would you say to Mrs. Martin?

   C. With whom would you discuss the situation?

   D. Where would you discuss the situation?

   E. What steps would you take to solve the problem?

4. Make flash cards of the prefixes, root words, and suffixes in Chapter 6. Write the meaning of each on the back of each flash card. Use the flash cards to help you study and learn medical terms. Work alone, with a classmate, or with a friend.

CROSSWORD

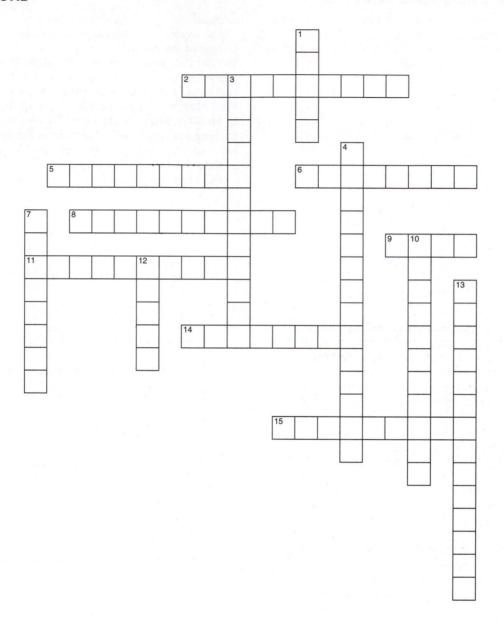

Across

2. Involves measuring if the goals in the planning step of the nursing process were met
5. Data (information) that are seen, heard, felt, or smelled
6. Subjective data
8. Data (things) a person tells you about that you cannot observe through your senses
9. The word element, which contains the basic meaning of the word
11. Involves collecting information about the person
14. A clash between opposing interests or ideas
15. The written account of care and observations

Down

1. Another term for the medical record
3. A shortened form of a word or phrase
4. Carrying out or performing the nursing measures in the care plan
7. Setting priorities and goals
10. Using the senses of sight, hearing, touch, and smell to collect information
12. Objective data
13. The method nurses use to plan and deliver nursing care

7 UNDERSTANDING THE PERSON

MATCHING

Match each term with the correct definition.

1. _____ Any lost, absent, or impaired physical or mental function
2. _____ Being unable to respond to stimuli
3. _____ Something necessary or desired for maintaining life and mental well-being
4. _____ Messages sent through facial expressions, gestures, posture, hand and body movements, gait, eye contact, and appearance
5. _____ Spiritual beliefs, needs, and practices
6. _____ A concept that considers the whole person

A. Need
B. Disability
C. Body language
D. Comatose
E. Religion
F. Holism

FILL IN THE BLANKS

7. The _____ or _____ is the most important person in the agency.

8. The whole person has _____, _____, _____, and _____ parts.

9. Define a need. _____ _____ _____

10. List the basic needs for life as described by Abraham Maslow (from the lowest level to the highest level).

    A. _____
    B. _____
    C. _____
    D. _____
    E. _____

11. Persons in hospitals and nursing centers feel safer and more secure if they know what will happen. For every task, the person should know:

    A. _____
    B. _____
    C. _____
    D. _____

12. A person's culture influences health _____ and _____.

13. Where will you find information about the person's cultural and religious practices?

    _____

14. Religion relates to _____ _____.

15. _____ communication involves the spoken word.

16. A nursing center resident has difficulty hearing. The person also has poor vision. The nurse tells you to write messages to communicate. When writing messages, you need to:

    A. _____
    B. _____
    C. _____

17. _____ communication does not use words.

18. The meaning of touch depends on _____, _____, _____, and _____.

19. You may use touch to communicate. Touch should be _____, not _____, _____, or _____.

20. Body language sends messages through

A. _____

B. _____

C. _____

D. _____

E. _____

F. _____

G. _____

21. Listening requires that you care and have interest. You need to follow these guidelines.

A. _____

B. _____

C. _____

D. _____

E. _____

22. Giving opinions is a communication barrier.

Opinions involve _____

_____.

23. Failure to listen is a communication barrier because

_____

_____

_____

_____.

24. How might illness and disability affect communication? _____

_____

_____.

25. A patient has visitors. You need to give care. What should you do?

_____

_____

_____

_____

_____

26. List 5 causes of anger.

A. _____

B. _____

C. _____

D. _____

E. _____

27. List six nonverbal signs of anger.

A. _____

B. _____

C. _____

D. _____

E. _____

F. _____

28. Causes of demanding behavior include:

A. _____

B. _____

C. _____

D. _____

MULTIPLE CHOICE

Circle the BEST answer.

29. Communication that uses written or spoken words is
    A. Holism
    B. Verbal communication
    C. Body language
    D. A direct question

30. Which action shows respect for the whole person?
    A. Addressing the person using his or her title
    B. Addressing the person using his or her first name
    C. Calling an older person Grandma or Grandpa
    D. Calling a person Honey or Sweetheart

31. Which needs are the most important for survival?
    A. Self-esteem
    B. Safety and security
    C. Physical
    D. Love and belonging

32. Which needs relate to feeling safe from harm, danger, and fear?
    A. Physical
    B. Safety and security
    C. Love and belonging
    D. Self-esteem

33. Many people find comfort and strength from religion during illness.
    A. True
    B. False

34. A nursing center resident stays in his room most of the day. He does not attend activities. He does not talk to his family when they visit. This behavior is
    A. Self-centered behavior
    B. Demanding behavior
    C. Withdrawal
    D. Anger

35. Inappropriate sexual behavior is always on purpose.
    A. True
    B. False
36. A person with aggressive behavior
    A. Is critical of others
    B. May swear, bite, hit, pinch, scratch, or kick
    C. Has little or no contact with others
    D. Has dementia
37. You are giving a patient a complete bed bath. She complains about how you are giving the bath. She also tells you that her breakfast was terrible. She tells you: "Nobody knows what they are doing and nobody cares about me." Which action is *not* helpful?
    A. Explaining that you are giving her bath in the right way and you do know what you are doing
    B. Listening and using silence; letting her express her feelings
    C. Staying calm and professional
    D. Discussing the situation with the nurse
38. Which action will *not* promote effective communication?
    A. Respecting the person's religion and culture
    B. Giving the person time to process information
    C. Telling the person that you are repeating information
    D. Asking questions to see if the person understood you
39. Which is *correct,* when using verbal communication?
    A. Look away from the person.
    B. Speak clearly, slowly, and distinctly.
    C. Use slang or vulgar words.
    D. Shout to be heard.
40. A person for whom you are caring cannot speak or read. How should you communicate with the person?
    A. Use gestures.
    B. Use nods and blinks.
    C. Follow the care plan.
    D. Use touch.
41. Nonverbal messages more truly reflect a person's feelings than words do.
    A. True
    B. False
42. You must never control your body language.
    A. True
    B. False
43. Which communication method focuses on certain information?
    A. Listening
    B. Open-ended questions
    C. Clarifying
    D. Direct questions
44. Using silence shows the person that
    A. You are uncomfortable
    B. You care and respect the person's feelings
    C. You are being rude
    D. You are not listening

45. Which is *not* a communication barrier?
    A. Using touch
    B. Giving opinions
    C. Giving pat answers
    D. Changing the subject
46. When communicating with foreign-speaking persons, which is *not* helpful?
    A. Speaking loudly
    B. Speaking distinctly
    C. Keeping messages short and simple
    D. Using gestures and pictures
47. You ask a person: "How do you feel about being here?" Which communication method have you used?
    A. A direct question
    B. Clarifying
    C. Silence
    D. An open-ended question
48. A person may acquire a disability any time from birth through old age.
    A. True
    B. False
49. Which means being unable to respond to verbal stimuli?
    A. Comatose
    B. Disability
    C. Nonverbal
    D. Holism
50. A patient for whom you are caring is comatose. When giving care, do the following *except*
    A. Explain care measures step-by-step as you do them
    B. Tell the person when you are finishing care
    C. Avoid touching the person when possible
    D. Tell the person when you are leaving the room
51. The presence or absence of family or friends affects the person's quality of life.
    A. True
    B. False
52. You give visitors support by answering their questions about the person's condition.
    A. True
    B. False
53. You observe that a patient's visitor is upsetting him. Which action is *correct?*
    A. Ask the visitor to leave.
    B. Report your observation to the nurse.
    C. Ask the person if you can help.
    D. Do nothing. It is none of your business.
54. Often the person who is comatose can hear and can feel touch and pain.
    A. True
    B. False
55. Which is ethical behavior?
    A. Insulting a person's health care beliefs
    B. Arguing with a person about religious beliefs
    C. Trying to force your views on another person
    D. Respecting a person's cultural practices

CASE STUDY

Mrs. Sarah Stein was admitted to Pine Crest Nursing Center today. She is an 80-year-old widow of Jewish religion. She came to the United States from Germany with her parents when she was 12 years old. She speaks German and English fluently. She was a college professor and taught at the local university for 20 years. She was married for 55 years. Her husband died 2 years ago. Mrs. Stein has difficulty hearing and wears eyeglasses. She walks with a cane. Before coming to Pine Crest Nursing Center, she lived with her married daughter for 2 years. Her daughter felt it was no longer safe for her mother to live with her because her mother was by herself most of the day. Mrs. Stein has fallen twice during the past month and has lost 5 pounds.

Answer the following questions:

1. What characteristics make Mrs. Stein unique?

2. How might her culture and religion affect her care plan?

3. How might the RN use the nursing process to help the nursing team meet Mrs. Stein's needs?

4. What feelings might Mrs. Stein have about moving to Pine Crest Nursing Center?
   A. What measures might help her adjust?

5. What needs might Mrs. Stein's daughter have?
   A. What measures might help her adjust?

ADDITIONAL LEARNING ACTIVITIES

1. Review the Caring About Culture boxes in Chapter 7 in the textbook.
   A. List some ways that knowing about a person's cultural and religious practices might help you give better care.

   B. Do you have cultural and/or religious beliefs that are important to you? Explain.

      (1) How do these beliefs influence your health practices?

2. Observe the nonverbal communication during social contacts with family and friends.
   A. Are you aware of your nonverbal communication? Explain.

   B. How do others communicate with you using nonverbal communication?

   C. Do you ever receive mixed messages from a person's verbal and nonverbal communication? Explain.

CROSSWORD

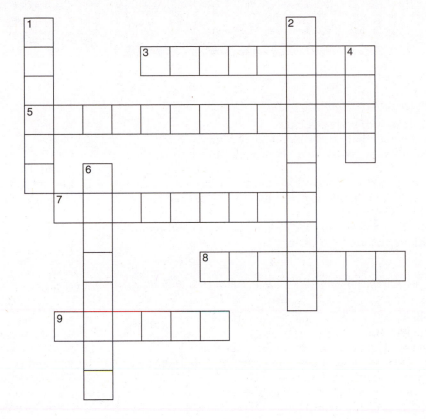

Across
3. Spiritual beliefs, needs, and practices
5. Messages sent through facial expressions, gestures, posture, hand and body movements, gait, eye contact, and appearance
7. Communication that does not use words
8. The characteristics of a group of people passed from one generation to the next
9. A concept that considers the whole person; the whole person has physical, social, psychological, and spiritual parts that are woven together and cannot be separated

Down
1. Communication that uses written or spoken words
2. Any lost, absent, or impaired physical or mental function
4. Something necessary or desired for maintaining life and mental well-being
6. Being unable to respond to verbal stimuli

MATCHING

Match each term with the correct definition.

1. _____ The basic unit of body structure
2. _____ A blood vessel that carries blood away from the body
3. _____ The point where two or more bones meet to allow movement
4. _____ A blood vessel that returns blood to the heart
5. _____ The substance in red blood cells that carries oxygen and gives blood its color
6. _____ The process of supplying the cells with oxygen and removing carbon dioxide from them

A. Artery
B. Vein
C. Cell
D. A joint
E. Respiration
F. Hemoglobin

The following terms relate to the immune system. Match each term with the correct definition.

7. _____ The body's reaction to a certain threat
8. _____ Normal body substances that are involved in destroying abnormal or unwanted substances
9. _____ Substances that can cause an immune response
10. _____ White blood cells that digest and destroy microorganisms and other unwanted substances
11. _____ White blood cells that produce antibodies
12. _____ The body's reaction to anything it does not recognize as a normal body substance
13. _____ Cells that destroy invading cells
14. _____ Cells that cause the production of antibodies that circulate in the plasma

A. B lymphocytes (B cells)
B. Antigens
C. Specific immunity
D. Nonspecific immunity
E. Antibodies
F. T lymphocytes (T cells)
G. Phagocytes
H. Lymphocytes

FILL IN THE BLANKS

15. Explain why you need to know the body's normal structure and function. _____

_____

_____

_____

_____

16. List and describe the basic structures of the cell.

A. _____

B. _____

C. _____

D. _____

17. Chromosomes are _____

_____

18. Cells reproduce by _____.

This process is called _____.

19. _____
tissue covers internal and external body surfaces.

20. _____ tissue
stretches and contracts to let the body move.

21. What is the function of nerve tissue? _____

_____

_____

22. The largest system is the _____

_____

23. _____ gives the skin
its color.

24. _____, _____,
    _____, and _____
    are skin appendages.

25. List three functions of the musculo-skeletal system.

    A. _____

    B. _____

    C. _____

26. Name the types of bones and their function.

    A. _____

    _____

    B. _____

    _____

    C. _____

    _____

    D. _____

    _____

27. A membrane called _____
    covers bones.

28. _____ acts as a
    lubricant so that the joint can move smoothly.

29. Describe the movement of each type of joint.

    A. Ball-and-socket _____

    _____

    B. Hinge _____

    _____

    C. Pivot _____

    _____

30. _____
    muscles can be consciously controlled.

31. List the three functions of muscles.

    A. _____

    B. _____

    C. _____

32. Strong, tough connective tissues called
    _____ connect muscles to bones.

33. The _____
    controls, directs, and coordinates body functions.

34. Name and describe the two main divisions of the
    nervous system.

    A. _____

    _____

    _____

    B. _____

    _____

    _____

35. The three main parts of the brain are:

    A. _____

    B. _____

    C. _____

36. The outside of the cerebrum is called the

    _____.

    It controls _____

    _____.

37. The brainstem contains the _____,

    _____, and

    _____.

38. The _____
    lies within the spinal column. It contains
    pathways that conduct messages to and from
    the brain.

39. What is the function of the cerebrospinal fluid?

    _____

    _____

    _____

    _____

40. The peripheral nervous system has 12 pairs of

    _____ and

    31 pairs of _____.

41. Some peripheral nerves form the

    _____

    This system controls _____

    _____

42. The autonomic nervous system is divided into the

    _____ and the

    _____

43. Name the five senses.

    A. _____

    B. _____

    C. _____

    D. _____

    E. _____

44. Where are touch receptors located?

    _____

    _____

45. The _____ gives the eye its color.

46. _____

    varies with the amount of light entering the eye.

47. The ear functions in _____

    and _____.

48. The circulatory system is made up of the

    _____, _____,

    and _____.

49. List five functions of the circulatory system.

    A. _____

    _____

    B. _____

    _____

    C. _____

    _____

    _____

    D. _____

    _____

    _____

    E. _____

    _____

    _____

50. The blood consists of _____

    _____.

51. _____

    are needed for blood clotting.

52. The _____ is the
    thick, muscular part of the heart.

53. Name and describe the two phases of heart action.

    A. _____

    _____

    _____

    B. _____

    _____

    _____

54. The three groups of blood vessels are:

    A. _____

    B. _____

    C. _____

55. The largest artery is the _____.

56. Arterial blood is rich in _____.

57. The two main veins are:

    A. _____

    B. _____

58. List three functions of the lymphatic system.

    A. _____

    _____

    B. _____

    _____

    C. _____

    _____

59. The _____ is the
    largest structure in the lymphatic system.

60. List four functions of the spleen

    A. _____

    B. _____

    C. _____

    D. _____

61. The respiratory system brings _____

    into the lungs and removes _____

    _____.

62. Respiration involves _____ and

    _____.

63. The _____ is a long tube that extends from the mouth to the anus.

64. List the accessory organs of digestion.

    A. _____

    B. _____

    C. _____

    D. _____

    E. _____

    F. _____

65. The waste products of digestion are called

    _____.

66. What are the four functions of the urinary system?

    A. _____

    B. _____

    C. _____

    D. _____

67. Human reproduction results from _____

    _____.

68. The male sex glands are _____.

69. The female sex glands are _____.

70. The female hormones secreted by the ovaries are

    _____ and

    _____.

71. The uniting of a sperm and ovum into one cell is

    called _____.

72. _____ regulate the activities of other organs and glands in the body.

73. Where is the pituitary gland located? _____

    _____

    _____

74. Thyroid-stimulating hormone (TSH) is needed for

    _____.

75. Adrenocorticotropic hormone (ACTH) stimulates the _____.

76. _____ causes uterine muscles to contract during childbirth.

77. The thyroid gland secretes thyroid hormone.

    It regulates _____.

78. List the three groups of hormones secreted by the adrenal cortex.

    A. _____

    B. _____

    C. _____

79. _____ is needed for sugar to enter the cells.

80. The _____ system protects the body from disease and infection.

81. Write the meanings of the following abbreviations:

    A. GI _____

    B. WBC _____

    C. RBC _____

MULTIPLE CHOICE

*Circle the **BEST** answer.*

82. Which part of the cell controls cell reproduction?
    A. The cell membrane
    B. Protoplasm
    C. The nucleus
    D. Cytoplasm

83. Genes control
    A. Traits children inherit from their parents
    B. The shape and size of the cell
    C. The function of the cell
    D. Cell division

84. Which type of tissue lines the nose and mouth?
    A. Epithelial
    B. Connective
    C. Muscle
    D. Nerve

85. The inner layer of the skin is the
    A. Epithelium
    B. Epidermis
    C. Dermis
    D. Nerve layer

86. Which is *not* a function of the skin?
    A. Preventing microbes from entering the body
    B. Protecting organs from injury
    C. Regulating body temperature
    D. Maintaining posture

87. Ligaments and tendons are
    A. Muscle tissue
    B. Nerve tissue
    C. Epithelial tissue
    D. Connective tissue

88. The vertebrae in the spinal column are
    A. Irregular bones
    B. Short bones
    C. Flat bones
    D. Long bones
89. The connective tissue at the end of long bones is
    A. The synovial membrane
    B. Cartilage
    C. Ligaments
    D. Joints
90. Blood cells are formed in the
    A. Periosteum
    B. Bone marrow
    C. Synovial membrane
    D. Irregular bone
91. Which are involuntary muscles?
    A. Arm muscles
    B. Leg muscles
    C. Finger muscles
    D. Stomach muscles
92. Which part of the brain regulates and coordinates body movements?
    A. Cerebellum
    B. Pons
    C. Midbrain
    D. Cerebrum
93. The center of thought and intelligence is the
    A. Spinal column
    B. Brainstem
    C. Cerebrum
    D. Medulla
94. Which part of the brain connects the cerebrum to the spinal cord?
    A. The cerebral cortex
    B. The cerebrum
    C. The myelin sheath
    D. The brainstem
95. The brain and spinal cord are covered by connective tissue called
    A. The medulla
    B. Meninges
    C. The arachnoid
    D. The cortex
96. The sympathetic nervous system
    A. Controls hearing and vision
    B. Causes muscles to relax
    C. Speeds up functions
    D. Slows down functions
97. Which layer of the eye has receptors for vision and the nerve fibers of the optic nerve?
    A. The sclera
    B. The choroid
    C. The pupil
    D. The retina
98. Light enters the eye through the
    A. Cornea
    B. Lens
    C. Optic nerve
    D. Aqueous chamber

99. Which structure separates the external and middle ear?
    A. The pinna
    B. The auditory canal
    C. Cerumen
    D. The tympanic membrane
100. Red blood cells are called
    A. Plasma
    B. Erythrocytes
    C. Hemoglobin
    D. Leukocytes
101. The outer layer of the heart is the
    A. Pericardium
    B. Heart sac
    C. Myocardium
    D. Endocardium
102. Which chamber of the heart receives blood from the lungs?
    A. The right atrium
    B. The left atrium
    C. The right ventricle
    D. The left ventricle
103. The smallest branch of an artery is
    A. A capillary
    B. A venule
    C. An arteriole
    D. The vena cava
104. Lymph nodes are *not* found in the
    A. Neck
    B. Chest
    C. Abdomen
    D. Hand
105. T lymphocytes (T cells) are developed in the
    A. Thyroid
    B. Thymus
    C. Tonsils
    D. Lungs
106. The tonsils and adenoids trap microorganisms in the mouth and nose to help prevent infection.
    A. True
    B. False
107. The lungs are separated from the abdominal cavity by a muscle called the
    A. Alveoli
    B. Diaphragm
    C. Pleura
    D. Rib cage
108. Where does digestion begin?
    A. In the esophagus
    B. In the stomach
    C. In the large intestine
    D. In the mouth

109. In the stomach, food is mixed and churned with gastric juices to form a semiliquid substance called
   A. Chyme
   B. Bile
   C. Peristalsis
   D. Saliva
110. The basic working unit of the kidney is the
   A. Glomerulus
   B. Nephron
   C. Renal pelvis
   D. Ureter
111. Urine is stored in the
   A. Bladder
   B. Kidney
   C. Nephron
   D. Urethra
112. Male sex cells are called
   A. Semen
   B. Prostate
   C. Sperm
   D. Testosterone
113. The female sex cell is called a(n)
   A. Progesterone
   B. Cervix
   C. Ovum
   D. Vagina
114. The male hormone is
   A. Estrogen
   B. Progesterone
   C. Sperm
   D. Testosterone

115. The tissue lining the uterus is the
   A. Menstruation
   B. Cervix
   C. Fundus
   D. Endometrium
116. Female external genitalia are called the
   A. Labia
   B. Hymen
   C. Uterus
   D. Vulva
117. Which gland is called the "master gland"?
   A. Pituitary
   B. Thyroid
   C. Adrenal
   D. Parathyroid
118. Insulin is secreted by the
   A. Thyroid
   B. Pancreas
   C. Gonads
   D. Pituitary
119. If there is too little insulin, sugar cannot enter the cells. Excess amounts of sugar build up in the blood. This condition is called
   A. Blood sugar
   B. Glucocorticoid
   C. Diabetes
   D. Epinephrine

LABELING

120. Label the three types of joints.

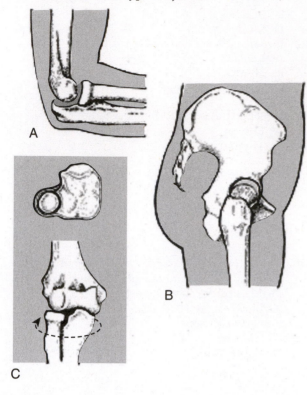

121. Label the major parts of the central nervous system.

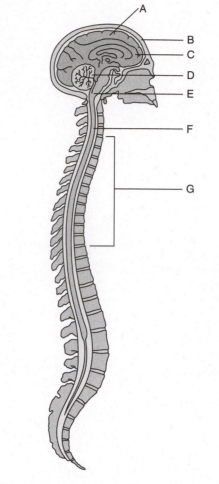

A. _____

B. _____

C. _____

A. _____

B. _____

C. _____

D. _____

E. _____

F. _____

G. _____

122. Label the structures of the heart.

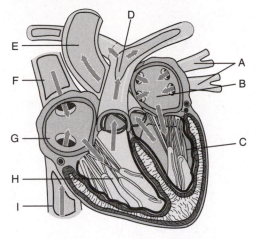

A. _____

B. _____

C. _____

D. _____

E. _____

F. _____

G. _____

H. _____

I. _____

123. Label the structures of the male reproductive system.

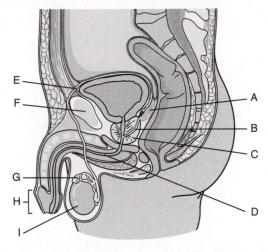

A. _____

B. _____

C. _____

D. _____

E. _____

F. _____

G. _____

H. _____

I. _____

124. Label the structures of the female external genitalia.

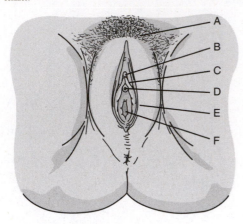

A. _____

B. _____

C. _____

D. _____

E. _____

F. _____

125. Label the glands of the endocrine system.

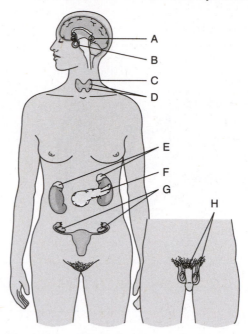

A. _____

B. _____

C. _____

D. _____

E. _____

F. _____

G. _____

H. _____

CASE STUDY

This chapter provides the student with a basic knowledge of body structure and function. The body is made up of systems. The systems are related to and depend on each other for proper function and survival. Injury or disease of one part affects the whole body. Basic knowledge of the body's structure and function should result in safe and dignified care.

Answer the following questions:
1. How might a basic knowledge of body structure and function help you:
   A. Meet the person's physical needs?

   B. Meet the person's safety and security needs?

   C. Understand the reasons for the care you give?

   D. Treat the person and the person's body with dignity and respect?

   E. Make accurate observations about the person?

ADDITIONAL LEARNING ACTIVITIES

1. List and define the three layers of connective tissue that line the brain and spinal cord. (See p. 85 in the textbook.)

2. Describe how the sympathetic nervous system and the parasympathetic nervous system balance each other. (See p. 85 in the textbook.)

3. Explain how the eye uses light to see. (See p. 86 in the textbook.)

4. Outline how the blood flows through the circulatory system. (See p. 87 in the textbook.)

5. Outline the process of respiration. (See pp. 89–90 in the textbook.)

6. Outline the process of digestion. (See p. 90 in the textbook.)

7. Explain how urine is formed and how it passes through the urinary system. (See p. 91 in the textbook.)

9. Outline the process of fertilization. (See p. 93 in the textbook.)

8. Outline the process of menstruation. (See p. 93 in the textbook.)

10. If available in your school or class site, use anatomical models to practice identifying body structures. Also, practice locating the body structures on your own body.

CROSSWORD

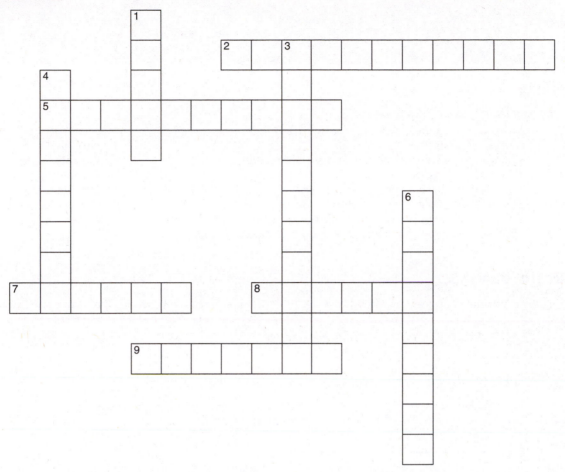

Across
2. Involuntary muscle contractions in the digestive system that move food through the alimentary canal
5. The burning of food for heat and energy by the cells
7. Organs that work together to perform special functions
8. A group of cells with similar functions
9. A chemical substance secreted by the endocrine glands into the bloodstream

Down
1. Groups of tissues with the same function
3. The process of supplying the cells with oxygen and removing carbon dioxide from them
4. Protection against a disease or condition; the person will not get or be affected by the disease
6. The process of physically and chemically breaking down food so that it can be absorbed for use by the cells

9 THE OLDER PERSON

MATCHING

Match each term with the correct definition.

1. _____ The physical changes that are measured and that occur in a steady, orderly manner
2. _____ Changes in mental, emotional, and social function
3. _____ The care of aging people
4. _____ The study of the aging process
5. _____ The time when menstruation stops and menstrual cycles end
6. _____ The physical, emotional, social, cultural, and spiritual factors that affect a person's feelings and attitudes about his or her sex

A. Menopause
B. Growth
C. Geriatrics
D. Sexuality
E. Development
F. Gerontology

FILL IN THE BLANKS

7. With aging, normal changes occur in body

   _____ and

   _____ .

   These changes increase the risk for

   _____, _____,

   and _____ .

8. Growth is _____

   _____

   _____

9. Development relates to _____

   _____

   _____ .

10. Growth and development occur in a

    _____, _____,

    and _____ .

11. A developmental task is _____

    _____

    _____ .

12. List five social changes that occur with aging.

    A. _____

    B. _____

    C. _____

    D. _____

    E. _____

13. When a person's partner dies, the person loses

    a _____, _____,

    _____, and _____ .

14. List six age-related changes in the musculo-skeletal system.

    A. _____

    B. _____

    C. _____

    D. _____

    E. _____

    F. _____

15. List three measures that help prevent bone loss and loss of muscle strength.

    A. _____

    B. _____

    C. _____

16. _____,
_____, and
_____
help prevent respiratory complications from
bedrest.

17. Persons with _____ or
_____
often need foods providing soft bulk, such as
whole grains and cooked fruits and vegetables.

18. List four age-related changes in the digestive
system.

    A. _____

    B. _____

    C. _____

    D. _____

19. As a result of age-related changes in the
digestive system, _____
foods are hard to chew and irritate the intestines.

20. List four age-related changes in the male reproductive system.

    A. _____

    B. _____

    C. _____

    D. _____

21. Nursing centers are options for _____
_____
_____.

22. The person needing nursing center care may
suffer some or all of the following losses. Loss of:

    A. _____

    B. _____

    C. _____

    D. _____

    E. _____

23. The losses listed in Question 22 may cause the
person to feel _____,
_____, and _____.

24. Frequency of sexual activity decreases for many
men and women. Reasons for this include:

    A. _____

    B. _____

    C. _____

    D. _____

    E. _____

25. You are giving a male resident a bed bath. You
notice that he is becoming aroused. What actions
should you take? _____
_____
_____
_____

26. A nursing center provides a temporary or permanent
residence for some persons. The setting must be
_____
_____
_____.

MULTIPLE CHOICE

*Circle the **BEST** answer.*

27. Which activity will help prevent loneliness in the
older person?
    A. Watching television in their bedroom alone
    B. Playing solitaire with cards
    C. Attending religious events
    D. Exercising alone

28. The older person is at a greater risk for burns
because of
    A. Increased fatty tissue layer
    B. Increased circulation
    C. Decreased blood vessels
    D. Decreased ability to feel hot and cold

29. Reduced blood flow to the brain because of aging
results in
    A. Quicker reflexes
    B. Slower reflexes
    C. Increased forgetfulness
    D. Longer memory

30. Which statement about retirement is *correct?*
    A. All people enjoy retirement.
    B. Retirement usually means increased income.
    C. All people retire because they want to.
    D. Some people retire because of poor health or
disability.

31. Most older people have regular contact with family and friends.
    A. True
    B. False
32. Some children care for older parents. Which statement is *incorrect?*
    A. This helps some older persons feel secure.
    B. Tensions may occur.
    C. Some older persons lose dignity and self-respect.
    D. This is always a good arrangement for the parent and the child.
33. Changes in the integumentary system include the following *except*
    A. The skin loses its elasticity
    B. The skin loses its fatty tissue layer
    C. Oil and sweat secretion increases
    D. The skin has fewer nerve endings
34. Changes in the skin occur with aging. Care measures include the following *except*
    A. Using mild soaps or soap substitutes
    B. A daily bath
    C. Using lotions, oils, and creams to prevent drying
    D. Protecting the person from drafts
35. A resident complains of cold feet. Which care measure is *correct?*
    A. Soaking the person's feet in very warm water
    B. Providing the person with socks
    C. Giving the person a bath
    D. Providing the person with a heating pad
36. Age-related changes in the musculo-skeletal system cause bones to break easily. Which measure is *not* helpful?
    A. Turning and moving the person gently
    B. Helping the person to get out of bed
    C. Helping the person to walk
    D. Keeping the person in bed as much as possible
37. Which is *not* a result of age-related nervous system changes?
    A. More sleep is needed.
    B. Blood flow to the brain is decreased.
    C. Reflexes slow.
    D. Memory is shorter.
38. Painful injuries or diseases may go unnoticed by an older person because
    A. Older persons are confused
    B. Hearing and vision losses occur
    C. Touch and sensitivity to pain and pressure are reduced
    D. Activity is decreased
39. Changes in the circulatory system result in
    A. Loss of appetite
    B. Poor circulation in many parts of the body
    C. Decreased ability to sleep
    D. Agitation and restlessness

40. Which measure does *not* promote normal breathing?
    A. Placing heavy bed linens over the person's chest
    B. Assisting with turning, repositioning, and deep breathing
    C. Positioning the person in Semi-Fowler's position
    D. Encouraging the person to be as active as possible
41. Which is *not* a result of age-related changes in the digestive system?
    A. Improved taste and smell
    B. Flatulence and constipation
    C. Indigestion
    D. Swallowing problems
42. Changes in the urinary system result in
    A. Less concentrated urine
    B. Urinary frequency and urgency
    C. Decreased risk for urinary tract infections
    D. Blood in the urine
43. Which measure will help reduce the need to urinate during the night?
    A. Limiting fluid intake to 1000 mL daily
    B. Taking all fluids before 1300 (1:00 PM)
    C. Drinking only water after 12:00 noon
    D. Taking most fluids before 1700 (5:00 PM)
44. Older persons are at risk for urinary tract infections.
    A. True
    B. False
45. Which is *not* an age-related change in the female reproductive system?
    A. Orgasm is less intense.
    B. Vaginal walls become thinner and drier.
    C. The ovaries and uterus increase in size.
    D. External genitalia shrink and lose elastic tissue.
46. Mr. and Mrs. Adams have been married for 52 years. They no longer have sexual intercourse. Which statement is *correct?*
    A. They are too old for sexual intercourse.
    B. They have lost sexual needs and desires.
    C. They can express closeness and intimacy in other ways.
    D. They no longer love one another.
47. A resident makes sexual advances toward you. Which action is *correct?*
    A. Refusing to care for the person
    B. Telling the person's family
    C. Discussing the matter with the nurse
    D. Ignoring the matter
48. Love, affection, and intimacy are needed throughout life.
    A. True
    B. False
49. Married couples living in nursing centers are allowed to share the same room.
    A. True
    B. False

50. Ms. Irma Adams and Mr. John Moore are nursing center residents. You see them kissing in Mr. Moore's private room. What should you do?
    A. Tell the nurse at once.
    B. Close the door for privacy.
    C. Escort Ms. Adams to her room.
    D. Discuss what you saw with co-workers in the lunchroom.
51. Which measure promotes sexuality?
    A. Letting the person practice grooming routines
    B. Choosing clothing for the person
    C. Judging the person's sexual relationships
    D. Entering the person's room without knocking
52. Sexually aggressive behaviors are always intentional.
    A. True
    B. False
53. A person you are caring for touches you in a sexual way. Which action is *incorrect*?
    A. Asking the person not to touch you and stating the places you were touched
    B. Telling the person that the behavior makes you uncomfortable
    C. Discussing the matter with the nurse
    D. Telling the person that you will report the behavior to the ombudsman

CASE STUDY

Mrs. June Chaney and Mr. Warren Anderson live at Green Acres Nursing Center. They have both been widowed for several years. Since moving to Green Acres, they have developed a relationship. They attend the same activities, eat at the same table in the dining room, and sit side by side in the recreation room. They are frequently seen holding hands and kissing. Sometimes they are together in Mrs. Chaney's room with the door closed. Mr. Anderson's son tells you that he is not happy about the relationship and wants you to keep his father and Mrs. Chaney apart.

Answer the following questions.
1. How are Mr. Anderson and Mrs. Chaney expressing their sexuality?

2. Should Mr. Anderson and Mrs. Chaney be allowed to continue their relationship? Explain your answer.

3. How might you address the concerns expressed by Mr. Anderson's son?

ADDITIONAL LEARNING ACTIVITIES

1. Ask an older relative, friend, or neighbor if you can interview him or her. Ask the person:
   A. What physical, social, and emotional changes have you experienced over the past 10 to 20 years?
   B. What support systems have helped you adjust to the changes?
   C. What brings meaning and quality to your life?

2. Read about the changes that occur as people age. Think about how these changes might affect you and your lifestyle as you age.
   A. Do you have fears or concerns? Explain.

B. How might you adjust to the changes?

3. List some ways you can help persons you care for express their sexuality.

C. What can you do now to slow or decrease the effects of aging?

4. You may have to deal with persons who are sexually aggressive toward you.
A. How do you feel about this?

D. Which people and what possessions might you have the most difficulty giving up? Explain.

B. How might you handle these uncomfortable situations?

10 SAFETY NEEDS

MATCHING

Match each term with the correct definition.

1. _____ A sudden catastrophic event in which many people are injured and killed and property is destroyed
2. _____ A state of being unaware of one's surroundings and being unable to react or respond to people, places, or things
3. _____ The loss of cognitive and social function caused by changes in the brain
4. _____ Any chemical in the workplace that can cause harm
5. _____ Violent acts directed toward persons at work or while on duty
6. _____ When breathing stops from the lack of oxygen

A. Dementia
B. Suffocation
C. Workplace violence
D. Disaster
E. Hazardous substance
F. Coma

FILL IN THE BLANKS

7. Where will you find the safety measures needed

   by the person? _____

8. List 8 factors that increase the risk of accidents and injuries.

   A. _____
   B. _____
   C. _____
   D. _____
   E. _____
   F. _____
   G. _____
   H. _____

9. List 6 drug side effects that increase a person's risk for accidents and injuries.

   A. _____
   B. _____
   C. _____
   D. _____
   E. _____
   F. _____

10. To identify the person before giving care, use the

    _____ .

11. Explain why calling the person by name is *not* a safe way to identify the person.

    _____

    _____

    _____

12. When comparing the identification (ID) bracelet with the assignment sheet, you need to check the

    person's full name carefully because _____

    _____

    _____ .

13. An alert and oriented nursing center resident chooses not to wear an ID bracelet. What is the correct procedure for identifying the person before giving care?

    _____

    _____

14. You notice that a patient's ID bracelet is too tight.

    What should you do? _____

15. List 4 common causes of burns.

    A. _____
    B. _____
    C. _____
    D. _____

16. List 5 common causes of suffocation.

    A. _____

    B. _____

    C. _____

    D. _____

    E. _____

17. The most common cause of choking is _____

    _____ .

18. With_____ ,

    you should stay with the person and encourage
    the person to keep coughing to expel the object.

19. _____
    is often called the "universal sign of choking."

20. Describe the signs and symptoms of severe airway

    obstruction. _____

    _____

    _____

    _____

    _____

    _____

21. _____ are
    used to relieve severe airway obstruction.

22. When is equipment unsafe?

    A. _____

    B. _____

    C. _____

23. Frayed cords and overloaded electrical outlets

    can cause _____ ,

    _____ ,

    and _____ .

24. List 7 warning signs of a faulty electrical item.

    A. _____

    B. _____

    C. _____

    D. _____

    E. _____

    F. _____

    G. _____

25. Where should you connect bed power cords?

    _____

    _____

26. Explain why you should turn off equipment before

    unplugging it. _____

    _____

    _____

27. Exposure to hazardous chemicals can occur from
    the release of a hazard into the workplace.
    Workplace hazards include:

    A. _____

    B. _____

    C. _____

28. Every hazardous substance has a material safety
    data sheet (SDS). You need to check the SDS
    before:

    A. _____

    B. _____

    C. _____

29. List the 3 things needed for a fire.

    A. _____

    B. _____

    C. _____

30. The word RACE will help you remember what to
    do first if a fire occurs. What do the letters
    R-A-C-E stand for?

    A. **R** _____

    B. **A** _____

    C. **C** _____

    D. **E** _____

31. You answer the phone at the nurses' station. The
    caller tells you that there is a bomb in the hospital.

    What should you do? _____

    _____

32. _____ is when
    a patient or resident leaves the agency without

    staff knowledge. _____

33. Explain why nurses and nursing assistants are at risk for workplace violence. _____

   _____

   _____

34. _____ involves identifying and controlling risks and safety hazards affecting the agency.

35. The intent of risk management is to:

   A. _____

   B. _____

   C. _____

   D. _____

36. The purpose of color-coded wristbands is to

   _____

   _____

37. To safely use color-coded wristbands:

   A. _____

   B. _____

   C. _____

   D. _____

   E. _____

38. Errors in care must be reported at once. Errors in care include:

   A. _____

   B. _____

   C. _____

39. Write the meaning for the following abbreviations:

   A. AED _____

   B. CPR _____

   C. PASS _____

   D. SDS _____

MULTIPLE CHOICE

*Circle the **BEST** answer.*

40. Cognitive relates to
   A. Dementia
   B. Impaired hearing
   C. Knowledge
   D. Balance and coordination

41. Loss of muscle function, loss of sensation, or loss of both muscle function and sensation is
   A. Dementia
   B. Paralysis
   C. Coma
   D. Suffocation

42. When identifying the person, which is *incorrect?*
   A. Use at least one identifier.
   B. Compare identifying information on the assignment sheet with that on the ID bracelet.
   C. Call the person by name when you check the ID bracelet.
   D. Carefully check all the information.

43. Safety measures to prevent burns include the following *except*
   A. Do not allow smoking in bed
   B. Do not allow smoking near oxygen equipment
   C. Measure bath water temperature before the person gets into the tub
   D. Turn on hot water first, then cold water

44. To prevent poisoning, do which of the following?
   A. Remove all personal care items from the person's room
   B. Inspect the person's drawers every shift
   C. Follow agency policy for storing personal care items
   D. Remind patients and residents not to drink shampoo, mouthwash, or lotion

45. Which measure helps prevent suffocation?
   A. Leaving a person alone in the bathtub
   B. Giving small amounts of oral foods and fluids to persons with feeding tubes
   C. Using bed rails for all patients and residents
   D. Reporting loose teeth or dentures to the nurse

46. Which method is used to relieve choking in the very obese and in pregnant women?
   A. The Heimlich maneuver
   B. Chest thrusts
   C. Back blows
   D. Abdominal thrusts

47. Which action will *not* help prevent equipment accidents?
   A. Inspecting power cords for damage
   B. Using two-pronged plugs on all electrical devices
   C. Keeping electrical items away from water
   D. Turning off equipment before unplugging it

48 You find a bottle of liquid in the tub room without a label. Which action is *correct?*
   A. Open the bottle to see what is inside.
   B. Leave the bottle and get the nurse.
   C. Take the bottle to the nurse and explain the problem.
   D. Ask a co-worker what is in the bottle.

49. When must you check material safety data sheets (SDSs)?
    A. Before using a hazardous substance
    B. Before cleaning up a leak or spill
    C. Before disposing of a hazardous substance
    D. All of the above are correct
50. Which is *not* a fire prevention measure?
    A. Following safety measures for oxygen use
    B. Supervising persons who smoke
    C. Emptying ashtrays into metal wastebaskets lined with plastic bags
    D. Storing flammable liquids in their original containers
51. The first thing you must do when a fire occurs is
    A. Pull the fire alarm
    B. Rescue persons in immediate danger
    C. Get the fire extinguisher
    D. Turn off electrical equipment
52. Do *not* use elevators if there is a fire.
    A. True
    B. False
53. A patient is receiving oxygen therapy. Which is *incorrect*?
    A. A NO SMOKING sign is placed on the person's door and near his bed.
    B. Smoking materials are kept in the person's bedside stand.
    C. The person and his visitors cannot smoke in the person's room.
    D. Materials that ignite easily are removed from the person's room.
54. Safety measures are needed where oxygen is used and stored.
    A. True
    B. False
55. The resident you are caring for has on a yellow wristband. What does this mean?
    A. Allergy alert
    B. Falls risk
    C. Do Not Resuscitate
    D. Limb alert

56. You are caring for a person who becomes agitated and aggressive. Which measure promotes safety?
    A. Using touch to calm the person
    B. Keeping your hands free
    C. Telling the person to calm down
    D. Standing close to the person
57. Which measure will help keep a patient's personal belongings safe?
    A. Sending all personal belongings home with the family
    B. Completing a personal belongings list
    C. Locking all personal belongings in the safe
    D. Keeping all personal belongings in the person's closet
58. In nursing centers, shoes and clothing are labeled with the person's name.
    A. True
    B. False
59. Accidents and errors in care are reported only if someone is injured.
    A. True
    B. False
60. Which is any event that has harmed or could harm a patient, resident, visitor, or staff member?
    A. Hazard
    B. Disaster
    C. Risk factor
    D. Incident
61. You notice that a light bulb has burned out in a resident's bathroom. Which action is *correct*?
    A. Get a new light bulb and change the light bulb.
    B. Do nothing. Assume the nurse already knows about the problem.
    C. Tell the resident to be extra careful when using the bathroom.
    D. Follow agency policy for reporting such problems.

CASE STUDY

Mr. John Wilson is 80 years old. He is a resident at Pine View Nursing Center. He is recovering from surgery to repair a fractured right leg. He is learning to use a walker. He is receiving oxygen for a chronic lung disease. He wears eyeglasses and has very poor vision without his glasses. Mr. Wilson has smoked a pack of cigarettes a day for the past 60 years. He is alert and oriented and able to make his needs known.

Answer the following questions:
1. What accident risk factors does Mr. Wilson have?

2. What types of accidents or injuries is Mr. Wilson at risk for?

3. What nursing measures might help decrease Mr. Wilson's risks for accidents and injury?

4. What is your role in providing a safe setting for Mr. Wilson?

ADDITIONAL LEARNING ACTIVITIES

1. Carefully review the safety measures to prevent burns, poisoning, and suffocation.
   A. List the safety measures you practice in your home related to each.

   B. List the safety measures you practice in your workplace related to each.

   C. Do you have a fire safety plan in your home? Explain.

   D. If you do not already have one, develop an evacuation plan for your home. Make sure that there are at least two possible exits from each room. Schedule regular fire drills with your family.

2. Make a list of emergency phone numbers (Poison Control, Police, Ambulance, Hospital, and Doctor). Keep the list by each phone in your home. Make sure all family members know where the list is.

3. Carefully review the procedure for relieving choking—adult or child (over 1 year of age).
   A. Under the supervision of a qualified instructor, practice the procedure. Use the procedure checklist on pp. 192-193 as a guide.

4. Carefully review the procedure for using a fire extinguisher.
   A. Under the supervision of your instructor, practice the procedure. Use the procedure checklist on p. 194 as a guide.

11 PREVENTING FALLS

FILL IN THE BLANKS

1. Where do most falls occur?

   _____

   _____

2. According to the Centers for Disease Control and Prevention, why are nursing center residents at an increased risk for falls?

   A. _____

   _____

   B. _____

   _____

   C. _____

   _____

3. List 5 bathroom and shower/tub room safety measures to prevent falls.

   A. _____

   _____

   B. _____

   _____

   C. _____

   _____

   D. _____

   _____

   E. _____

   _____

4. Explain why wheeled equipment is pulled, not pushed, through doorways.

   _____

   _____

   _____

5. Why should you do a safety check of the person's room after visitors leave?

   _____

   _____

   _____

   _____

6. A resident's care plan states that he needs bed rails. When must his bed rails be up?

   _____

   _____

7. Bed rails cannot be used unless _____

   _____ .

   They must be_____

   _____ .

8. How will you know which patients or residents use bed rails?

   _____

   _____

   _____

   _____

9. If the person uses bed rails, you need to:

   A. _____

   _____

   B. _____

   _____

   C. _____

   _____

10. A patient does not use bed rails. How will you promote the person's safety when giving care?

   _____

   _____

   _____

   _____

11. What is the purpose of hand rails in hallways and stairways?

   _____

   _____

12. What is the purpose of grab bars in bathrooms and shower/tub rooms?

   _____

   _____

13. Bed wheels have locks to prevent the bed from moving. You need to lock bed wheels when:

    A. _____

    B. _____

14. To use a transfer belt safely, follow _____

    _____

15. While assisting a person with ambulation, the person starts to fall. Explain why you should ease the person to the floor (not try to prevent the fall).

    _____

    _____

    _____

MULTIPLE CHOICE

*Circle the **BEST** answer.*

16. A history of falls increases the risk of falling again.
    A. True
    B. False
17. Persons older than 65 years are at risk for falling.
    A. True
    B. False
18. Which is a factor increasing the risk of falls?
    A. Wearing eyeglasses
    B. Wearing hearing aids
    C. Living in one's own home
    D. Foot problems
19. A patient is incontinent of urine. The person is at increased risk of falling.
    A. True
    B. False
20. Which is *not* a safety measure to prevent falls?
    A. The bed is kept in the highest horizontal position.
    B. Furniture is placed for easy movement.
    C. Bed wheels are locked for transfers.
    D. Crutches, canes, and walkers have nonskid tips.
21. Which statement about bed rails is *incorrect*?
    A. Bed rails are considered restraints.
    B. Bed rails are necessary for all nursing center residents.
    C. A person can get trapped or entangled in bed rails.
    D. The person or legal representative must give consent for raised bed rails.

22. A patient uses bed rails. You promote the person's comfort by
    A. Making sure needed items are within reach
    B. Keeping the bed in the highest horizontal position
    C. Raising both bed rails when giving care
    D. Leaving the person alone when the bed is raised
23. Bed wheels must be locked at all times except when moving the bed.
    A. True
    B. False
24. A transfer belt is unsafe for persons with certain conditions involving the chest or abdomen.
    A. True
    B. False
25. Transfer belts are always applied over clothing.
    A. True
    B. False
26. You are applying a transfer belt on a woman. Which is *incorrect*?
    A. Apply the belt around the woman's waist over clothing.
    B. You should be able to slide your open, flat hand under the belt.
    C. Make sure the woman's breasts are not caught under the belt.
    D. Secure the buckle over the woman's spine.
27. A person starts to fall while you are assisting her with ambulation. You ease the person to the floor. The person is confused and tries to get up. You should force the person to remain on the floor until the nurse arrives.
    A. True
    B. False
28. You must complete an incident report after a patient or resident falls.
    A. True
    B. False
29. Which is *not* a safety measure to prevent falls?
    A. Meeting fluid needs
    B. Placing bed rails on all beds
    C. Wiping up spills at once
    D. Responding to alarms at once

CASE STUDY

Miss Lynn Adams is a new nursing center resident. She is 86 years old. Miss Adams wears eyeglasses and a hearing aid in her right ear. She has arthritis and high blood pressure. In report, the nurse tells you that Miss Adams has been a little confused since admission to the nursing center 2 days ago.

Answer the following questions:
1. What factors increase Miss Adams's risk for falling?

2. What safety measures might help prevent Miss Adams from falling?

ADDITIONAL LEARNING ACTIVITIES

1. Review the safety measures to prevent falls in Box 11-2 on p. 124 in the textbook.
   A. List the safety measures you practice in your home.

   B. List the safety measures you practice in your workplace.

2. Review the procedures for:
   A. Applying a transfer/gait belt
   B. Helping the falling person
      Under the supervision of your instructor, practice each procedure. Use the procedure checklists on pp. 195–197 as a guide.

12 RESTRAINT ALTERNATIVES AND RESTRAINTS

MATCHING

Match each term with the correct definition.

1. _____ A device that limits freedom of movement but is used to promote independence, comfort, or safety

2. _____ An indication or characteristic of a physical or psychological condition

3. _____ Any change in place or position for the body or any part of the body that the person is physically able to control

4. _____ Any drug used for discipline or convenience and not required to treat medical symptoms

A. Freedom of movement
B. Medical symptom
C. Chemical restraint
D. Enabler

FILL IN THE BLANKS

5. _____ have rules for using restraints. Like the Omnibus Budget Reconciliation Act of 1987 (OBRA), these rules protect _____.

6. Restraints may be used only to _____ _____ or _____ _____ .

7. List 7 risks of restraint use.

   A. _____
   B. _____
   C. _____
   D. _____
   E. _____
   F. _____
   G. _____

8. Restraints cannot be used for staff convenience. Convenience is any action that:

   A. _____
   B. _____
   C. _____

9. The nurse restrains a resident to the chair in the person's room so that he can make rounds without being interrupted. This action is unacceptable because it is for _____ .

10. According to the Centers for Medicare & Medicaid Services, physical restraints include these points:

   A. _____
   _____
   B. _____
   _____
   C. _____
   _____
   D. _____
   _____

11. Drugs cannot be used if they _____ _____ .

12. List 9 mental effects of restraint use.

   A. _____
   B. _____
   C. _____
   D. _____
   E. _____
   F. _____
   G. _____
   H. _____
   I. _____

13. List 6 legal aspects of restraint use.

   A. _____

     _____

   B. _____

     _____

   C. _____

     _____

   D. _____

     _____

   E. _____

     _____

   F. _____

     _____

14. A resident's doctor writes an order for a restraint. What information does the doctor's order include?

   A. _____

   B. _____

   C. _____

   D. _____

15. The nurse tells you to apply a wrist restraint to a patient's right wrist. You do not understand why the restraint is being used. What should you do? Explain. _____

   _____

   _____

   _____

16. Explain why you should never secure restraints to the bed rails. _____

   _____

   _____

   _____

17. You apply a belt restraint to a resident in a wheelchair. What information must you report to the nurse?

   A. _____

   B. _____

   C. _____

   D. _____

   E. _____

   F. _____

   G. _____

   H. _____

   I. _____

   J. _____

   K. _____

   L. _____

   M. _____

18. You are applying a belt restraint to a patient. The person is confused and resists your efforts. What should you do? _____

   _____

   _____

   _____

19. Before you apply any restraint, what information do you need from the nurse and the care plan?

   A. _____

   B. _____

   C. _____

   D. _____

   E. _____

   F. _____

   G. _____

   H. _____

   I. _____

   J. _____

   K. _____

   L. _____

   M. _____

   N. _____

20. A patient has a wrist restraint on his right wrist. You are checking the circulation in the person's right wrist. What signs and symptoms must you report to the nurse at once?

   A. _____

   _____

B. _____

_____

C. _____

_____

D. _____

_____

21. What is the purpose of bed rail covers and gap

protectors? _____

_____

_____

22. When applying a restraint to a person's chest, you

must _____

_____

_____

_____ .

23. Criss-crossing vest restraints in back can cause

_____ .

24. You must remove a restraint at least every
2 hours. What care measures do you need to
perform before you reapply the restraint?

A. _____

B. _____

C. _____

D. _____

E. _____

F. _____

G. _____

25. Define *remove easily.* _____

_____

_____

_____ .

26. Write the meaning of the following abbreviations:

A. CMS _____

B. FDA _____

C. TJC _____

MULTIPLE CHOICE

Circle the **BEST** *answer.*

27. Knowing and treating the cause of certain behaviors
can prevent restraint use.
A. True
B. False

28. Physical restraints
A. Restrict freedom of movement or normal
access to one's body
B. Must be used to control a person's behavior
C. Are effective in preventing falls
D. Should never be used

29. Which is a physical restraint?
A. The person is moved closer to the nurses'
station.
B. The person is taken to a supervised activity.
C. The person wears padded hip protectors
under his or her clothing.
D. The person's chair is placed so close to the
wall that the person cannot move.

30. The most serious risk from restraints is
A. Loss of dignity
B. Fractured hip
C. Increased agitation
D. Death from strangulation

31. Which is *not* a restraint alternative?
A. An exercise program is provided.
B. A floor cushion is placed next to the person's
bed.
C. The person's bed sheets are tucked in so
tightly that the person cannot move.
D. Extra time is spent with the restless person.

32. Which of the following measures is a restraint
alternative?
A. The person is kept in his or her room with the
door closed.
B. The person is allowed to wander in a safe area.
C. The person's wheelchair is placed tight against
a table. The wheelchair wheels are locked.
D. Bed rails are used to keep the person in bed.

33. Restraints cannot be used without consent.
A. True
B. False

34. A resident is confused. The person cannot give
informed consent for restraint use. Who does so
for the person?
A. The doctor
B. The RN
C. The agency's administrator
D. The person's legal representative

35. You may need to apply restraints or care for persons who are restrained. Which action is *unsafe?*
    A. Using the restraint noted in the person's care plan
    B. Using only restraints that have manufacturer's instructions and warning labels
    C. Using a restraint to position a person on the toilet
    D. Padding bony areas and skin

36. For safe use of restraints
    A. Keep bed rails down when using vest, jacket, or belt restraints
    B. Position the person in the supine position when using vest, jacket, or belt restraints
    C. Tie restraints according to agency policy
    D. Secure restraints to the bed rail

37. A belt restraint is used to restrain a person on the toilet.
    A. True
    B. False

38. How often do you need to check the person's circulation if mitt, wrist, or ankle restraints are used?
    A. At least every 15 minutes
    B. At least every 30 minutes
    C. Every hour
    D. Every 2 hours

39. Restraints can increase confusion and agitation.
    A. True
    B. False

40. Which restraints limit arm movement?
    A. Mitt restraints
    B. Wrist restraints
    C. Belt restraints
    D. Vest restraints

41. Which type of restraint is the *most* restrictive?
    A. A mitt restraint
    B. A wrist restraint
    C. A belt restraint
    D. A vest restraint

42. You are applying a wrist restraint. The person is in bed. Where should you tie the straps?
    A. To the headboard
    B. To the bed rail out of the person's reach
    C. To the footboard
    D. To the movable part of the bed frame out of the person's reach

CASE STUDY

Mr. Howard Hein is a 76-year-old man in the hospital. He is recovering from abdominal surgery. Mr. Hein has a large abdominal dressing. He is receiving intravenous (IV) therapy (receiving nutrition and medications through a catheter in his vein). The IV catheter is in his left arm. He receives pain medication every 4 hours.

Mr. Hein is very restless and moves around a lot in bed. He is agitated at times. He has removed his abdominal dressing and pulled the IV catheter from his arm. The RN has scheduled an emergency care planning conference.

Mr. Hein has a daughter, a son, and two adult grandchildren who visit daily. The daughter and son will be attending the care planning conference.

Answer the following questions:

1. What safety risk factors does Mr. Hein have?

2. What behaviors does Mr. Hein have that interfere with his treatment?

3. What are possible causes for Mr. Hein's behaviors?

4. What restraint alternatives might the health team try?

5. Before the doctor orders a restraint, what must he or she do?

6. If a restraint is ordered:
   A. What are the risk factors?

   B. What safety measures must be followed?

C. What must be reported and recorded about the restraint?

D. How will you provide for Mr. Hein's basic needs?

E. How will you provide for Mr. Hein's quality of life?

ADDITIONAL LEARNING ACTIVITIES

1. You are caring for a person who is restrained. List some things you can do to protect the person's quality of life. Discuss how you would want to be treated.

2. Under the supervision of your instructor, practice with a classmate the procedure for applying restraints.
   A. Use the procedure checklist on pp. 198–201. Remember that restraints can cause serious injury and even death. They must always be applied correctly.

3. Under the supervision of your instructor, allow a classmate to practice applying restraints to you. Discuss how it feels to be restrained. Answer these questions:
   A. Did you feel safe? Explain.

   B. Did you feel comfortable? Explain.

C. Did you feel in control? Explain.

4. Imagine that you are in a nursing center or hospital. You are having a lot of pain. You do not know the staff. The medication you are taking makes you drowsy. You are not sure what day it is. You have an IV in your right arm and a tube in your nose. You are frightened.
   A. What behaviors might you have?

   B. What could be some reasons for your behaviors?

   C. Might the staff believe that you are confused? Explain.

D. Would you feel safer and less fearful if you were restrained?

E. What measures might make you feel safe and less fearful?

5. View the following video clips on the Evolve companion site to help you learn and practice the procedures:
   A. Offering Diversions

   B. Using a Jacket Restraint

13 PREVENTING INFECTION

MATCHING

Match each term with the correct definition.

1. _____ Items contaminated with blood, body fluids, secretions, or excretions
2. _____ A disease caused by pathogens that spread easily; a contagious disease
3. _____ The process of killing pathogens
4. _____ A human or animal that is a reservoir for microbes but does not develop the infection
5. _____ The process of destroying all microbes
6. _____ Practices used to reduce the number of microbes and prevent their spread from one person or place to another person or place; clean technique
7. _____ A microbe that does not usually cause an infection
8. _____ A small living thing seen only with a microscope

A. Carrier
B. Microorganism (a microbe)
C. Sterilization
D. Biohazardous waste
E. Medical asepsis
F. Disinfection
G. Nonpathogen
H. Communicable disease

FILL IN THE BLANKS

9. Where are microbes found? _____

10. Microbes need a _____ to live and grow.

11. _____ organisms can resist the effects of antibiotics.

12. A _____ is in a body part. A _____ involves the whole body.

13. The chain of infection is a process. Describe the process.

_____

_____

_____

_____

_____

_____

_____

_____

_____

14. List the portals of exit and portals of entry used by pathogens to leave and enter the body.

A. _____

B. _____

C. _____

D. _____

E. _____

F. _____

15. In medical asepsis, an item or area is _____ when it is free of pathogens.

16. A resident with dementia does not understand aseptic practices. When do you need to assist the person with hand washing?

A. _____

B. _____

C. _____

D. _____

17. Explain why hand lotions or hand creams are applied to the hands after practicing hand hygiene.

_____

_____

_____

18. List 2 aseptic measures that help protect the susceptible host.

A. _____

_____

_____

B. _____

_____

_____

19. Isolation precautions are based on _____ and _____ . Clean areas are not _____ or _____ .

20. _____ are used for all persons whenever care is given.

21. Standard Precautions prevent the spread of infection from:

A. _____

B. _____

C. _____

D. _____

22. The personal protective equipment needed for Standard Precautions depends on:

A. _____

_____

_____

B. _____

_____

_____

23. _____ are always worn when gowns are worn.

24. List the 3 types of Transmission-Based Precautions.

A. _____

B. _____

C. _____

25. To provide care for a patient, the nurse tells you that you need to wear gloves, a mask, goggles, and a gown. List the order in which you should apply this attire.

A. _____

B. _____

C. _____

D. _____

26. Wear gloves whenever contact with _____ , _____ , _____, _____, _____, and _____ is likely.

27. You notice an itchy rash on your hands after you remove your gloves. What should you do?

_____

_____

28. Some patients and residents are allergic to latex. Where will you find this information? _____

_____

_____

29. Which part of a mask is contaminated?

_____

30. You need to wear a mask to provide care. When should you practice hand hygiene?

_____

_____

31. Which parts of goggles and face shields are considered clean?

_____

_____

32. Explain how contaminated items are removed from the person's room.

_____

_____

_____

_____

33. Double-bagging of items is *not* needed unless

_____

_____

_____

34. Masks, gowns, goggles, and face shields can change how you look. This can cause fear and agitation in some persons. Before putting on personal protective equipment (PPE), you need to do the following.

    A. _____

    _____

    B. _____

    _____

    C. _____

    _____

    D. _____

    _____

    E. _____

    _____

    F. _____

    _____

    G. _____

    _____

35. _____
    protects against exposure to the human immunodeficiency virus and the hepatitis B virus.

36. Bloodborne pathogens are spread to others by

    _____ and

    _____.

37. You need to discard contaminated needles and sharp instruments in containers that are

    _____,

    _____, and

    _____.

    These containers are color-coded in _____

    and have the _____ symbol.

38. List the times you need to decontaminate work surfaces.

    A. _____

    B. _____

    C. _____

39. What should you use to clean up broken glass?

    _____

    _____

40. An exposure incident is _____

    _____.

41. Parenteral means _____

    _____.

42. The source individual is _____

    _____

    _____.

43. Write the meaning of the following abbreviations.

    A. AIIR _____

    B. HAI _____

    C. MRSA _____

    D. OPIM _____

    E. TB _____

    F. VRE _____

    G. OSHA _____

MULTIPLE CHOICE

*Circle the **BEST** answer.*

44. Microbes are destroyed by
    A. Water
    B. A warm environment
    C. A dark environment
    D. Heat and light

45. A carrier can pass a pathogen to others.
    A. True
    B. False

46. Health care–associated infections are prevented by the following *except*
    A. Medical asepsis
    B. The immune system
    C. Standard Precautions
    D. The Bloodborne Pathogen Standard

47. Which of the following is *not* a sign or symptom of infection?
    A. Fever
    B. Increased appetite
    C. Pain and tenderness
    D. Redness and swelling

48. The most important measure to prevent the spread of infection is
    A. Sterilization of equipment
    B. Hand hygiene
    C. Surgical asepsis
    D. Isolation precautions

49. An alcohol-based hand rub can be used to decontaminate your hands
    A. When they are visibly dirty or soiled with blood, body fluids, secretions, or excretions
    B. Before eating
    C. After using the restroom
    D. After removing gloves

50. Which is *not* a rule for hand washing with soap and water?
    A. Wash your hands under warm running water.
    B. Stand away from the sink.
    C. Keep your hands and forearms higher than your elbows.
    D. Rub your palms together to work up a good lather.

51. Single-use equipment items are discarded after 1 use.
    A. True
    B. False

52. When cleaning equipment, do the following *except*
    A. Wear personal protective equipment
    B. Rinse the item in hot water first
    C. Wash the item with soap and hot water
    D. Scrub thoroughly using a brush if necessary

53. Disposable gloves are worn when using chemical disinfectants.
    A. True
    B. False

54. All nonpathogens and pathogens are destroyed by
    A. Disinfection
    B. Cleaning
    C. Sterilization
    D. Hand hygiene

55. Which aseptic measure controls reservoirs?
    A. Washing the over-bed table with soap and water before placing a meal tray on it
    B. Wearing personal protective equipment as needed
    C. Holding soiled linens away from your uniform
    D. Providing good skin care

56. Which aseptic measure controls a portal of entry?
    A. Cleaning away from your body
    B. Providing perineal care after bowel elimination
    C. Emptying urinals promptly
    D. Cleaning and disinfecting the shower after use

57. Which is an aseptic practice?
    A. Taking equipment from one person's room to another
    B. Holding equipment and linen close to your uniform
    C. Covering your nose and mouth when coughing or sneezing
    D. Shaking linen to remove wrinkles

58. You help prevent the spread of infection by
    A. Cleaning toward your body
    B. Using leak-proof plastic bags for soiled linens
    C. Holding equipment and linens against your uniform
    D. Cleaning from the dirtiest area to the cleanest area

59. Which is *not* a rule for isolation precautions?
    A. Collect all needed items before entering the room.
    B. Use paper towels to handle contaminated items.
    C. Do not touch any clean area or object if your hands are contaminated.
    D. Wear gloves to turn faucets on and off.

60. Which statement about wearing gloves is *correct*?
    A. Gloves are easier to put on when hands are wet.
    B. Remove a torn glove when you complete the task.
    C. The same pair of gloves is worn for persons in the same room.
    D. Change gloves when moving from a contaminated body site to a clean body site.

61. Gloves are removed so that the inside part is on the outside. The inside is clean.
    A. True
    B. False

62. Which statement is *correct*?
    A. A gown must completely cover you from your neck to your knees.
    B. The gown opens in the front.
    C. Gowns are used more than once.
    D. Gowns are clean on the outside.

63. A wet or moist mask is contaminated.
    A. True
    B. False

64. The Bloodborne Pathogen Standard is a regulation of
    A. OBRA
    B. Medicare
    C. OSHA
    D. Medicaid

65. Hepatitis B is spread by
    A. The fecal-oral route
    B. Blood and sexual contact
    C. Contaminated water
    D. Coughing and sneezing

66. Which statement about the hepatitis B vaccine is *incorrect*?
    A. You can receive the vaccination within 10 working days of being hired.
    B. You can refuse the vaccination.
    C. If you refuse the vaccination, you can have it at a later time.
    D. You pay for the vaccination.

67. Which work practice is required by OSHA?
    A. Store food and drinks where blood or other potentially infectious materials (OPIM) are kept.
    B. Practice hand hygiene before removing gloves.
    C. Wash hands as soon as possible after skin contact with blood or OPIM.
    D. Recap and remove needles by hand.

68. Which is *not* a safety measure for using PPE?
    A. Remove PPE when a garment becomes contaminated.
    B. Wash and decontaminate disposable gloves for reuse.
    C. Place used PPEs in marked areas or containers.
    D. Wear gloves when you expect contact with blood or OPIM.

69. OSHA requires the following measures for contaminated laundry *except*
    A. Handle it as little as possible
    B. Wear gloves or other needed OPIM
    C. Bag contaminated laundry in the dirty utility room
    D. Place wet, contaminated laundry in leak-proof containers before transport
70. When do you need to report an exposure incident?
    A. At once
    B. At the end of your shift
    C. Only if you request blood testing
    D. When you have time
71. Persons requiring isolation precautions may feel lonely. You can help the person by doing the following *except*
    A. Encouraging family to stay away to prevent the spread of microbes
    B. Providing hobby materials if possible
    C. Organizing your work so that you can stay to visit with the person
    D. Saying "hello" from the doorway often

72. Your co-worker's patient requires droplet precautions. Your co-worker asks you to help answer the call lights of her other patients while she is in the person's room. You should
    A. Do so willingly and pleasantly
    B. Tell your co-worker that you have your own work to do
    C. Report your co-worker's behavior to the nurse
    D. Ignore the request and complete your own assignment

CASE STUDY

Miss Joan McMillan is a 50-year-old patient. She was admitted to the hospital with severe acute respiratory syndrome (SARS). She is in an airborne infection isolation room (AIIR). She is on airborne precautions. Miss McMillan is hard of hearing. She has difficulty seeing without her eyeglasses. She has very few visitors. She lives in her own home in a small rural town about 50 miles from the hospital.

Answer the following questions:
1. What precautions are required when providing care for Miss McMillan?

2. What guidelines will you follow if you need to transport Miss McMillan to another area of the hospital for tests?

3. What measures might help prevent Miss McMillan from feeling lonely?

ADDITIONAL LEARNING ACTIVITIES

1. List the measures you practice in your personal life to prevent infection.

2. List the special care needs of the person requiring isolation precautions. Describe how you can help meet the person's needs.

3. View the following video clips on the Evolve companion site to help you learn and practice the procedures:
   A. Removing Gloves
   B. Using Alcohol-Based Hand Rub

4. Review the procedures described in Chapter 13. Using the procedure checklists provided on pp. 202–205:
   A. Practice the procedures for hand washing, using an alcohol-based hand sanitizer, and donning and removing PPE.
   B. Observe a classmate performing the procedures.

CROSSWORD

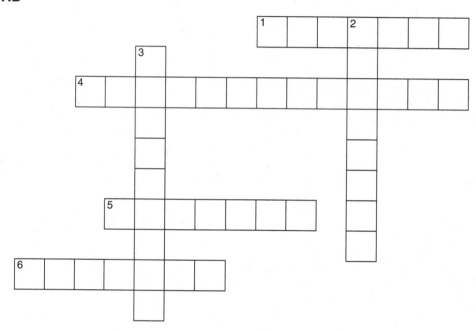

Across

1. Being free of disease-producing microbes
4. The process of becoming unclean
5. The absence of all microbes
6. A microorganism

Down

2. A microbe that is harmful and can cause an infection
3. A disease state resulting from the invasion and growth of microbes in the body

14 BODY MECHANICS

MATCHING

Match each term with the correct definition.

1. _____ The back-lying or supine position
2. _____ The way the head, trunk, arms, and legs are aligned with one another
3. _____ Using the body in an efficient and careful way
4. _____ A semisitting position; the head of the bed is raised between 45 and 60 degrees
5. _____ The person lies on one side or the other; the side-lying position
6. _____ The area on which an object rests
7. _____ The amount of physical effort needed to perform a task
8. _____ Body alignment
9. _____ Lying on the abdomen with the head turned to one side
10. _____ The lateral position
11. _____ A left side-lying position in which the upper leg is sharply flexed so that it is not on the lower leg and the lower arm is behind the person
12. _____ The science of designing a job to fit the worker

A. Body mechanics
B. Force
C. Base of support
D. Sims' position
E. Body alignment
F. Dorsal recumbent position
G. Fowler's position
H. Posture
I. Side-lying position
J. Ergonomics
K. Prone position
L. Lateral position

FILL IN THE BLANKS

13. _____, _____, and _____ can result from improper use and positioning of the body during activity or rest.

14. _____ lets the body move and function with strength and efficiency.

15. Your strongest and largest muscles are in the _____, _____, _____, and _____.

16. For good body mechanics, you need to _____ _____ to lift a heavy object.

17. For good body mechanics, hold items _____ to your body and base of support.

18. The goal of ergonomics is to _____ _____ _____.

19. Work-related musculo-skeletal disorders (MSDs) are _____ _____ _____ _____.

20. Early signs and symptoms of MSDs include _____ _____ _____.

21. Describe these risk factors for MSDs in nursing team members.

    A. Repeating action _____

    _____

    _____

    B. Awkward postures _____

    _____

    _____

22. Signs and symptoms of back injury include:

    A. _____

    B. _____

    C. _____

23. _____ are serious threats from lying or sitting too long in one place.

24. A contracture is _____

    _____

    _____

25. _____

    _____

    help prevent contractures.

26. You are positioning a person in Fowler's position. For good alignment, you need to:

    A. _____

    B. _____

    C. _____

27. You have positioned a person in the prone position. Where should you place small pillows?

    _____

    _____

28. You are positioning a person in a chair. For good alignment you need to:

    A. _____

    _____

    B. _____

    _____

    C. _____

    _____

MULTIPLE CHOICE

*Circle the **BEST** answer.*

29. Which is *not* involved in good body mechanics?
    A. Keep objects close to your body when you lift, move, or carry them.
    B. Push, slide, or pull heavy objects.
    C. Work with sudden motions.
    D. Turn your whole body when changing the direction of your movement.
30. To pick up a box using good body mechanics, which is *correct*?
    A. Use the muscles of the lower back.
    B. Bend your hips and knees.
    C. Hold the box away from your body.
    D. Stand with your feet very close together.
31. After helping move a patient up in bed, you feel pain in your lower back. When should you report this?
    A. As soon as possible
    B. Only if the pain gets worse
    C. Before your next scheduled break
    D. At the end of your shift
32. Which is *not* a rule for body mechanics?
    A. Use an upright working posture.
    B. Bend your back, not your legs.
    C. Keep objects close to your body when you lift, move, or carry them.
    D. Avoid unnecessary bending and reaching.
33. Regular position changes and good alignment promote the following *except*
    A. Comfort and well-being
    B. Breathing
    C. Circulation
    D. Contractures and pressure ulcers
34. Whether in bed or in a chair, the person is repositioned
    A. Every hour
    B. At least every 2 hours
    C. At least every 4 hours
    D. Every shift and when the person requests it
35. Which will *not* promote comfort and safety when moving the person?
    A. Providing for privacy
    B. Telling the person what you are going to do before and during the procedure
    C. Moving the person with quick, firm movements
    D. Using pillows as directed by the nurse for support and alignment
36. Before repositioning the person, you need the following information from the nurse and the care plan *except*
    A. How to use body mechanics
    B. How many staff members need to help you
    C. What assist devices to use
    D. What observations to report and record

37. A person is positioned in a chair. If restraints are used, a pillow must be used behind the person's back.
    A. True
    B. False
38. Which action promotes the person's independence?
    A. Positioning the person's wheelchair so that the person can see outside
    B. Letting the person stay in the same position for up to 4 hours
    C. Letting the person help as much as safely possible
    D. Arranging the person's room for your convenience

39. Transferring and positioning a person should be done by one worker whenever possible.
    A. True
    B. False

LABELING

Label each position.

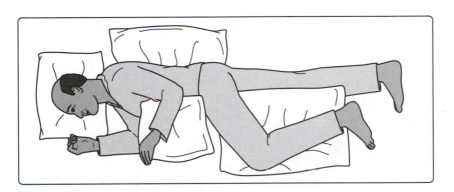

40. _____

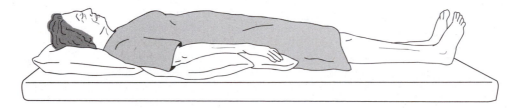

41. _____

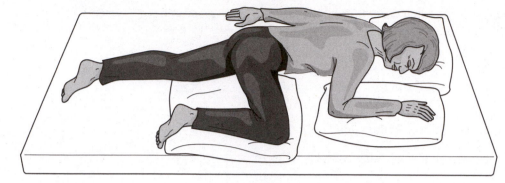

42. _____

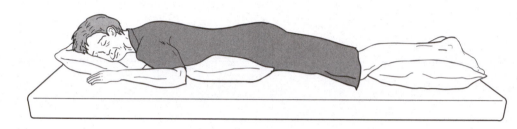

43. _____

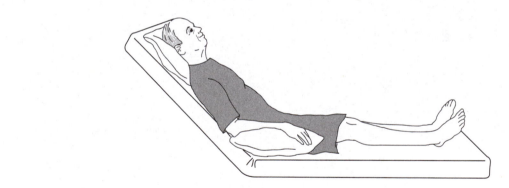

44. _____

CASE STUDY

The nurse asks you to assist a resident to move up in bed. The person is an 85-year-old woman. She is weak. You know that the person has osteoporosis and arthritis.

Answer the following questions:

1. What information do you need from the nurse and the care plan before you assist the person to turn in bed?

2. What measures can you take to avoid causing pain when repositioning the person?

3. How can you ensure that the person is comfortable after you have moved her up in bed?

ADDITIONAL LEARNING ACTIVITIES

1. Review the rules for body mechanics.
   A. Do you practice these rules in your daily activities? Explain.

   B. Do you practice these rules in your work activities? Explain.

   C. Are there ways you can change how you move and work to decrease your risk for injury?

2. List the measures needed for good alignment for each of the following positions (see pp. 178-182 in the textbook).
   A. Fowler's position

   B. Supine position

   C. Lateral position

   D. Sims' position

   E. Chair position

3. Practice proper positioning (Fowler's, supine, prone, lateral, and Sims') with a classmate or family member. Use pillows to promote comfort and body alignment. Assume each position yourself.

15 MOVING THE PERSON

MATCHING

Match each term with the correct definition.

1. _____ Sitting on the side of the bed
2. _____ The rubbing of one surface against another
3. _____ How a person moves to and from a lying position, turns from side to side, and repositions in a bed or other furniture
4. _____ Turning the person as a unit, in alignment, with one motion
5. _____ When skin sticks to a surface while muscles slide in the direction the body is moving

A. Bed mobility
B. Logrolling
C. Dangling
D. Shearing
E. Friction

FILL IN THE BLANKS

6. Many older persons have fragile bones and joints. To prevent injuries:

   A. _____

   B. _____

   C. _____

   D. _____

   E. _____

7. To promote mental comfort when moving a person, you must always:

   A. _____

   _____

   _____

   B. _____

   _____

   _____

   _____

8. You are getting ready to move a person up in bed. The person can be without a pillow. Why should you place the pillow upright against the headboard?

   _____

   _____

   _____

9. To prevent work-related injuries; what information do you need from the nurse and the care plan?

   A. _____

   B. _____

   C. _____

   D. _____

   E. _____

   F. _____

   G. _____

   H. _____

   I. _____

   J. _____

   K. _____

   L. _____

10. These measures reduce friction and shearing.

    A. _____

    B. _____

11. Explain how you would move each of the following persons.

    A. A male resident with a dependence level 4: Total

       Dependence _____

       _____

       _____

       _____

    B. A female resident with a dependence level 2:

       Limited Assistance _____

       _____

       _____

       _____

12. After moving a person up in bed, what observations do you need to report and record?

    A. _____

    B. _____

    C. _____

    D. _____

    E. _____

13. It is best to have help and to use an assist device when moving persons up in bed. You can perform this procedure alone *only if:*

    A. _____

    B. _____

    C. _____

    D. _____

    E. _____

    F. _____

    G. _____

14. Explain why assist devices are used to move persons up in bed. _____

    _____

    _____

    _____

15. Some incontinence products are used as assist devices. For use as assist devices, incontinence products must:

    A. _____

       _____

    B. _____

       _____

    C. _____

       _____

16. You are moving a patient up in bed using an assist device. How should you stand?

    _____

    _____

    _____

17. Explain why you need to move the person to the side of the bed before turning him or her.

    _____

    _____

    _____

18. You are moving a person to the side of the bed. You need to use a mechanical lift or assist device method following Occupational Safety and Health Administration guidelines and for the following persons.

    A. _____

    B. _____

    C. _____

19. You will move a resident in segments. Which part of the person's body do you need to move first?

    _____

20. What information do you need from the nurse and the care plan before turning a person?

    A. _____

    B. _____

    C. _____

    D. _____

    E. _____

    F. _____

    G. _____

    H. _____

    I. _____

    J. _____

    K. _____

21. To safely turn a person, do the following.

    A. _____

    B. _____

    C. _____

22. Logrolling is used to turn the following persons.

    A. _____

    B. _____

    C. _____

    D. _____

23. You are assisting a patient to dangle. The person complains of feeling dizzy. What should you do?

    _____

24. You are assisting a patient to dangle. After the person is in the sitting position, you need to check the person's condition by:

    A. _____

    B. _____

    C. _____

    D. _____

25. List 4 measures to promote pride and independence while handling, moving, and transferring a person.

    A. _____

    B. _____

    C. _____

    D. _____

MULTIPLE CHOICE

Circle the **BEST** *answer.*

26. You need to reposition an older person in bed. Which will *not* help prevent injuries?
    A. Following the rules for body mechanics
    B. Trying to move the person by yourself
    C. Keeping the person in good alignment
    D. Making sure the person's face is not obstructed by a pillow or other device

27. Before moving a person, you need the following information from the nurse and the care plan *except*
    A. The person's height and weight
    B. The person's dependence level
    C. If the person has a weak side
    D. The person's age

28. A lift sheet is used to move a person up in bed. Which is *incorrect?*
    A. Two workers are needed.
    B. Shearing and friction are reduced.
    C. Place the sheet under the person from her waist to her knees.
    D. Roll the sides of the lift sheet up close to the person.

29. You need to move a person in segments. Which helps protect you from injury?
    A. Move the person toward you.
    B. Move the person away from you.
    C. Use a mechanical lift.
    D. Have two co-workers help you.

30. Two or three staff members are needed to logroll a person.
    A. True
    B. False

31. A 90-year-old resident has arthritis. Before turning the person, you need to move her to the side of bed. You need to move her in segments.
    A. True
    B. False

32. You are helping a patient to dangle. Which is *incorrect?*
    A. Provide support if necessary.
    B. Ask the person how she feels.
    C. Check the person's pulse and respirations.
    D. Leave the person alone if she tells you she is okay.

33. When preparing to dangle a person, the head of the bed should be
    A. As flat as possible
    B. Slightly raised
    C. Raised to a sitting position
    D. In the position the person prefers

34. You are repositioning a patient in the wheelchair. The person is able to assist. Which is *correct?*
    A. Stand behind the person.
    B. Ask the person to place his folded hands in his lap.
    C. Position the person's feet on the footplates.
    D. Lock the wheelchair wheels.

35. Which action promotes the person's independence?
    A. Focusing on the person's disabilities
    B. Letting the person stay in the same position for up to 4 hours
    C. Letting the person help as much as safely possible
    D. Positioning the person's wheelchair farther away from the bed than necessary

CASE STUDY

You are caring for an 82-year-old resident living at Pine View Nursing Center. The person is 5 feet, 11 inches tall and weighs 190 pounds. The person cannot walk. He uses a wheelchair. He cannot stand without assistance. The person's right side is his strong side. He needs help to change positions when in bed.

Answer the following questions:
1. For what skin problems is the person at risk?

2. How can you protect the person from friction and shearing during moving him in bed?

3. How often do you need to help with repositioning?

ADDITIONAL LEARNING ACTIVITIES

1. Review the procedures described in Chapter 15.
   A. Under the supervision of your instructor, practice each procedure.
      (1) Use the procedure checklists provided on pp. 206–217.
      (2) Take your turn being the patient or resident.
      (3) Discuss the experience with your classmates and instructor. Answer these questions:
         A. Were your safety needs met?

   B. Were your comfort needs met?

16 TRANSFERRING THE PERSON

FILL IN THE BLANKS

1. A transfer is how a person moves _____
   _____ .

2. To protect yourself and the person from injury,
   _____
   _____ .

3. Many older persons have fragile bones and joints.
   To prevent injuries:_____
   A. _____
   B. _____
   C. _____
   D. _____

4. To promote mental comfort when handling, moving,
   or transferring a person, you must always:
   A. _____
      _____
      _____
      _____
   B. _____
      _____
      _____
   C. _____
      _____
      _____

5. Pivot means to _____
   _____ .

6. A stand-and-pivot transfer is used if:
   A. _____
   B. _____
   C. _____

7. To safely transfer the person, what information do
   you need from the nurse and the care plan?
   A. _____
   B. _____
   C. _____
   D. _____
   E. _____
   F. _____
   G. _____
   H. _____
   I. _____
   J. _____

8. Explain how you would transfer each of the
   following persons.
   A. A male resident with a dependence level 4: Total
      Dependence _____
      _____
      _____
      _____
   B. A female resident with a dependence level 2:
      Limited Assistance _____
      _____
      _____
      _____

9. After transferring a person using a stand-and-
   pivot procedure, what observations do you need
   to report and record?
   A. _____
   B. _____
   C. _____
   D. _____
   E. _____
   F. _____

10. Explain why you need to know about areas of weakness before you transfer a person.

    _____

    _____

    _____

    _____

    _____

11. The person wears _____ footwear for transfers.

12. Transfer belts are used to:

    A. _____

    B. _____

    C. _____

13. A person's left side is weak. When transferring the person, which side moves first?

    _____

14. You are transferring a person from the chair to the bed. The number of staff members needed for a transfer depends on the person's

    _____ ,

    _____ ,

    and _____ .

15. You are preparing to transfer a resident from the wheelchair to the bed. The person's left side is her weak side. How will you position the wheelchair for the transfer? _____

    _____

    _____

16. Bed and wheelchair wheels are _____ for a safe transfer.

17. Using the bathroom for elimination promotes

    _____, _____, _____,

    and _____. _____

18. How is the wheelchair positioned for wheelchair-to-toilet transfers? _____

    _____

    _____

    _____

19. The nurse tells you to transfer a resident using a mechanical lift. You have not used the lift before. What should you do?

    _____

    _____

    _____

20. How will you promote the person's mental comfort when using a mechanical lift to transfer him or her?

    _____

    _____

    _____

21. When performing a procedure, you must give step-by-step directions. When giving directions, you need to:

    A. _____

    B. _____

    C. _____

    D. _____

    E. _____

    F. _____

    G. _____

MULTIPLE CHOICE

Circle the ***BEST*** *answer.*

22. A person with dementia resists your efforts to transfer her from the bed to the chair. Which will *not* prevent work-related injuries?
    A. Proceeding quickly and forcefully
    B. Using a calm and pleasant voice
    C. Diverting the person's attention
    D. Getting a co-worker to help you

23. Before transferring a person, you need the following information from the nurse and the care plan *except*
    A. The person's height and weight
    B. The person's dependence level
    C. If the person has a weak side
    D. The person's age

24. You are transferring a person from the bed to the chair. Which is *correct?*
    A. The person wears nonskid footwear.
    B. The person is helped out of bed on her weak side.
    C. The bed is kept in the high position.
    D. The person places her arms around your neck.

25. You are assisting a patient transfer from the bed to the wheelchair. You must do the following *except*
    A. Lock the wheelchair wheels
    B. Make sure the wheelchair footplates are down
    C. Remove or swing the front rigging out of the way
    D. Lower the bed to its lowest position

26. Before transferring a person to the toilet, you need to
    A. Practice hand hygiene
    B. Remove the elevated toilet seat
    C. Check the towel bar to make sure it is secure
    D. Have the person wear warm slippers

27. Which statement about mechanical lifts is *incorrect*?
    A. Persons who cannot help themselves are transferred with mechanical lifts.
    B. The slings, straps, hooks, and chains must be in good repair.
    C. The person's weight must not exceed the lift's capacity.
    D. If you know how to use one type of lift, you know how to use all types.

28. You are using a mechanical lift to transfer a resident. You should instruct the person to hold on to the swivel bar.
    A. True
    B. False

29. A stand-assist lift is used for persons who
    A. Cannot assist with transfers
    B. Are heavy
    C. Can follow directions
    D. Are unable to bear weight

30. The sling used depends on the lift type and the person's
    A. Age
    B. Size
    C. Gender
    D. Race

31. To avoid injury during a transfer
    A. Move all persons by yourself
    B. Use broken equipment
    C. Position the chair away from the bed
    D. Do not exceed equipment weight limits

CASE STUDY

You are caring for a 92-year-old resident living at Valley View Nursing Center. The person is 5 feet, 9 inches tall and weighs 180 pounds. The person cannot walk. He uses a wheelchair. He cannot stand without assistance. He is able to bear some weight on his legs to assist with transfers from his bed to the wheelchair and from the wheelchair onto the toilet. The person's right side is his strong side.

Answer the following questions:

1. How can you protect the person from injury during transfers?

2. When assisting the person with transfers, which side will you move first?

ADDITIONAL LEARNING ACTIVITIES

1. View the following video clips on the Evolve companion site to help you learn and practice the procedures:
   A. Equipment Preparation for a Transfer
   B. Lowering the Person to the Chair
   C. Transferring to the Stretcher

2. Review the procedures described in Chapter 16.
   A. Under the supervision of your instructor, practice each procedure.
      (1) Use the procedure checklists provided on pp. 218–228.

      (2) Take your turn being the patient or resident.

(3) Discuss the experience with your classmates and instructor. Answer these questions:
   A. Were your safety needs met?

   B. Were your comfort needs met?

30. Why is it important to follow Standard Precautions and the Bloodborne Pathogen Standard when removing linen from the person's bed?

_____

_____

_____

31. After making a bed, you must _____

_____

_____

_____ .

32. You are putting the top sheet on a closed bed. The hem stitching should face _____

_____

_____ .

33. Describe how you should place the pillow on the person's bed. _____

_____

_____

34. A closed bed becomes an open bed by _____

_____ .

35. A surgical bed is also called _____

_____ .

36. A patient received a strong pain-relief drug. You must practice these safety measures.

    A. _____

    B. _____

    C. _____

    D. _____

37. A patient received a pain-relief drug. How long do you need to wait before giving care?

    _____

38. List 7 factors that affect pain.

    A. _____

    B. _____

    C. _____

    D. _____

    E. _____

    F. _____

    G. _____

39. Before giving a back massage, you need to observe the skin for:

    A. _____

    B. _____

    C. _____

    D. _____

40. List 3 methods used to warm lotion before applying it.

    A. _____

    B. _____

    C. _____

41. Back massages are dangerous for persons with certain:

    A. _____

    B. _____

    C. _____

    D. _____

42. Which position is best for giving a back massage?

    _____

43. You need to give a back massage to a 90-year-old resident. The person has arthritis in her hips and knees. Which position will likely be most comfortable for the person?

    _____

44. List 7 factors that affect the amount and quality of sleep.

    A. _____

    B. _____

    C. _____

    D. _____

    E. _____

    F. _____

    G. _____

45. Sleep disorders involve _____

    _____

    _____ .

46. List 3 things you can do to help reduce noise in patient and resident areas.

   A. _____

   _____

   B. _____

   _____

   C. _____

   _____

MULTIPLE CHOICE

*Circle the **BEST** answer.*

47. To maintain the person's unit, you need to
   A. Adjust the temperature so that it is comfortable for you
   B. Arrange personal items the way you prefer
   C. Keep the call light within the person's reach at all times
   D. Empty the person's wastebasket weekly
48. You are assisting a patient with a bath. You notice many small scraps of paper with notes on them lying on the person's bedside stand. You can throw them in the trash to keep the unit neat and clean.
   A. True
   B. False
49. Which room temperature range is usually comfortable for most healthy people?
   A. 65°F to 68°F
   B. 68°F to 74°F
   C. 72°F to 82°F
   D. 82°F to 90°F
50. Which action will *not* help reduce odors?
   A. Dispose of incontinence products at the end of your shift.
   B. Check incontinent persons often.
   C. Keep laundry containers closed.
   D. Provide good hygiene.
51. To reduce odors, you need to
   A. Change wet or soiled linens every 4 hours
   B. Empty, clean, and disinfect bedpans promptly
   C. Use a room deodorizer every 4 hours
   D. Dispose of ostomy products at the end of your shift
52. A person has dementia. Which statement is *incorrect*?
   A. The person may not understand the meaning of sounds.
   B. The person may have extreme reactions to sounds.
   C. The person's reactions to sound are less severe at night.
   D. A strange room can make the person's reactions to sounds worse.

53. Good lighting is needed for safety and comfort. Which is *correct*?
   A. Provide bright light to help the person relax.
   B. Provide dim lighting during the night.
   C. Adjust lighting the way visitors request.
   D. Keep light controls within the person's reach.
54. Which bed positions require a doctor's order?
   A. Flat and Fowler's
   B. Fowler's and semi-Fowler's
   C. Semi-Fowler's and reverse Trendelenburg's
   D. Trendelenburg's and reverse Trendelenburg's
55. A resident tells you that he does not like his mattress because it is too hard. What should you do?
   A. Tell the person that it is the only mattress available.
   B. Call maintenance and ask for a new mattress.
   C. Tell the nurse about the person's complaint.
   D. Ask the person's family to bring a more comfortable mattress.
56. Which item *cannot* be placed on the over-bed table?
   A. A bedpan
   B. The water pitcher
   C. A box of tissues
   D. A book
57. Where should you store the person's bedpan and toilet paper?
   A. On the over-bed table
   B. On the lower shelf in the bedside stand
   C. In the person's closet
   D. In the person's bathroom
58. Each person's unit must have at least one chair. The chair must
   A. Be a reclining chair
   B. Be a straight-back chair
   C. Not move or tip during transfers
   D. Be provided by the person or family
59. The privacy curtain must be pulled completely around the person's bed
   A. Always when giving care
   B. Only when the person's roommate is present
   C. Only when the room door is open
   D. Only if the person requests it to be
60. Persons who are confused do not need call lights.
   A. True
   B. False
61. For the person's safety, you must
   A. Keep the call light within the person's reach
   B. Place the call light on the person's weak side
   C. Remind the person to use the call light only in emergencies
   D. Take the call light away from a person if he or she uses it too often
62. CMS requires closet space for each nursing center resident.
   A. True
   B. False

63. To keep beds neat and clean, you need to
    A. Straighten linens whenever loose or wrinkled and at bedtime
    B. Check for and remove food and crumbs once each shift
    C. Straighten linens whenever they become wet, soiled, or damp
    D. Change all linens daily

64. This type of bed is made for persons who are out of bed for a short time.
    A. A closed bed
    B. An occupied bed
    C. An open bed
    D. A surgical bed

65. You are making a closed bed for a new resident. Which piece of linen is placed on the bed first?
    A. Bottom sheet
    B. Cotton drawsheet
    C. Mattress pad
    D. Pillowcase

66. This type of bed is made after a person is discharged.
    A. An open bed
    B. A closed bed
    C. An occupied bed
    D. A surgical bed

67. You are making an occupied bed. Which is *incorrect*?
    A. Keep the bed in the lowest position.
    B. If the person uses bed rails, the far bed rail is up.
    C. Keep the person in good alignment.
    D. After making the bed, lock the bed wheels.

68. You have finished making a surgical bed for a resident arriving by stretcher. After making the bed, you should leave the bed in its highest position.
    A. True
    B. False

69. Wear gloves when removing linen from the person's bed.
    A. True
    B. False

70. Which is a rule for bedmaking?
    A. Shake linens to remove wrinkles.
    B. Hold linens against your uniform.
    C. Place dirty linen on the floor.
    D. Follow the rules of medical asepsis.

71. You brought an extra pillowcase into a patient's room. What should you do?
    A. Take it back to the linen closet.
    B. Put it in the dirty laundry.
    C. Use it for another patient.
    D. Put it in the patient's closet.

72. Which statement about pain is *incorrect*?
    A. Pain can cause anxiety.
    B. Pain seems worse when a person is tired.
    C. Dealing with pain is often easier when family and friends offer support.
    D. Pain affects all persons in the same way.

73. Changes in usual behavior may signal pain in persons with dementia.
    A. True
    B. False

74. When giving a back massage, do the following *except*
    A. Warm the lotion before applying it
    B. Use firm strokes
    C. Always keep your hands in contact with the person's skin
    D. Massage bony areas that are reddened

75. A back massage is safe for all persons.
    A. True
    B. False

76. When giving a back massage, use fast movements to relax the person.
    A. True
    B. False

77. After giving a back massage, what do you need to report and record?
    A. The type of lotion used
    B. How you warmed the lotion
    C. How long the massage lasted
    D. Breaks in the skin and reddened areas

78. Which occurs during sleep?
    A. Stress and tension increase.
    B. The body uses more energy than when awake.
    C. Tissue healing and repair occur.
    D. Body functions speed up.

79. Sleep problems are *uncommon* in persons with Alzheimer's disease and other dementias.
    A. True
    B. False

80. Which of these measures will *not* promote sleep?
    A. Giving a back massage
    B. Reducing noise
    C. Keeping the room cool and well lighted
    D. Positioning the person in good alignment

81. A resident asks for a bedtime snack. Which will *not* help promote sleep?
    A. Coffee and a brownie
    B. Milk
    C. Toast
    D. Crackers and milk

CASE STUDY

Ms. Angela Lopez and Ms. Lois Green share a room at Pine View Nursing Center.

Ms. Lopez has the bed by the window. She likes to sleep with the window open. She likes the privacy curtain between her bed and Ms. Green's bed to be open so that she can see out the door. Family and friends visit Ms. Lopez often. They often bring her ethnic foods. She sometimes hides food in her drawers and closet.

Ms. Green is a very private person. She chills easily. She likes to go to bed early. Listening to opera music helps her fall asleep. Ms. Green has many figurines, which she likes to display in a cabinet she brought from home. She worries about them getting broken. She also brought her own reclining chair from home.

Answer the following questions:

1. What challenges does the interdisciplinary health team have in meeting the needs of each resident?

2. How can the rights of each resident be promoted?

3. How can the interdisciplinary health team promote each person's comfort and quality of life?

ADDITIONAL LEARNING ACTIVITIES

1. Discuss the importance of personal space in your daily life. Answer the following questions:
   A. How would you feel about sharing a room with another person?

   B. How would you decide what items to take with you and what items to leave behind?

2. Make a list of factors that affect your ability to sleep. Answer the following questions:
   A. What temperatures are most comfortable for you? How do you adapt to changes in temperature?

   B. Are there certain odors that prevent sleep? How do you control the odors in your environment?

   C. How do noises and sounds affect your ability to sleep? What sounds keep you awake? Are there sounds that help you relax?

   D. How do you control the light in your environment to help you sleep?

E. Do you have certain rituals that help you sleep? Explain.

F. How might you use what you know about your personal comfort needs to help you provide better care?

3. How much sleep do you need to feel rested?
    A. How does lack of sleep affect your daily activities?

4. Practice gathering linen in the correct order for bedmaking. List the correct order on an index card. Carry the card with you until you have the order memorized.

5. View the video clips on the Evolve companion site to help you learn and practice the procedures.

6. Practice the procedures in Chapter 17. Use the procedure checklists provided on pp. 229–237.

7. Observe classmates performing the procedures in Chapter 17. Use the procedure checklists provided on pp. 229–237.

18 HYGIENE NEEDS

MATCHING

Match each term with the correct definition.

1. _____ Routine care given before breakfast
2. _____ Routine hygiene done after lunch and before the evening meal
3. _____ Breathing fluid, food, vomitus, or an object into the lungs
4. _____ Care given at bedtime
5. _____ Mouth care
6. _____ Cleaning the genital and anal areas
7. _____ Care given after breakfast

A. Morning care
B. Oral hygiene
C. Evening care (PM care)
D. Early morning care (AM care)
E. Afternoon care
F. Aspiration
G. Perineal care (pericare)

FILL IN THE BLANKS

8. The _____ defends the body against disease.

9. Intact skin prevents _____ from entering the body.

10. You will assist patients and residents with personal hygiene. You need to protect the person's right to

_____ and

_____.

11. Oral hygiene does the following.

A. _____

B. _____

C. _____

D. _____

E. _____

12. You assist the person with oral hygiene. What observations do you need to report and record?

A. _____

B. _____

C. _____

D. _____

E. _____

F. _____

13. Explain why you need to follow Standard Precautions and the Bloodborne Pathogen Standard when giving oral hygiene.

_____

_____

_____

_____

_____

14. Many people brush their own teeth. You may have to brush the teeth of persons who:

A. _____

B. _____

C. _____

15. Explain why flossing is done.

_____

_____

_____

16. You are giving oral care to an unconscious person. To prevent aspiration, you need to:

A. _____

_____

B. _____

_____

C. _____

_____

17. You are using a sponge swab to give oral hygiene to an unconscious person. Explain why you need to make sure the sponge is tight on the stick.

    _____

    _____

18. A _____ is an artificial tooth or a set of artificial teeth.

19. A resident removed her dentures and placed them under her pillow. While you were straightening the person's pillow, the dentures fell off the bed and broke. What should you do?

    _____

20. A patient wears an upper denture. You need to remove the denture for the person. Explain how

    you would do so. _____

    _____

    _____

    _____

21. List 8 benefits of bathing.

    A. _____

    B. _____

    C. _____

    D. _____

    E. _____

    F. _____

    G. _____

    H. _____

22. The bathing method for each person depends on:

    A. _____

    B. _____

    C. _____

23. You are giving a person a tub bath. What observations do you need to report and record?

    A. _____

    B. _____

    C. _____

    D. _____

    E. _____

    F. _____

    G. _____

    H. _____

    I. _____

    J. _____

    K. _____

    L. _____

24. Do not use powder near persons with respiratory

    disorders because _____

    _____

    _____.

25. To safely apply powder, you need to:

    A. _____

    B. _____

    C. _____

    D. _____

26. Explain why you should allow the person to use the bathroom, commode, bedpan, or urinal

    before bathing. _____

    _____

    _____

    _____

27. You are giving a patient a complete bed bath. Why should you wait to remove the person's gown or pajamas until after you wash his face, ears, and neck?

    _____

    _____

    _____

28. Bed baths are usually needed by persons who are:

    A. _____

    B. _____

    C. _____

    D. _____

29. A partial bath involves bathing the

    _____ ,

    _____ ,

    _____ ,

    _____ ,

    _____ , and

    _____ .

30. You protect the person's privacy during a shower by:

    A. _____

    B. _____

    C. _____

31. Before assisting with a shower or tub bath, what information do you need from the nurse and the care plan?

    A. _____

    B. _____

    C. _____

    D. _____

    E. _____

    F. _____

    G. _____

    H. _____

32. Perineal care involves _____

    _____

33. Explain why perineal care is given. _____

    _____

    _____

34. When is perineal care given?

    A. _____

    B. _____

35. When giving perineal care, work from

    _____ to

    _____ .

36. When giving perineal care, what observations do you need to report and record?

    A. _____

    B. _____

    C. _____

    D. _____

37. You are giving perineal care to a male patient. Explain how you will clean the tip of his penis.

    _____

    _____

    _____

    _____

    _____

    _____

    _____

    _____

    _____

38. Perineal care is very important for persons who:

    A. _____

    B. _____

    C. _____

    D. _____

    E. _____

39. Provide the abbreviation for each of the following words.

    A. Centigrade _____

    B. Fahrenheit _____

    C. Identification _____

MULTIPLE CHOICE

Circle the BEST answer.

40. Before giving oral hygiene, you need the following information from the nurse and the care plan *except*
    A. The type of oral hygiene to give
    B. The type of toothbrush to use
    C. If flossing is needed
    D. How much help the person needs

41. Which action is *incorrect* when flossing the person's teeth?
    A. Hold the floss between the middle fingers of each hand.
    B. Start at the upper back tooth on the right side.
    C. Move the floss gently up and down between the teeth.
    D. Use a new piece of floss for each tooth.

42. When providing mouth care to the unconscious person, which is *correct*?
    - A. Use your fingers to hold the mouth open.
    - B. Position the person on his or her back.
    - C. Use a hard-bristled toothbrush.
    - D. Explain what you are doing step-by-step.
43. How often is mouth care given to unconscious persons?
    - A. At least every 2 hours
    - B. At least every 4 hours
    - C. Every 6 hours
    - D. Twice a day
44. You are giving mouth care to an unconscious person. Which action is *incorrect*?
    - A. Provide for privacy.
    - B. Place a towel under the person's face.
    - C. Place a kidney basin under the chin.
    - D. With the tongue blade, use force to separate the upper and lower teeth.
45. When cleaning dentures, which is *correct*?
    - A. Use hot water.
    - B. Firmly hold them over a basin of water lined with a towel.
    - C. Use a sponge swab to clean them.
    - D. Store them dry in a container with a lid.
46. Which is *not* a rule for bathing?
    - A. Follow the care plan for bathing method.
    - B. Allow personal choice whenever possible.
    - C. Cover the person for warmth and privacy.
    - D. Briskly rub the person dry with a clean towel.
47. Which is *not* a rule for bathing?
    - A. Protect the person from falling.
    - B. Use good body mechanics at all times.
    - C. Use hot water and soap.
    - D. Keep bar soap in the soap dish between latherings.
48. A person with dementia becomes agitated when you try to give him a tub bath. Which measure might be helpful?
    - A. Trying to hurry the person to get the bath over with as soon as possible
    - B. Explaining to the person that there is nothing to be afraid of
    - C. Trying the bath later
    - D. Getting help to force the person into the tub
49. Persons with dementia may feel threatened by bathing procedures.
    - A. True
    - B. False
50. Water temperature for a complete bed bath is usually between:
    - A. 95°F and 100°F
    - B. 100°F and 110°F
    - C. 110°F and 115°F
    - D. 115°F and 120°F

51. When giving a complete bed bath, do the following *except*
    - A. Place the bed in the lowest horizontal position
    - B. Lower the head of the bed
    - C. Cover the person for warmth
    - D. Change the water if it is soapy or cool
52. To wash around the person's eyes
    - A. Use warm soapy water
    - B. Wipe from the outer to the inner aspect of the eye
    - C. Clean around the near eye first
    - D. Use a clean part of the washcloth for each stroke
53. Risks from tub baths and showers include
    - A. Falls, chilling, and burns
    - B. Dementia, confusion, and restlessness
    - C. Skin breakdown and infection
    - D. Hypertension and shortness of breath
54. You are giving a resident a tub bath. Which is *correct*?
    - A. The bath should last 30 minutes.
    - B. The tub bath may cause the person to feel faint and weak.
    - C. Use bath oils in the water.
    - D. Drain the tub after the person gets out of the tub.
55. Shower chair wheels are locked during the shower.
    - A. True
    - B. False
56. Which is *not* a safety measure for tub baths and showers?
    - A. Clean and disinfect the tub or shower before and after use.
    - B. Place needed items within the person's reach.
    - C. Place the call light within the person's reach.
    - D. Have the person use the towel bars for support.
57. When giving a shower, turn hot water on first, then the cold water.
    - A. True
    - B. False
58. Fill the tub before the person gets into it.
    - A. True
    - B. False
59. A resident can bathe alone in the tub. How often do you need to check on the person?
    - A. At least every 5 minutes
    - B. At least every 15 minutes
    - C. Whenever you have time
    - D. Only when the person turns on the call light

60. When giving perineal care, which action is *correct*?
    A. Cover the person with a drawsheet.
    B. Use hot water.
    C. Rinse thoroughly.
    D. Rub the area dry after rinsing.
61. When giving perineal care, you need to use a clean part of the washcloth for each stroke.
    A. True
    B. False

62. You protect the person's right to privacy by
    A. Exposing the person during bathing procedures
    B. Allowing visitors to stay in the room when giving care
    C. Providing care with the room door open
    D. Covering persons who are taken to and from tubs and shower rooms

CASE STUDY

A resident of Pine View Nursing Center is alert and can make her needs known. The person is continent of bowel and bladder. You are assigned to care for the person today. Your assignment sheet tells you that the person:

- Uses a wheelchair to get around
- Eats all of her meals in the dining room
- Has an upper and lower denture
- Needs a whirlpool tub bath today
  - Likes her bath at 10 AM
- Gets a back massage after her bath

Answer the following questions:

1. What care do you need to give the person before breakfast?

2. What care do you need to give the person after breakfast?

3. Before assisting the person with a bath, what information do you need from the nurse and the care plan?

4. When assisting the person with a bath, what observations do you need to make?

5. How will you promote the person's right to privacy?

6. How will you promote the person's right to personal choice?

ADDITIONAL LEARNING ACTIVITIES

1. Discuss the importance of hygiene and cleanliness in your personal life.
   A. Explain how important it is for you to feel clean and free from unpleasant odors when you are around other people.

   B. List the personal care routines you practice daily to promote cleanliness.

2. Has illness ever prevented you from carrying out your daily hygiene routines? Explain.
   A. Discuss how this affected your personal comfort.

3. To help you learn and practice the procedures, view the following video clips on the Evolve companion site:
   A. Brushing the Person's Teeth
   B. Removing Dentures
   C. Cleaning with Soap
   D. Washing the Face
   E. Cleaning the Penis Using a Circular Motion
   F. Helping to Dry the Person

4. The procedures in this chapter require you to provide personal care to another person. The procedures must be performed in a way that respects the person's privacy and dignity. It will help you understand how the person feels if you practice the procedures with a classmate. Take your turn being the patient or resident. Under the supervision of your instructor, use the procedure checklists provided on pp. 238–258 to practice the procedures in Chapter 18. Use a simulator to practice female and male perineal care.
   A. After practicing each procedure, discuss your experience.

19 GROOMING NEEDS

MATCHING

Match each term with the correct definition.

1. _____ Hair loss
2. _____ Excessive amounts of dry, white flakes from the scalp
3. _____ Excessive body hair
4. _____ A skin disorder caused by a female mite
5. _____ Being in or on a host
6. _____ Infestation with wingless insects; lice
7. _____ Prevents or slows down blood clotting

A. Hirsutism
B. Alopecia
C. Anticoagulant
D. Pediculosis
E. Dandruff
F. Infestation
G. Scabies

FILL IN THE BLANKS

8. The nursing process reflects the person's:

A. _____

B. _____

C. _____

D. _____

E. _____

9. Hirsutism results from _____

_____

_____ .

10. Lice spread to others through:

A. _____

B. _____

C. _____

D. _____

E. _____

F. _____

G. _____

H. _____

11. Common sites for scabies are _____

_____

_____ .

Other sites include _____

_____ .

12. Brushing and combing hair are part of

_____ ,

_____ , and

_____ care.

13. _____
chooses how to brush, comb, and style hair.

14. You have finished brushing a resident's hair. What observations do you need to report and record?

A. _____

B. _____

C. _____

D. _____

E. _____

F. _____

G. _____

H. _____

15. Describe the following.

A. Nits (lice eggs attached to hair shafts)

_____

_____

B. Lice

_____

_____

_____

16. A resident is dressed for the day. The person asks you to brush her hair. Explain why you should place a towel across the person's back and shoulders before you begin.

    _____

    _____

    _____

17. The nurse tells you which shampoo method to use. The shampoo method depends on:

    A. _____

    B. _____

    C. _____

18. List 3 shampoo methods.

    A. _____

    B. _____

    C. _____

19. You have finished shampooing a patient's hair. What observations do you need to report and record?

    A. _____

    B. _____

    C. _____

    D. _____

    E. _____

    F. _____

    G. _____

    H. _____

20. A patient uses medicated shampoo. When you are finished shampooing the person's hair, what should you do with the shampoo?

    _____

    _____

    _____

21. You need to shampoo a resident's hair. The person has scalp sores. You need to wear _____.

22. An 80-year-old resident cannot tip his head back. You are shampooing the person's hair in the tub. How would you keep shampoo out of the person's eyes while shampooing his hair?

    _____

    _____

    _____

    _____

23. What type of shaver is used for a person taking an anticoagulant drug?

    _____

    _____

24. When using a safety razor, shave in the direction of hair growth when shaving _____

    _____

    _____.

25. Explain why you should not use a safety razor to shave a person with dementia.

    _____

    _____

    _____

    _____

26. When shaving a person, what observations do you need to report at once?

    A. _____

    B. _____

    C. _____

27. Where are used razor blades and disposable shavers disposed of?

    _____

    _____

28. Never trim or shave a beard or mustache without

    _____.

29. When giving foot care, what observations do you need to report and record?

    A. _____

    B. _____

    C. _____

    D. _____

    E. _____

    F. _____

30. You do not cut or trim toenails if a person:

    A. _____

    B. _____

    C. _____

    D. _____

31. How are fingernails trimmed?

_____

_____

_____

32. List the rules to follow when changing clothes and hospital gowns.

A. _____

_____

B. _____

_____

C. _____

_____

D. _____

_____

E. _____

_____

F. _____

_____

G. _____

_____

H. _____

_____

33. Before assisting with dressing, what information do you need from the nurse and the care plan?

A. _____

B. _____

C. _____

D. _____

E. _____

F. _____

34. Before changing a gown, what information do you need from the nurse and the care plan?

A. _____

B. _____

35. Write the meaning of the following abbreviations.

A. IV _____

B. C _____

C. ID _____

MULTIPLE CHOICE

*Circle the **BEST** answer.*

36. Infestation of the scalp with lice is
    A. Pediculosis capitis
    B. Pediculosis pubis
    C. Pediculosis corporis
    D. Dandruff
37. Brushing and combing hair is
    A. Done whenever needed
    B. Done when you have time
    C. Not your responsibility
    D. Always done by the patient or resident
38. When giving hair care, which action is *correct*?
    A. You decide how to style the hair.
    B. Brush or comb from the scalp to the hair ends.
    C. Cut matted and tangled hair.
    D. Braid long hair to keep it neat.
39. Before shampooing a person's hair, you need the following information from the nurse and the care plan *except*
    A. When to shampoo the person's hair
    B. What method to use
    C. The person's position restrictions or limits
    D. How long the person's hair is
40. A patient has limited range of motion in her neck. The person is not shampooed
    A. In bed
    B. In the shower
    C. In the tub
    D. At the sink or on a stretcher
41. A person receives a cut during shaving. Which action is *correct*?
    A. Apply aftershave lotion to the cut.
    B. Apply direct pressure to the cut.
    C. Put a dressing on the cut.
    D. Put a piece of tissue on the cut.
42. A resident has a beard. Which action is *incorrect*?
    A. Wash and comb the beard daily.
    B. Ask the person how to groom his beard.
    C. Trim the person's beard once a week.
    D. Wash the beard whenever mouth or nose drainage is present.
43. Use nail clippers to cut fingernails. Never use scissors.
    A. True
    B. False
44. Nails are easier to trim and clean
    A. In the morning
    B. Before the bath
    C. Right after soaking or bathing
    D. At bedtime
45. When trimming fingernails, which action is *correct*?
    A. Let the fingernails soak for 30 minutes before starting.
    B. Clip the fingernails in a curved shape.
    C. Shape the nails with an emery board or a nail file.
    D. Use scissors.

46. Feet are soaked for
    A. 5 to 10 minutes
    B. 15 to 20 minutes
    C. 25 to 30 minutes
    D. 30 minutes
47. You are assisting a person with dementia to dress. Which action is *not* helpful?
    A. Let the person choose what to wear from two or three outfits.
    B. Choose clothing that is easy to get on and off.
    C. Stack clothes in the order that they will be put on.
    D. Dress the person as quickly as possible.
48. You must allow for personal choice and independence when assisting with dressing and undressing.
    A. True
    B. False

49. If there is injury or paralysis, the gown is removed from
    A. The strong side first
    B. The weak side first
    C. The right side first
    D. The left side first
50. You need to follow the person's grooming routines whenever possible.
    A. True
    B. False
51. You promote courteous and dignified care by
    A. Combing the person's hair the way you like it
    B. Making sure clothing is properly fastened
    C. Encouraging a man to shave off his beard
    D. Exposing the person when changing garments

CASE STUDY

A patient is recovering from surgery on her right knee. Today is the person's bath day. She also wants her hair shampooed. The person has thick, long curly hair, which she usually wears up. She dresses in regular clothes during the day and wears a nightgown to bed. The person needs some assistance with dressing and undressing.

Answer the following questions:

1. Before you assist the person to shampoo her hair, what information do you need from the nurse and the care plan?

2. When assisting the person with shampooing, what safety measures will you practice?

3. How will you brush or comb the person's hair?

4. Who will choose what the person wears?

ADDITIONAL LEARNING ACTIVITIES

1. List the grooming activities you perform every day. Answer these questions:
   A. How important are your grooming routines?

   B. When you are performing your grooming activities, how important is personal choice?

   C. When you are performing your grooming activities, how important is privacy?

   D. How might you feel if you were unable to perform your grooming activities?

   (1) How would you want to be treated?

2. View the following video clips on the Evolve companion site to help you learn and practice the procedures:
   A. Brushing Tangled Hair
   B. Shampooing Hair in Bed
   C. Cleaning Under Fingernails
   D. Using a Safety Razor
   E. Removing Pullover Shirts
   F. Sliding Gown Over/Under IV Fluids

3. Carefully review the procedures in Chapter 19. Under the supervision of your instructor, use the procedure checklists on pp. 259–273 to practice each procedure.
   A. Practice dressing and undressing procedures with classmates or family members.
      (1) Use different types of clothing (e.g., clothes that open in front and clothes that open in back, button and pullover shirts, pants with zippers and buttons, and pants that pull on.)
      (2) Role-play weakness on one side of the body.
      (3) Role-play that the person is not able to help.
      (4) Take your turn being the patient or resident.

   B. Did you feel safe and secure during the procedures?

   C. How might your experience affect how you help others with grooming and dressing activities?

20 URINARY NEEDS

MATCHING

Match each term with the correct definition.

1. _____ Small amounts of urine leak from a full bladder
2. _____ Urine is lost at predictable intervals when the bladder is full
3. _____ When urine leaks during exercise and certain movements that cause pressure on the bladder
4. _____ The loss of urine is in response to a sudden, urgent need to void
5. _____ The need to void at once
6. _____ The person has bladder control but cannot use the toilet in time
7. _____ Voiding at frequent intervals
8. _____ The involuntary loss or leakage of urine

A. Overflow incontinence
B. Urinary frequency
C. Functional incontinence
D. Urinary urgency
E. Stress incontinence
F. Reflex incontinence
G. Urge incontinence
H. Urinary incontinence

FILL IN THE BLANKS

9. The urinary system removes _____ from the blood and maintains the body's
_____

10. List seven factors that affect urine production.

    A. _____
    B. _____
    C. _____
    D. _____
    E. _____
    F. _____
    G. _____

11. When assisting with urination, you need to observe urine for:

    A. _____
    B. _____
    C. _____
    D. _____
    E. _____
    F. _____

12. A patient is recovering from hip replacement surgery. What type of bedpan will the person use?

    _____

13. Explain how you will promote safety when handling bedpans and their contents.

    A. _____
    _____
    B. _____
    _____

14. A resident cannot assist in getting on the bedpan. How will you give the person the bedpan?

    A. _____
    B. _____
    C. _____
    D. _____
    E. _____

15. A person you assist with the bedpan is unable to clean her genital area. Describe how you will clean the person's genital area.

    _____
    _____
    _____
    _____

16. Men use _____ to void.

17. Before assisting with urinals, what information do you need from the nurse and the care plan?

A. _____

_____

B. _____

_____

C. _____

_____

D. _____

_____

E. _____

_____

F. _____

_____

G. _____

_____

H. _____

_____

18. Explain why you need to empty urinals promptly.

_____

_____

_____

_____

_____

19. A resident stands to use the urinal. How will you give him the urinal?

A. _____

B. _____

C. _____

D. _____

20. A _____ is a chair or wheelchair with an opening for a container.

21. When assisting with commodes, what information do you need from the nurse and the care plan?

A. _____

B. _____

C. _____

D. _____

E. _____

F. _____

G. _____

22. After you transfer a person to the commode, how can you provide warmth and promote privacy?

_____

_____

23. List seven causes of functional incontinence.

A. _____

B. _____

C. _____

D. _____

E. _____

F. _____

G. _____

24. A person has stress incontinence and urge incontinence. This is called _____.

25. What should you do if incontinence is a new problem for a patient or resident?

_____

26. A resident is incontinent of urine. You help prevent urinary tract infections by:

A. _____

B. _____

C. _____

D. _____

27. To promote dignity and self-esteem, use the following terms for incontinence products

A. _____

B. _____

C. _____

28. Before applying an incontinence product, what information do you need from the nurse and the care plan?

A. _____

B. _____

C. _____

D. _____

E. _____

F. _____

29. What is the goal of a bladder training program?

_____

MULTIPLE CHOICE

*Circle the **BEST** answer.*

30. How much urine does the healthy adult produce each day?
    A. About 500 mL
    B. About 700 mL
    C. About 1500 mL
    D. About 3000 mL
31. Which is *not* a rule for normal elimination?
    A. Follow Standard Precautions and the Bloodborne Pathogen Standard.
    B. Limit the amount of fluid intake to 1500 mL daily.
    C. Follow the person's voiding routines and habits.
    D. Help the person to the bathroom when the request is made.
32. You promote normal elimination by
    A. Setting new voiding routines
    B. Asking the person to hurry
    C. Providing only small amounts of fluid
    D. Providing privacy
33. Normal urine
    A. Is pale yellow, straw colored, or amber
    B. Does not have an odor
    C. Is cloudy
    D. Contains particles
34. Hematuria is
    A. Scant amount f urine
    B. An abnormally large amounts of urine
    C. Painful or difficult urination
    D. Blood in the urine
35. To place a fracture pan correctly, the smaller end is placed under the buttocks.
    A. True
    B. False

36. Before assisting with the bedpan, you need the following information from the nurse and the care plan *except*
    A. How to position the bedpan
    B. If you can leave the room
    C. If the nurse needs to observe the results
    D. What observations to report
37. Remind men to place urinals on the over-bed table after use.
    A. True
    B. False
38. Nervous system disorders and injuries are common causes of
    A. Stress incontinence
    B. Urge incontinence
    C. Functional incontinence
    D. Reflex incontinence
39. Which is *not* a nursing measure for persons with urinary incontinence?
    A. Increase fluid intake at bedtime.
    B. Provide good skin care.
    C. Answer call lights promptly.
    D. Observe for signs of skin breakdown.
40. You feel impatient when caring for a person with incontinence. Which action is *correct*?
    A. Tell a co-worker to take care of the person for you.
    B. Wait to provide care until you feel less stressed.
    C. Talk to the nurse at once.
    D. Tell the person how you feel.
41. You observe a resident with dementia urinating in the trash can. Which action is *correct*?
    A. Remove the trash can from the person's room.
    B. Tell the person to urinate in the bathroom.
    C. Tell the person to empty the trash can into the toilet.
    D. Check with the nurse and the care plan for measures to help the person.
42. When a person has dementia, which measure can help keep the person clean and dry?
    A. Remind the person where the bathroom is.
    B. Provide all fluids before 5:00 PM.
    C. Follow the person's bathroom routine as closely as possible.
    D. Tell the person to ask to use the bathroom when the urge to void is felt.
43. What observations do you need to report to the nurse when changing a brief?
    A. Pale yellow urine
    B. A faint odor
    C. Blood in the urine
    D. Properly fitting product
44. The abbreviation for milliliter is
    A. ML
    B. Ml
    C. ml
    D. mL

CASE STUDY

A 70-year-old hospital patient has functional incontinence and dementia. The person is alert but cannot assist with her daily care. She wears a brief. The person walks with a walker and is out of bed most of the day. Her husband visits every day at 1300.

Answer the following questions:

1. Before applying an incontinence product, what information do you need from the nurse and the care plan?

2. When giving incontinence care, what observations do you need to report and record?

3. What safety measures do you need to practice when applying incontinence products?

4. How often do you need to provide perineal care?

5. How will you protect the person's right to privacy?

ADDITIONAL LEARNING ACTIVITIES

1. Think of your personal voiding patterns.
   A. List the factors that affect your daily patterns.

   B. Discuss how changes in your personal patterns affect your comfort.

2. View the following video clips on the Evolve companion site to help you learn and practice the procedures:
   A. Applying a Brief in Bed
   B. Rolling the Person on to the Bedpan
   C. Transfer to the Bedside Commode
   D. Using a Self-Adhering Condom Catheter
   E. Using the Urinal in Bed

3. Carefully review and practice the procedure for giving the bedpan. Work with a classmate. Use a regular bedpan and a fracture pan.
   A. Use the procedure checklist provided on pp. 274–276 as a guide.
   B. Wear clothing to practice. Take your turn being the patient or resident. Discuss your experience.

   (1) Did you have concerns about dignity and privacy?

   (2) Was the experience physically comfortable? Explain.

(3) Was it difficult to position the bedpan correctly? Explain.

4. Carefully review and practice all the procedures in this chapter. Use a simulator when appropriate. Use the procedure checklists provided on pp. 274–282. If you are embarrassed by any of these procedures, discuss your feelings with your instructor or a nurse.

(4) How might it feel to be left on a bedpan for 15 minutes or longer?

CROSSWORD

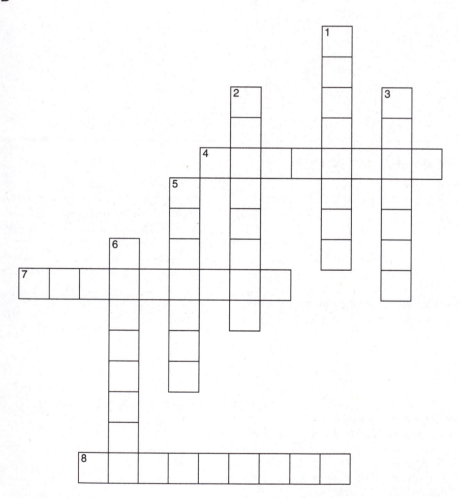

Across
4. Scant amount of urine
7. Blood in the urine
8. The process of emptying urine from the bladder

Down
1. Frequent urination at night
2. Abnormally large amounts of urine
3. Urination
5. Painful or difficult urination
6. A tube used to drain or inject fluid through a body opening

21 URINARY CATHETERS

MATCHING

Match each term with the correct definition.

1. _____ A catheter that drains the bladder and then is removed
2. _____ The process of inserting a catheter
3. _____ A tube used to drain or inject fluid through a body opening
4. _____ A soft sheath that slides over the penis and is used to drain urine
5. _____ A catheter left in the bladder so that urine drains constantly into a drainage bag

A. Indwelling catheter
B. Catheterization
C. Condom catheter
D. Catheter
E. Straight catheter

FILL IN THE BLANKS

6. _____ is the process of inserting a catheter.

7. This type of urinary catheter is left in the bladder.

_____

_____

8. Persons with catheters are at risk for _____.

9. Indwelling catheters are used for:

A. _____

B. _____

C. _____

D. _____

E. _____

F. _____

10. A resident has an indwelling catheter. Why do you need to keep the drainage bag below the person's bladder?

_____

_____

11. What information do you need from the nurse and the care plan before providing catheter care?

A. _____

B. _____

C. _____

D. _____

E. _____

F. _____

G. _____

H. _____

I. _____

12. After giving catheter care, what observations do you need to report and record?

A. _____

B. _____

C. _____

D. _____

E. _____

F. _____

G. _____

H. _____

13. The catheter must not _____ at the insertion site. This causes _____ and

_____.

14. Explain why a closed drainage system is used for an indwelling catheter.

_____

_____

_____

_____

15. What should you do if a urinary drainage system is accidentally disconnected?

    A. _____

    B. _____

    C. _____

    D. _____

    E. _____

    F. _____

    G. _____

16. You empty a person's urinary drainage bag at the end of your shift. What observations do you need to report and record?

    A. _____

    B. _____

    C. _____

    D. _____

    E. _____

    F. _____

    G. _____

17. A patient is embarrassed about having a catheter. What measures can help promote the person's mental comfort?

    _____

    _____

    _____

    _____

    _____

18. A _____ is a soft sheath that slides over the penis.

19. Never use adhesive tape to secure a condom catheter because

    _____

    _____

    _____.

20. You should not apply a condom catheter if

    _____

    _____.

21. You are applying a condom catheter. The man becomes aroused. What should you do?

    _____

    _____

    _____

    _____

    _____

MULTIPLE CHOICE

*Circle the **BEST** answer.*

22. Catheters are used for the following reasons *except*
    A. As a first choice to treat incontinence
    B. For persons who are too weak or disabled to use the bedpan, urinal, commode, or toilet
    C. To protect wounds and pressure ulcers from urine
    D. To allow hourly urinary output measurements

23. You are assisting the nurse with inserting a straight catheter. You know this type of catheter will
    A. Remain in the bladder
    B. Drain the bladder and be removed
    C. Empty stomach contents
    D. Slide over the tip of the penis

24. When caring for a person with an indwelling catheter, you need to do the following *except*
    A. Keep the catheter connected to the drainage tubing
    B. Attach the drainage bag to the bed rail
    C. Coil the drainage tubing on the bed and secure it to the bottom linen
    D. Report leaks to the nurse at once

25. When providing catheter care, you observe blood in the drainage bad. What do you do?
    A. Notify the person's doctor
    B. Notify the person's son
    C. Nothing, this is normal
    D. Notify the nurse

26. When repositioning the person in bed, you notice the catheter tubing is under a leg. You know this can cause
    A. Increased urine flow
    B. Increased circulation
    C. Increased comfort
    D. Increased risk for skin breakdown

27. To properly perform catheter care
    A. Pull on the catheter
    B. Clean down the catheter at least 2 inches
    C. Clean and rinse downward, away from the meatus
    D. Pat dry at insertion site only

28. A standard drainage bag holds less urine than a leg bag
    A. True
    B. False

29. When emptying a drainage bag
    A. Use a wash basin
    B. Use a graduate placed directly on the floor
    C. Use a graduate placed on a paper towel on the floor
    D. Use a cup
30. Condom catheters are also called which of the following:
    A. Arizona catheter
    B. Texas catheter
    C. Internal catheter
    D. Ohio catheter
31. To apply a condom catheter correctly, you need to do the following *except*
    A. Roll the sheath onto the penis
    B. Leave a 1-inch space between the penis and the end of the catheter
    C. Apply tape completely around the penis
    D. Make sure the condom is not twisted
32. You do not know how to apply the condom catheter used at your agency. What should you do?
    A. Ask the patient or resident how to apply it.
    B. Read the instructions before you apply it.
    C. Ask the nurse to show you the correct application.
    D. Use an incontinence product for the person instead.

CASE STUDY

A 60-year-old hospital patient has an indwelling catheter. The person is alert and can assist with her daily care. She likes to make her own decisions. The person walks with a walker and is out of bed most of the day. Her husband visits every day at 1300.

Answer the following questions.

1. Before giving catheter care, what information do you need from the nurse and the care plan?

2. When giving catheter care, what observations do you need to report and record?

3. What safety measures do you need to practice?

4. How often do you need to give catheter care?

5. How will you protect the person's right to privacy?

6. How will you promote the person's independence?

ADDITIONAL LEARNING ACTIVITIES

1. View the following video clips on the Evolve companion site to help you learn and practice the procedures:
   A. Positioning the Graduate
   B. Connecting Drainage Bag Tubing
   C. Cleaning Catheter with Soap

2. Carefully review and practice all the procedures in this chapter. Use a simulator when appropriate. Use the procedure checklists provided on pp. 283–288. If you are embarrassed by any of these procedures, discuss your feelings with your instructor or a nurse.

BOWEL NEEDS

MATCHING

Match each term with the correct definition.

1. _____ The inability to control the passage of feces and gas through the anus
2. _____ The process of excreting feces from the rectum through the anus (bowel movement)
3. _____ The prolonged retention and buildup of feces in the rectum
4. _____ The semi-solid mass of waste products in the colon that is expelled through the anus
5. _____ The excessive formation of gas or air in the stomach and intestines
6. _____ Excreted feces

A. Flatulence
B. Stool
C. Fecal impaction
D. Fecal incontinence
E. Defecation
F. Feces

FILL IN THE BLANKS

7. Stools are normally _____,

   _____,

   _____,

   _____,

   and _____.

   They normally have an _____.

8. _____

   _____

   causes black or tarry stools.

9. What observations about stools do you need to report to the nurse?

   A. _____

   B. _____

   C. _____

   D. _____

   E. _____

   F. _____

   G. _____

   H. _____

   I. _____

10. List nine factors that affect the frequency, consistency, color, and odor of stools.

    A. _____

    B. _____

    C. _____

    D. _____

    E. _____

    F. _____

    G. _____

    H. _____

    I. _____

11. Explain why providing privacy is important when meeting the person's elimination needs.

    _____

    _____

    _____

    _____

12. Explain how aging affects bowel elimination.

    _____

    _____

    _____

    _____

    _____

    _____

13. _____
results if constipation is not relieved.

14. You are caring for a person with diarrhea. You need to:

A. _____

B. _____

C. _____

D. _____

15. Causes of diarrhea include _____
_____.

16. *Clostridium difficile (C. difficile)* is _____
_____
_____.

17. How can you spread *C. difficile?*
_____
_____
_____
_____
_____.

18. List 11 causes of fecal incontinence.

A. _____

B. _____

C. _____

D. _____

E. _____

F. _____

G. _____

H. _____

I. _____

J. _____

K. _____

19. The person with fecal incontinence may need the following.

A. _____

B. _____

C. _____

D. _____

20. List six causes of flatulence.

A. _____

B. _____

C. _____

D. _____

E. _____

F. _____

21. What are the two goals of bowel training?

A. _____

B. _____

22. Doctors order enemas to _____
_____
_____.

23. Describe the following types of enemas.

A. Tap water enema _____
_____
_____

B. Saline enema _____
_____
_____

C. Soapsuds enema _____
_____
_____

D. Small-volume enema _____
_____
_____

E. Oil-retention enema _____
_____
_____

24. You are giving a cleansing enema. You need to stop tube insertion if:

A. _____

B. _____

C. _____

25. After giving a saline enema, what do you need to report and record?

    A. _____

    B. _____

    C. _____

    D. _____

    E. _____

    F. _____

    G. _____

26. Enemas are dangerous for _____ _____ _____.

27. To prevent cramping when giving an enema, you need to:

    A. _____

    B. _____

28. The doctor orders *enemas until clear*. This means _____ _____ _____.

29. To give a small-volume enema, squeeze and roll up the plastic bottle from the bottom. You should not release pressure on the bottle because _____ _____ _____.

30. After giving an oil retention enema, you need to do the following.

    A. _____ _____ _____

    B. _____ _____ _____

    C. _____ _____ _____

    D. _____ _____

31. Describe the following.

    A. A permanent colostomy _____ _____ _____

    B. A temporary colostomy _____ _____ _____

32. If a colostomy is near the end of the colon, stools are _____.

33. List five measures that help prevent ostomy pouch odors.

    A. _____

    B. _____

    C. _____

    D. _____

    E. _____

34. A resident wears an ostomy pouch. You need to assist the person with a tub bath. Why should you delay the bath for 1 to 2 hours after applying a new pouch? _____ _____

35. Write the meanings of the following abbreviations.

    A. BM _____

    B. oz _____

MULTIPLE CHOICE

*Circle the **BEST** answer.*

36. Normal stools are
    A. Black in color
    B. Soft, formed, and moist
    C. Hard and marble-sized
    D. Liquid and pale in color

37. Safety and comfort during bowel elimination are promoted by the following *except*
    A. Positioning the person in a normal sitting or squatting position
    B. Covering the person for warmth and privacy
    C. Allowing time for a BM
    D. Allowing visitors to stay in the room

38. Which will *not* promote safety and comfort during bowel elimination?
    A. Follow Standard Precautions and the Blood-borne Pathogen Standard.
    B. Place the call light and toilet tissue within the person's reach.
    C. Leave the room. Check on the person in 15 minutes.
    D. Dispose of stools promptly.
39. Warm fluids decrease peristalsis.
    A. True
    B. False
40. A patient's stool is black in color and has a tarry consistency. What should you do?
    A. Ask if the person has had anything unusual to eat.
    B. Ask the nurse to observe the stool.
    C. Dispose of the stool and report the color to the nurse.
    D. Ask a co-worker if this is normal for the person.
41. You need to follow Standard Precautions and the Bloodborne Pathogen Standard when in contact with stools.
    A. True
    B. False
42. Which is a common cause of constipation?
    A. A high-fiber diet
    B. Regular exercise
    C. Increased fluid intake
    D. Ignoring the urge to have a BM
43. Which is a sign of fecal impaction?
    A. Liquid feces seeping from the anus
    B. Black, tarry stools
    C. Increased flatulence
    D. Frequent passage of soft stools
44. *Clostridium difficile* is a microbe found in
    A. Water
    B. Food
    C. Feces
    D. The air
45. A resident has fecal incontinence. Which statement is *correct?*
    A. The person has dementia.
    B. A bowel training program will cure the person's incontinence.
    C. You need to provide good skin care.
    D. The person has an intestinal disease.
46. Which action will *not* help produce flatus?
    A. Lying quietly in the supine position
    B. Walking
    C. Moving in bed
    D. The left side-lying position

47. Which measure does *not* promote comfort and safety when giving an enema to an adult?
    A. Have the person void first.
    B. Lubricate the enema tip before inserting it.
    C. Insert the enema tubing 6 inches.
    D. Give the solution slowly.
48. The preferred position for giving enemas is
    A. Fowler's or Semi-Fowler's
    B. The left side-lying or Sims'
    C. Prone
    D. Dorsal recumbent
49. All states and agencies allow nursing assistants to give enemas.
    A. True
    B. False
50. The doctor orders *enemas until clear.* You need to ask the nurse how many enemas to give.
    A. True
    B. False
51. After giving an oil retention enema, do the following *except*
    A. Position the person in the supine position
    B. Urge the person to retain the enema for the time ordered
    C. Place extra waterproof pads on the bed if needed
    D. Check the person often while the person retains the enema
52. A resident has a colostomy. Which statement is *incorrect?*
    A. Good skin care is very important.
    B. Colostomies can be permanent or temporary.
    C. Feces and flatus pass through a stoma located on the abdominal wall.
    D. The entire large intestine has been removed.
53. A resident has an ileostomy. Which statement is *correct?*
    A. Part of the colon is removed.
    B. Stool consistency ranges from liquid to solid.
    C. A skin barrier is not needed around the stoma.
    D. Good skin care is required.
54. Ostomy pouches are changed
    A. When completely full
    B. Every shift and when they leak
    C. Every 3 to 7 days and when they leak
    D. After each meal
55. Used ostomy pouches are flushed down the toilet.
    A. True
    B. False
56. Leaving a person sitting in feces is neglect. It is a form of physical abuse.
    A. True
    B. False

CASE STUDY

A 50-year-old patient in Valley View Hospital is scheduled for bowel radiographs in the morning. The person's doctor ordered saline enemas until clear. The RN has delegated the task of giving the enemas to you.

Answer the following questions:

1. How is a saline enema prepared?

2. How will you promote the person's safety and comfort?

3. How will you protect the person's right to privacy?

4. After giving the enema, what measures do you need to take to promote the person's safety and comfort?

ADDITIONAL LEARNING ACTIVITIES

1. Think of your personal elimination routines.
   A. Explain how important these routines are to your physical and psychological comfort.

   B. Are you aware of how your diet, fluid intake, and level of activity affect your bowel elimination routines? Explain.

   C. Have you had personal experience with constipation or diarrhea? How did the experience affect your comfort?

2. If available at your school or place of work, examine several types of colostomy and ileostomy pouches. Read the manufacturer's instructions. Practice handling the pouches and applying them on yourself and a willing classmate.
3. Handle the various types of enema equipment and become familiar with how each is used. This will increase your comfort and confidence.
4. Carefully review the procedure in Chapter 22.
   A. Under the supervision of your instructor, practice the procedure. Use a simulator when appropriate. Use the procedure checklist provided on pp. 289–290 as a guide.
   B. If this procedure embarrasses you, discuss your feelings with your instructor.

NOTE: Remember that some states and agencies do not allow nursing assistants to give enemas.

CROSSWORD

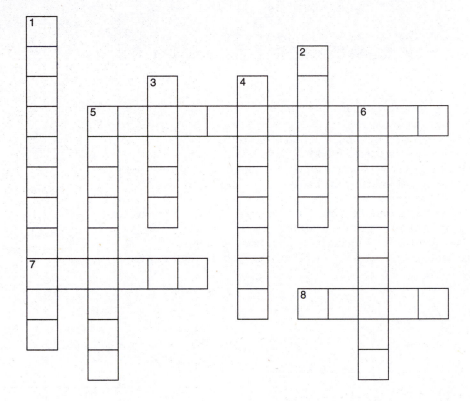

Across

5. The passage of a hard, dry stool
7. A surgically created opening
8. An opening

Down

1. A cone-shaped, solid drug that is inserted into a body opening; it melts at body temperature
2. Gas or air passed through the anus
3. The introduction of fluid into the rectum and lower colon
4. The frequent passage of liquid stools
5. A surgically created opening between the colon and abdominal wall
6. A surgically created opening between the ileum and the abdominal wall

NOTE: Remember that some states and agencies do not allow nursing assistants to give enemas.

23 NUTRITION NEEDS

MATCHING

Match each term with the correct definition.

1. _____ Difficulty swallowing
2. _____ Breathing fluid, food, vomitus, or an object into the lungs
3. _____ The fuel or energy value of food
4. _____ The processes involved in the ingestion, digestion, absorption, and use of foods and fluids by the body
5. _____ The loss of appetite
6. _____ Giving nutrients into the gastrointestinal tract through a feeding tube
7. _____ The process of giving a tube feeding
8. _____ The backward flow of stomach contents into the mouth
9. _____ A substance that is ingested, digested, absorbed, and used by the body

A. Gavage
B. Anorexia
C. Calorie
D. Regurgitation
E. Aspiration
F. Nutrition
G. Nutrient
H. Dysphagia
I. Enteral nutrition

FILL IN THE BLANKS

10. The person's diet affects _____

_____.

11. Good nutrition is needed for _____

_____.

12. Nutrients are grouped into _____,

_____, _____,

_____,

_____, and _____.

13. The MyPlate symbol encourages _____

_____

_____.

14. MyPlate helps you make wise food choices in the following ways:

A. Balancing calories by _____

_____

_____

B. Increasing certain foods by _____

_____

_____

C. Reducing certain foods by _____

_____

_____

15. The amount needed from each food group depends on

_____

_____.

16. _____ is the most important nutrient.

17. _____ provide energy and fiber for bowel elimination.

18. List 13 factors that affect nutrition and eating habits.

A. _____

B. _____

C. _____

D. _____

E. _____

F. _____

G. _____

H. _____

I. _____

J. _____

K. _____

L. _____

M. _____

19. Explain how illness can affect eating and nutrition.

   _____

   _____

   _____

   _____

   _____

   _____

20. What effect does aging have on the gastrointestinal system?

   A. _____

   B. _____

   C. _____

21. Doctors order special diets for the following reasons:

   A. _____

   B. _____

   C. _____

22. Explain what happens when there is too much sodium in the body. _____

   _____

   _____

   _____

23. Sodium-controlled diets involve:

   A. _____

   B. _____

   C. _____

   D. _____

24. _____ is produced and secreted by the pancreas. It lets the body use sugar.

25. Explain why it is important for persons with diabetes to eat at regular times each day.

   _____

   _____

26. You are feeding a person with dysphagia. What observations do you need to report at once?

   _____

   _____

27. To provide for comfort, the meal setting must be free of

   _____

   _____.

28. You are preparing a resident for breakfast. The person will eat breakfast in bed. After you assist with eyeglasses, hearing aids, oral hygiene, elimination, and hand washing, you need to:

   A. _____

   _____

   B. _____

   _____

   C. _____

   _____

29. Nursing centers have dining programs to meet resident needs. With _____, residents eat at a dining room table with four to six others. Food is served as in a restaurant. Residents are oriented and can feed themselves.

30. Describe low-stimulation dining. _____

   _____

   _____

31. Explain why it is important to prepare the person for a meal before serving the meal tray.

   _____

   _____

   _____

   _____

32. A person's food was not served within 15 minutes. What should you do?

   _____

   _____

   _____

   _____

   _____

116   Chapter 23

33. Before serving meal trays, what information do you need from the nurse and the care plan?

A. _____

B. _____

C. _____

D. _____

E. _____

F. _____

G. _____

34. After feeding a person, what observations do you need to report and record?

A. _____

B. _____

C. _____

D. _____

35. A resident eats slowly. The person complains that food will not go down. The person frequently coughs after swallowing. These are signs and

symptoms of _____.

36. A resident has finished eating. The nurse tells you to check for pocketing. You need to check:

A. _____

B. _____

C. _____

37. A patient has dysphagia. To prevent aspiration, the person is positioned in a chair or in the semi-

Fowler's position for at least _____ after eating.

38. When are snacks served? _____

_____

39. Define the following terms.

A. Nasogastric (NG) tube _____

_____

_____

B. Gastrostomy tube _____

_____

_____

40. _____,

_____,

_____, and

_____

are risks from enteral nutrition.

41. Why is it important for the RN to check tube placement before a tube feeding? _____

_____

_____

_____

_____

42. Why is the left side-lying position avoided after a

tube feeding?_____

_____

43. A patient is receiving nutrients through an NG tube. How often is oral hygiene provided?

_____

44. Explain why NG tubes are secured to the person's nose and to the person's garment.

_____

_____

_____

_____

_____

45. Write the meaning of the following abbreviations.

A. GI _____

B. ID _____

C. mg _____

D. NPO _____

LABELING

46. Using the numbers on a clock, describe each food item and where it is located on the plate.

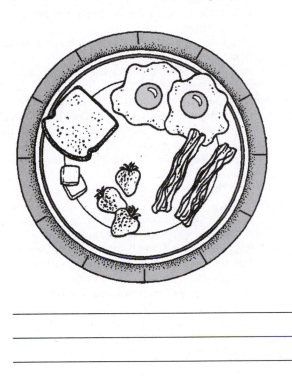

_____

_____

_____

_____

_____

_____

MULTIPLE CHOICE

Circle the **BEST** *answer.*

47. Poor diet and poor eating habits
    A. Decrease the risk for disease
    B. Cause healing problems
    C. Do *not* affect mental function
    D. Decrease the risk for accidents
48. One gram of protein has
    A. 4 calories
    B. 6 calories
    C. 8 calories
    D. 9 calories
49. One gram of fat has
    A. 4 calories
    B. 6 calories
    C. 8 calories
    D. 9 calories
50. Vegetables have the following health benefits *except*
    A. Most vegetables are low in fat and calories
    B. They contain no cholesterol
    C. They contain potassium and dietary fiber
    D. They help build and maintain bone mass

51. Which is a health benefit of milk?
    A. It contains no cholesterol.
    B. It reduces the risk of kidney stones.
    C. It helps build and maintain bone mass.
    D. It contains dietary fiber.
52. *Which is correct* when choosing foods from the meat and beans group?
    A. Choose lean and low-fat meat and poultry.
    B. Using fat for cooking decreases the caloric value of the food.
    C. Liver and other organ meats are low in cholesterol.
    D. Egg yolks are cholesterol free.
53. *Which is correct* when making oil choices?
    A. Vegetable oils are low in calories.
    B. The best oil choices are from fish, nuts, and vegetable oils.
    C. Oils from plant sources are high in cholesterol.
    D. Oils are a major source of vitamin C.
54. Protein is an important nutrient because
    A. It provides fiber for bowel elimination
    B. It is needed for tissue growth and repair
    C. It helps the body use certain vitamins
    D. It does not provide calories
55. Which vitamins are stored by the body?
    A. The B complex vitamins
    B. Vitamin C and the B complex vitamins
    C. Vitamins A, D, E, and K
    D. Vitamin B_{12} and the B complex vitamins
56. This nutrient is needed for all body processes.
    A. Water
    B. Protein
    C. Carbohydrate
    D. Fat
57. Which is *not* an OBRA requirement for food served in nursing centers?
    A. Food is nourishing and tastes good.
    B. Hot food is served hot, and cold food is served cold.
    C. Each person receives at least three meals and three snacks a day.
    D. The center provides needed assistive devices and utensils.
58. Diabetes is a chronic disease from a lack of insulin. Insulin lets the body use
    A. Sugar
    B. Fat
    C. Protein
    D. Minerals
59. To promote safety and comfort when feeding a person with dysphagia, you must
    A. Feed the person only liquids
    B. Position the person in the semi-Fowler's position in bed
    C. Give thickened liquids using a straw
    D. Feed the person according to the care plan

60. Food spills out of a person's mouth while eating. This is a sign of
    A. Dementia
    B. Toothache
    C. Infection
    D. Dysphagia
61. Which is *not* a sign or symptom of dysphagia?
    A. Food pockets in the person's cheeks.
    B. The person eats very fast.
    C. The person regurgitates food after eating.
    D. The person is hoarse after eating.
62. To prepare a person for meals, you need the following information from the nurse and the care plan *except*
    A. How much help the person needs
    B. Where the person will eat
    C. A list of the person's favorite foods
    D. How to position the person
63. Always check food temperature after reheating.
    A. True
    B. False
64. When feeding a person, do the following *except*
    A. Serve food and fluids in the order the person prefers
    B. Use a fork to feed the person
    C. Offer fluids during the meal
    D. Sit facing the person
65. When feeding a visually impaired person, you need to
    A. Tell the person what is on the tray
    B. Describe the aroma of each food item
    C. Describe the color and consistency of each food item
    D. Offer fluids only at the end of the meal
66. Aspiration precautions include
    A. Feeding the person liquids through a straw
    B. Positioning the person upright
    C. Checking the person's mouth before each meal for pocketing
    D. Positioning the person supine after each meal and snack

67. A calorie count is being kept for a patient. Which is *correct*?
    A. On a flow sheet, note what the person ate and how much.
    B. Weigh the food on the person's tray before and after eating.
    C. Measure the number of calories in each food item.
    D. Ask the dietitian to check the person's tray after each meal.
68. A resident is receiving nutrition through an NG tube. The person complains of nausea and discomfort during the tube feeding. What should you do?
    A. Measure the person's vital signs.
    B. Report the person's complaints to the nurse at once.
    C. Stop the tube feeding until the person feels better.
    D. Give the person cool water orally.
69. The OBRA survey team makes sure that
    A. Residents eat all meals in the dining room
    B. Needed help is provided during meals
    C. Tablecloths are used at all meals
    D. At least three menu choices are offered at each meal
70. A patient was served five baby carrots as part of his lunch. He ate only one of them. What percentage of the carrots did he finish?
    A. 50%
    B. 10%
    C. 30%
    D. 20%

CASE STUDY

An 80-year-old resident of Pine View Nursing Center with diabetes and high blood pressure needs assistance to get ready for meals. The person wears eyeglasses and a hearing aid in her right ear. She has upper and lower dentures, which she cares for herself. She is continent of bowel and bladder. She needs help with transfers to and from the toilet. She uses a wheelchair to get to the dining room and can push the wheelchair herself. She needs help preparing her food but can eat by herself. The person sits at a dining room table with three other residents. She always prays before meals.

The person requires diabetes meal planning.

You help her get ready for the noon meal and help prepare her food when she is in the dining room. She complains that her food is not appetizing. She tells you that her portions are too small. She also tells you that she had bread and dessert for every meal when she was doing her own cooking.

Answer the following questions:

1. What factors might affect the person's eating and nutrition?

2. What is involved in diabetes meal planning?

3. What information will you report to the nurse when the person is finished eating? Why is this information important?

4. To whom will you report the person's complaints? When will you report her complaints?

A. How might this information be used in the care planning process?

ADDITIONAL LEARNING ACTIVITIES

1. Discuss with a classmate the importance of food in your daily life. Besides meeting physical needs, what role does food play in your life?
   A. Discuss how your culture and religion affect the food you eat.

   B. Discuss the role food plays in your social life.

   C. Discuss why you enjoy some foods and dislike others.

2. Has illness ever affected your appetite or your ability to eat certain foods? Explain.

   A. Discuss your experience. How might your experience help you provide better care?

3. Review the MyPlate food guidance system (see p. 332 in the textbook).
   A. On the basis of the MyPlate food guidance system, are you making wise food choices?

4. Discuss the special needs of persons with dementia. List ways that you can help meet their nutritional needs.

5. View the following video clips on the Evolve companion site to help you learn and practice the procedures:
   A. Setting up a Bed Tray
   B. Sit Facing the Person
   C. Viewing at Eye-Level

6. Carefully review the procedures in Chapter 23.
   A. Use the procedure checklists on pp. 291–295 as a guide.
   B. Practice feeding a classmate using various food thicknesses.
   C. Take your turn being fed by a classmate. Discuss your experience. Answer these questions.

      (1) How does it feel to be fed by another person?

(2) Did you enjoy your meal? Explain.

(3) Were you fed too fast or too slow?

(4) Was the amount given with each bite right for you?

(5) Were liquids offered during the meal?

(6) Did your food remain at the right temperature throughout the meal?

(7) How might your experience affect the care you give?

24 FLUID NEEDS

MATCHING

Match each term with the correct definition.

1. _____ The swelling of body tissues with water
2. _____ The amount of fluid lost
3. _____ Having an adequate amount of water in body tissues
4. _____ Giving fluids through a needle or catheter inserted into a vein
5. _____ The amount of fluid taken in
6. _____ A decrease in the amount of water in body tissues
7. _____ The number of drops per minute (gtt/min) or milliliters per hour (mL/hr)
8. _____ A measuring container for fluid

A. Dehydration
B. Edema
C. Flow rate
D. Graduate
E. Hydration
F. Intake
G. Intravenous therapy
H. Output

FILL IN THE BLANKS

9. Water is needed to _____.

10. Water is lost through _____,

_____, and _____. It is

also lost through the _____ and the

_____.

11. Fluid balance involves

A. _____

B. _____

C. _____

D. _____

E. _____

12. List six common causes of dehydration.

A. _____

B. _____

C. _____

D. _____

E. _____

F. _____

13. An adult needs _____ mL of water daily to survive.

14. List four common fluid orders

A. _____

B. _____

C. _____

D. _____

15. Intake and output (I&O) records are used to

_____

_____.

They are also kept when _____

_____.

16. Output includes _____

_____.

17. A measuring container for fluids is called a

_____.

18. Measure intake as follows.

A. _____

_____

B. _____

_____

C. _____

_____

D. _____

_____

E. _____

_____

F. _____

_____

G. _____

_____

H. _____

_____

19. Before passing drinking water, what information do you need from the nurse and the care plan?

A. _____

B. _____

C. _____

20. List six ways to prevent the spread of microbes when providing drinking water in the person's mug

A. _____

B. _____

C. _____

D. _____

E. _____

F. _____

21. A patient is receiving IV therapy. When giving the person a bath, you check the flow rate. You need to tell the RN at once if:

A. _____

B. _____

C. _____

D. _____

22. Write the meaning of the following abbreviations.

A. gtt _____

B. I&O _____

C. mL _____

D. NPO _____

MULTIPLE CHOICE

*Circle the **BEST** answer.*

23. For normal fluid balance, how many mL of water are needed per day?
    A. 1000 to 1500
    B. 1500 to 2000
    C. 2000 to 2500
    D. 2500 to 3000

24. Signs and symptoms of dehydration include all of the following except:
    A. Low blood pressure
    B. Dark yellow urine
    C. Slow pulse
    D. Muscle cramps

25. Body water increases with age.
    A. True
    B. False

26. You notice an NPO sign above a patient's bed. This means
    A. All of the person's fluids are given with a straw
    B. The person cannot eat or drink anything
    C. Water is offered in small amounts
    D. The person cannot have solid food

27. A resident has an order for thickened liquids. This means that all liquids are thickened, including water.
    A. True
    B. False

28. While recording intake for your resident, which fluid would you not include in the total?
    A. Water
    B. IV fluids
    C. Custard
    D. Gelatin

29. For lunch your person drank 4 oz of orange juice and 250 mL of coffee. He also ate a 6-oz cup of ice cream. What would you chart for lunch intake?
    A. 260 mL
    B. 550 mL
    C. 15 oz
    D. 420 mL

30. When providing drinking water, which action is *incorrect*?
    A. Make sure the water pitcher is labeled with the person's name and room and bed numbers.
    B. Do not touch the rim or inside of the water cup or pitcher.
    C. Do not let the ice scoop touch the rim or inside of the water cup or pitcher.
    D. Keep the ice scoop in the ice container or dispenser.

31. You have an alarm on an IV infusion pump. What should you do?
    A. Turn the pump off.
    B. Adjust the controls on the pump.
    C. Close the regulator clamp.
    D. Tell the nurse at once.

32. You are *never* responsible for starting or maintaining IV therapy.
    A. True
    B. False
33. A patient complains of pain at the IV site. The area around the IV site is swollen. What should you do?
    A. Turn off the IV infusion pump.
    B. Place a dressing over the IV insertion site.
    C. Apply heat to the area.
    D. Tell the nurse at once.
34. How many milliliters is 14 ounces?
    A. 490
    B. 350
    C. 420
    D. 84

35. Your resident was given 5 oz of orange juice and 10 oz of water at breakfast. She drank 3 oz of orange juice and all of the water. How many millimeters would you chart as breakfast intake?
    A. 390
    B. 450
    C. 360
    D. 300
36. A patient was given 9 oz of juice with dinner. You measure 2 oz left in the cup. How many millimeters would you chart as dinner intake?
    A. 270
    B. 60
    C. 210
    D. 175

CASE STUDY

A 90-year-old resident of Valley Side Nursing Center with dementia needs reminders to drink water. She is incontinent of bowel and bladder. She is very confused most days and often refuses care. She is ambulatory on the unit and rarely sits down to relax.

Answer the following questions:
1. What factors might affect the person's hydration?

2. What information will you report to the nurse regarding hydration status?

3. How could you encourage fluids with this resident?

ADDITIONAL LEARNING ACTIVITIES

1. Record your intake for a 24-hour period. Calculate your daily total. Discuss with your classmates your findings.
   A. Are you getting enough fluids for normal body needs?

2. Carefully review the procedures in Chapter 24.
   A. Use the procedure checklists on pp. 296–299 as a guide.

   B. Do you need to alter your intake?

MATCHING

Match each term with the correct definition.

1. _____ The amount of heat in the body that is a balance between the amount of heat produced and the amount lost by the body
2. _____ Elevated body temperature
3. _____ A device used to measure temperature
4. _____ The pressure in the arteries when the heart is at rest
5. _____ Blood pressure measurements that remain above a systolic pressure of 140 mm Hg or a diastolic pressure of 90 mm Hg
6. _____ When the systolic blood pressure is below 90 mm Hg and the diastolic pressure is below 60 mm Hg
7. _____ The beat of the heart felt at an artery as a wave of blood passes through the artery
8. _____ The amount of force exerted against the walls of an artery by the blood
9. _____ The number of heartbeats or pulses felt in 1 minute
10. _____ Breathing air into (inhalation) and out of (exhalation) the lungs
11. _____ An instrument used to listen to the sounds produced by the heart, lungs, and other body organs
12. _____ Pressure in the arteries when the heart contracts
13. _____ Temperature, pulse, respirations, and blood pressure
14. _____ With a fever
15. _____ To ache, hurt, or be sore

A. Hypertension
B. Blood pressure
C. Respiration
D. Pulse
E. Stethoscope
F. Hypotension
G. Diastolic pressure
H. Thermometer
I. Pulse rate
J. Febrile
K. Vital signs
L. Pain
M. Body temperature
N. Systolic pressure
O. Fever

FILL IN THE BLANKS

16. Vital signs reflect these three body processes.

   A. _____

   B. _____

   C. _____

17. Accuracy is essential when you _____,

   _____, and

   _____

   vital signs.

18. Vital signs show even minor changes in a person's condition. They also tell about response to treatment and often signal life-threatening events. Therefore you must report the following at once.

   A. _____

   B. _____

19. List the sites for measuring body temperature.

   A. _____

   B. _____

   C. _____

   D. _____

   E. _____

20. List the normal range for body temperature for the:

   A. Rectal site _____

   B. Oral site _____

   C. Tympanic membrane site _____

   D. Axillary site _____

21. Oral temperatures are *not* taken if the person:

A. _____

B. _____

C. _____

D. _____

E. _____

F. _____

G. _____

H. _____

I. _____

J. _____

22. A patient has heart disease. Which temperature sites

can you use? _____

_____

_____

23. Which temperature site is *not* used for children

under 4 or 5 years of age? _____

24. Which temperature site is less reliable than the
other sites?

_____

25. How should you shake down a glass thermometer?

_____

_____

_____

_____

26. What do the short lines on a Fahrenheit thermo-

meter mean? _____

27. What does each long line on a centigrade thermo-

meter mean? _____

28. List four special measures needed when taking a
rectal temperature with a glass thermometer.

A. _____

_____

B. _____

_____

C. _____

_____

D. _____

_____

29. The covered probe of a tympanic membrane
thermometer is gently inserted into the

_____.

30. How is temperature measured using a temporal

artery thermometer? _____

_____

_____

31. _____ and

_____

thermometers are used to measure temperatures
for persons who are confused and resist care.

32. After measuring temperature, what observations
do you need to report and record?

A. _____

B. _____

33. When measuring using a rectal temperature, how

is the person positioned? _____

34. Which site is used most often for taking a pulse?

_____

35. Which pulse is taken with a stethoscope?

_____

36. To use a stethoscope, do the following.

A. _____

_____

_____

B. _____

_____

_____

C. _____

_____

_____

D. _____

_____

_____

E. _____

_____

_____

37. Stethoscope diaphragms tend to be _____.

    You need to _____ the diaphragm in your hand before applying it to the person.

38. The normal adult pulse rate is between _____ and _____ beats per minute.

39. The rhythm of the pulse should be regular. This means _____

    _____

    _____.

40. Where is the radial artery located? _____

    _____

41. You should not use your thumb to take a pulse because _____

    _____

    _____

    _____.

42. Apical pulses are taken for persons who:

    A. _____

    B. _____

    C. _____

43. Describe normal respirations. _____

    _____

    _____

44. The healthy adult has _____ respirations per minute.

45. When are respirations counted?

    _____

46. After counting respirations, what observations do you need to report and record?

    A. _____

    B. _____

    C. _____

    D. _____

    E. _____

    F. _____

47. Respirations are usually counted for 30 seconds. The number is multiplied by 2. You need to count respirations for 1 minute if:

    A. _____

    B. _____

    C. _____

    D. _____

48. _____ and

    are used to measure blood pressure.

49. Blood pressure is measured in _____

    _____.

50. What should you do if a mercury manometer breaks?

    _____

    _____

    _____

    _____

51. Before measuring blood pressure, what information do you need from the nurse and the care plan?

    A. _____

    B. _____

    C. _____

    D. _____

    E. _____

    F. _____

    G. _____

    H. _____

    I. _____

52. When measuring a blood pressure, how should you position the person's arm? _____

    _____

    _____

53. Describe the following types of pain.

A. Acute pain _____

_____

_____

_____

B. Chronic pain _____

_____

_____

_____

C. Radiating pain _____

_____

_____

_____

D. Phantom pain _____

_____

_____

_____

54. A resident complains of pain in her lower abdomen. What other information about the person's pain does the nurse need?

A. _____

B. _____

C. _____

D. _____

E. _____

F. _____

G. _____

55. Before measuring weight and height, what information do you need from the nurse and the care plan?

A. _____

B. _____

C. _____

D. _____

E. _____

56. Write the meanings of the following abbreviations.

A. C _____

B. Hg _____

C. mm _____

D. mm Hg _____

LABELING

57. Record the readings on the thermometers shown.

A. _____

B. _____

C. _____

58. Label the pulse sites.

A. _____

B. _____

C. _____

D. _____

E. _____

F. _____

G. _____

H. _____

I. _____

59. Label the parts of a stethoscope.

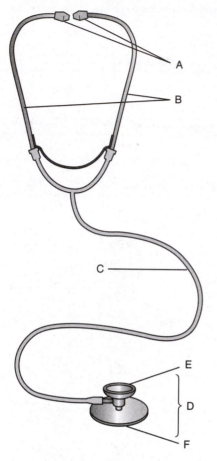

A. _____

B. _____

C. _____

D. _____

E. _____

F. _____

60. Place an **X** at the apical pulse site.

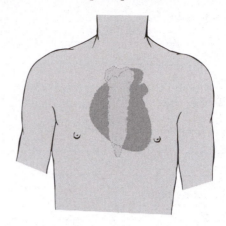

61. Fill in the drawing so that the dials show the correct blood pressure.

A. 152/86 mm Hg

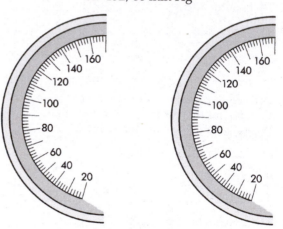

B. 104/68 mm Hg

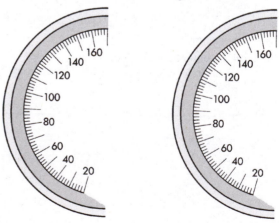

62. Fill in the drawing so that the mercury column shows the correct blood pressure.

A. 152/86 mm Hg

B. 198/100 mm Hg

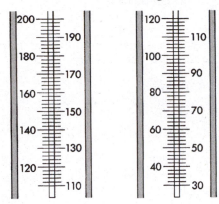 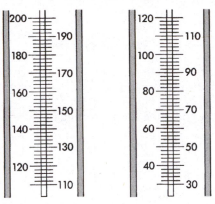

MULTIPLE CHOICE

*Circle the **BEST** answer.*

63. Unless otherwise ordered, vital signs are taken
    A. After the person's bath
    B. With the person at rest lying or sitting
    C. After breakfast
    D. After performing range-of-motion exercises
64. You are unsure of a person's pulse rate. What should you do?
    A. Ask the person what the usual rate is.
    B. Wait 15 minutes and take it again.
    C. Record a previous measurement.
    D. Ask the nurse to take the person's pulse again.
65. Do *not* take a rectal temperature if
    A. The person is unconscious
    B. The person has just had a bath
    C. The person is receiving oxygen
    D. The person has diarrhea
66. The least reliable temperature site is the
    A. Oral site
    B. Axillary site
    C. Tympanic membrane site
    D. Rectal site
67. When using a glass thermometer, which measure will help prevent infection?
    A. Use only the person's thermometer.
    B. Rinse the thermometer under warm running water.
    C. Dry the thermometer from the bulb to the stem with tissue.
    D. After cleaning, store the thermometer in the person's bedside stand.
68. You are taking a rectal temperature with a glass thermometer. Which is *incorrect*?
    A. Privacy is important.
    B. The thermometer is lubricated before insertion.
    C. The thermometer is held in place.
    D. The thermometer remains in the rectum for 1 minute.

69. Axillary temperatures
    A. Are more reliable than oral temperatures
    B. Are taken right after bathing the person
    C. Are taken for 3 minutes
    D. Are used when other routes cannot be used
70. The force of a pulse relates to
    A. How regular the pulse is
    B. The strength of the pulse
    C. The number of beats per minute
    D. The number of skipped beats
71. Which pulse rate would you report to the nurse at once?
    A. 60 beats per minute
    B. 72 beats per minute
    C. 90 beats per minute
    D. 104 beats per minute
72. The apical pulse is located
    A. In the middle of the sternum
    B. On the right side of the chest slightly above the nipple
    C. On the left side of the chest slightly below the nipple
    D. One inch below and to the left of the sternum
73. An apical pulse is counted for
    A. 30 seconds
    B. 1 minute
    C. 2 minutes
    D. 5 minutes
74. When counting respirations, count each rise of the chest as one respiration and each fall of the chest as one respiration.
    A. True
    B. False
75. The period of heart muscle contraction is called
    A. Systole
    B. Diastole
    C. Blood pressure
    D. Aneroid

76. The normal range for diastolic pressure is
    A. Greater than 80 mm Hg
    B. Less than 80 mm Hg
    C. Greater than 120 mm Hg
    D. Less than 120 mm Hg
77. The normal range for systolic pressure is
    A. Greater than 80 mm Hg
    B. Less than 80 mm Hg
    C. Greater than 120 mm Hg
    D. Less than 120 mm Hg
78. Which is *not* a guideline for measuring blood pressure?
    A. Avoid taking blood pressure on an injured arm.
    B. Let the person rest for 10 to 20 minutes before measuring blood pressure.
    C. Measure blood pressure with the person sitting or lying.
    D. Apply the cuff over clothing.
79. Blood pressure is normally measured
    A. In the radial artery
    B. At the apical site
    C. In the brachial artery
    D. In the popliteal artery
80. You are having problems hearing a person's blood pressure measurement. What should you do?
    A. Report what you think you heard.
    B. Ask a co-worker what the person's usual blood pressure is.
    C. Tell the nurse.
    D. Ask the person what his usual blood pressure is.
81. Pain is personal. It differs for each person.
    A. True
    B. False

82. Pain felt in a body part that is no longer there is
    A. Chronic pain
    B. Radiating pain
    C. False pain
    D. Phantom pain
83. Appetite changes and difficulty sleeping can suggest that a person is having pain.
    A. True
    B. False
84. One ounce (oz) equals
    A. 30 mL
    B. 50 mL
    C. 90 mL
    D. 100 mL
85. Which is *correct* when measuring weight and height?
    A. The person wears pajamas, a robe, and shoes for warmth and comfort.
    B. After breakfast is the best time to weigh the person.
    C. Balance the scale at zero before weighing the person.
    D. The person voids after being weighed.
86. When taking a patient's pulse, you counted 40 beats in 30 seconds. The pulse rate in beats per minute is
    A. 40
    B. 80
    C. 120
    D. 60

CASE STUDY

An 80-year-old resident of Valley View Nursing Center shares a room. The person is receiving continuous oxygen by mask. She has a dressing on her lower left arm. The person is able to communicate her needs. The nurse has delegated measuring and recording the person's vital signs to you. When you enter the person's room, you notice that she is drinking a cup of coffee.

Answer the following questions:

1. What sites can you use to measure the person's temperature?

2. Which arm will you use to measure the person's pulse and blood pressure?

3. What observations about the person's pulse do you need to report and record?

4. What pulse rates do you need to report at once?

6. How can you protect the person's right to privacy?

5. How can you promote the person's right to personal choice?

ADDITIONAL LEARNING ACTIVITIES

1. View the following video clips on the Evolve companion site to help you learn and practice the procedures:
   A. Correct Cuff Placement
   B. Counting the Pulse
   C. Pretending to Count Pulse
   D. Oral Temperature
   E. Stethoscope Placement on Chest
   F. Zeroing the Scale
2. Under the supervision of your instructor, practice the procedures in Chapter 25 with a classmate. Use the procedure checklists on pp. 300–311 as a guide. Practice with various partners. Take your turn being the patient or resident.
   Use a simulator for practicing rectal temperature.
   A. Temperature
      (1) Practice reading a glass thermometer.
      (2) If available, practice taking temperatures with different types of thermometers. Discuss the advantages and disadvantages of each.

   B. Pulse
      (1) Practice with various classmates. Locate the following pulse sites: carotid, apical, brachial, radial, femoral, popliteal, and dorsalis pedis.
      (2) Take radial pulses on various persons. Do you notice differences in rate, rhythm, and force?
      (3) Take a person's pulse before and after exercise. Notice and record the differences in rate, rhythm, and force.

   C. Respirations
      (1) Practice with various people. Note differences in respiratory rates. Do the respiratory rate and depth of respirations change with exercise?

   D. Blood pressure
      (1) Practice with various people.
      (2) Take and record blood pressures before and after exercise.
      (3) Take and record blood pressures with the person lying, sitting, and standing.
      (4) If available, practice using different types of blood pressure equipment.

26 COLLECTING SPECIMENS

MATCHING

Match each term with the correct definition.

1. _____ Sugar in the urine
2. _____ Blood in the urine
3. _____ Bloody sputum
4. _____ Samples collected and tested to prevent, detect, and treat disease
5. _____ A substance that appears in urine from rapid breakdown of fat for energy
6. _____ Mucus from the respiratory system that is expectorated through the mouth

A. Hematuria
B. Sputum
C. Glucosuria (glycosuria)
D. Hemoptysis
E. Acetone (ketone body or ketone)
F. Specimens

FILL IN THE BLANKS

7. All specimens sent to the laboratory require

_____.

8. Before collecting a urine specimen, what information do you need from the nurse and the care plan?

A. _____

B. _____

C. _____

D. _____

E. _____

F. _____

G. _____

H. _____

I. _____

9. To identify the person when collecting a

specimen, you need to _____

_____

_____

10. A _____ is collected for a routine urinalysis.

11. To help ensure accuracy, where should you label

the specimen container? _____

_____

12. The midstream specimen is also called

_____

_____.

13. The nurse asks you to collect a midstream specimen. Before going to the person's room, what equipment and supplies do you need to collect?

A. _____

B. _____

C. _____

D. _____

E. _____

F. _____

14. You are collecting a midstream urine specimen from a female. How is the person's perineal area

cleansed? _____

_____

_____

_____

_____

_____

_____

15. _____ measures if urine is acidic or alkaline.

16. A _____ specimen is needed to test urine pH.

17. Unseen blood is called _____.

18. When testing urine specimens, what observations do you need to report and record?

    A. _____

    B. _____

    C. _____

    D. _____

    E. _____

    F. _____

    G. _____

19. How can you make sure that you use reagent

    strips correctly? _____

    _____

    _____

20. What information do you need from the nurse before collecting a stool specimen?

    A. _____

    B. _____

    C. _____

    D. _____

    E. _____

    F. _____

    G. _____

21. When collecting specimens, you must follow:

    A. _____

    B. _____

    C. _____

22. Sputum specimens are studied for

    _____, _____,

    and _____.

23. Mouthwash is not used to rinse the mouth before collecting a sputum specimen because

    _____

    _____

24. The nurse asks you to collect a sputum specimen. What observations do you need to report and record?

    A. _____

    B. _____

    C. _____

    D. _____

    E. _____

    F. _____

    G. _____

    H. _____

    I. _____

25. When collecting a sputum specimen from a person who has or may have tuberculosis (TB), you need to follow Standard Precautions and the Blood-borne Pathogen Standard. The doctor may order

    _____.

26. When collecting specimens, you promote comfort and privacy by:

    A. _____

    _____

    B. _____

    _____

    C. _____

    _____

    D. _____

    _____

27. You made an error in procedure when collecting a stool specimen. What should you do?

    _____

    _____

    _____

28. Write the meaning of each of the following abbreviations.

    A. mL _____

    B. I&O _____

    C. oz _____

    D. TB _____

    E. U/A _____

MULTIPLE CHOICE

Circle the BEST answer.

29. Which is *not* a rule for collecting specimens?
    A. Follow the rules of medical asepsis.
    B. Use the correct container.
    C. Label the container accurately.
    D. Collect the specimen when you have time.
30. What type of specimen is collected for a routine urinalysis?
    A. A random specimen
    B. A midstream specimen
    C. A clean-catch specimen
    D. A 24-hour urine specimen
31. A random urine specimen is collected in the morning before breakfast.
    A. True
    B. False
32. A sterile container is used for a midstream specimen.
    A. True
    B. False
33. A 24-hour urine specimen is needed to test urine for occult blood.
    A. True
    B. False
34. The body needs insulin to
    A. Maintain fluid balance
    B. Use protein for tissue repair
    C. Produce urine
    D. Use sugar for energy

35. What kind of urine specimen is needed to test for blood?
    A. A clean-catch specimen
    B. A 24-hour urine specimen
    C. A routine specimen
    D. An early-morning specimen
36. The normal pH of urine is
    A. 2.0 to 3.5
    B. 4.6 to 8.0
    C. 10.2 to 10.8
    D. 10.5 to 12.2
37. When testing urine with reagent strips, you need to wear gloves.
    A. True
    B. False
38. Stool specimens must *not* be contaminated with urine.
    A. True
    B. False
39. Which statement about collecting sputum specimens is *incorrect*?
    A. The person coughs up sputum from the bronchi and trachea.
    B. The person rinses the mouth with water before coughing up sputum.
    C. Privacy is important.
    D. It is easier to collect a specimen in the evening.

CASE STUDY

You have been assigned to assist with the care of a 60-year-old patient. Your assignment includes collecting:
- A urine specimen to check for blood
- A stool specimen to check for occult blood

The person is able to assist in obtaining the specimens. The RN will test the urine and stool specimens.

Answer the following questions:

1. What information do you need from the nurse before collecting each specimen?

2. What safety measures do you need to practice when collecting each specimen?

3. What instructions do you need to give the person about the urine specimen?

4. What type of urine specimen do you need to collect?

ADDITIONAL LEARNING ACTIVITIES

1. The nurse asks you to collect a 24-hour urine specimen.
   A. What additional information do you need from the nurse before you collect the specimen?

   B. What equipment and supplies do you need to collect?

   C. How will you explain the procedure to the person?

   D. What are the steps involved in collecting the specimen?

   E. What observations do you need to report and record?

2. Under the supervision of your instructor, practice the procedures in Chapter 26. Use the procedure checklists on pp. 312–322 as a guide.

3. View the following video clips on the Evolve companion site to help you learn and practice the procedures:
   A. Container Filling and Storage
   B. Position Collection Container
   C. Obtaining Blood Sample
   D. Obtaining Expectorated Sample
   E. Using Test Card

27 EXERCISE AND ACTIVITY NEEDS

MATCHING

Match the following terms with the correct definitions.

1. _____ Moving a body part away from the midline of the body
2. _____ Moving a body part toward the midline of the body
3. _____ The lack of joint mobility caused by abnormal shortening of a muscle
4. _____ Turning the joint
5. _____ The foot is bent; bending the foot down at the ankle
6. _____ Turning the joint outward
7. _____ The act of walking
8. _____ Turning the joint upward
9. _____ The decrease in size or the wasting away of tissue
10. _____ Bending a body part
11. _____ Excessive straightening of a body part
12. _____ The foot falls down at the ankle; permanent plantar flexion
13. _____ Abnormally low blood pressure when the person suddenly stands up
14. _____ Straightening a body part
15. _____ Turning the joint downward
16. _____ The movement of a joint to the extent possible without causing pain
17. _____ Turning the joint inward
18. _____ Bending the toes and foot up at the ankle

A. Adduction
B. Dorsiflexion
C. Hyperextension
D. Orthostatic hypotension
E. Pronation
F. Internal rotation
G. Abduction
H. External rotation
I. Contracture
J. Flexion
K. Plantar flexion
L. Supination
M. Atrophy
N. Extension
O. Range of motion (ROM)
P. Rotation
Q. Footdrop
R. Ambulation

FILL IN THE BLANKS

19. Inactivity, whether mild or severe, affects

_____.

It also affects mental well-being.

20. A resident with dementia resists your efforts to assist with exercises. What should you do?

_____

_____

_____

_____

21. List 5 reasons why bedrest is ordered.

A. _____

B. _____

C. _____

D. _____

E. _____

22. Define these types of bedrest.

A. Strict bedrest _____

_____

_____

B. Bedrest _____

_____

_____

C. Bedrest with commode privileges

_____

_____

_____

D. Bedrest with bathroom privileges

_____

_____

_____

23. List 10 complications of bedrest.

A. _____

B. _____

C. _____

D. _____

E. _____

F. _____

G. _____

H. _____

I. _____

J. _____

24. Postural relates to _____.

25. _____
is key to preventing orthostatic hypotension.

26. To check for postural hypotension, ask the person these questions.

A. _____

B. _____

C. _____

D. _____

27. What is the purpose of footboards?

_____

_____

_____

28. Trochanter rolls prevent the hips and legs from

_____.

29. Hand rolls or hand grips prevent _____

_____

_____.

30. Splints keep the _____,

_____,

_____,

_____,

_____, and _____
in normal position.

31. _____ keep
the weight of top linens off the feet and toes.

32. _____ range-of-motion
exercises are done by the person.

33. You have been delegated range-of-motion exercises. What information do you need from the nurse and the care plan?

A. _____

B. _____

C. _____

D. _____

E. _____

F. _____

G. _____

34. When can you perform range-of-motion exercises to a person's neck? _____

_____

_____

35. List and describe the range-of-motion exercises performed to the forearms.

A. _____

B. _____

36. List and describe the range-of-motion exercises performed to the hips.

A. _____

B. _____

C. _____

D. _____

E. _____

F. _____

37. The nurse asks you to assist a patient with ambulation. The person is weak and unsteady. What safety measures are needed?

_____

_____

_____

_____

38. After assisting with ambulation, what observations do you need to report and record?

A. _____

B. _____

C. _____

D. _____

E. _____

39. Before assisting with ambulation, you need to talk to the person about the activity. Why is this important?

_____

_____

40. You will assist a patient with ambulation. How should you encourage the person to stand?

_____

_____

41. You are helping a resident walk. Where should you walk? _____

_____

_____

42. Explain why loose clothes are unsafe for a person using crutches. _____

_____

_____

_____

43. Canes help provide _____

and _____ .

44. A resident uses a cane for ambulation. The person's left leg is weak. In which hand is the cane held?

_____

45. Braces are used to:

A. _____

B. _____

C. _____

46. You are applying a knee brace to a patient's left knee. What observations do you need to report to the nurse at once?

A. _____

B. _____

47. The _____ tells you when to apply and remove a brace.

48. To promote the person's activity, exercise, and well-being, you can:

A. _____

_____

_____

B. _____

_____

_____

C. _____

_____

_____

D. _____

_____

_____

E. _____

_____

_____

49. Nursing center activity programs promote

_____

_____

_____ .

50. Write the meaning of each of the following abbreviations.

A. ID _____

B. ADL _____

C. ROM _____

MULTIPLE CHOICE

*Circle the **BEST** answer.*

51. Exercise and activity are promoted in all persons to the extent possible.
    A. True
    B. False

52. Complications of bedrest include the following *except*
    A. Pneumonia
    B. Muscle atrophy
    C. Pressure ulcers
    D. Dorsiflexion

53. Bed boards are used to
    A. Prevent the mattress from sagging
    B. Prevent plantar flexion
    C. Prevent orthostatic hypotension
    D. Strengthen the feet
54. Where are hip abduction wedges placed?
    A. At the foot of the bed
    B. Between the person's legs
    C. Alongside the person's body
    D. Under the mattress
55. Trochanter rolls prevent
    A. Plantar flexion
    B. Footdrop
    C. External rotation of the hips
    D. Contractures of the knees
56. Who performs active-assistive range-of-motion exercises?
    A. The person
    B. The person with some help from another person
    C. A health team member
    D. The physical therapist
57. You are assisting a patient with range-of-motion exercises. Which is *incorrect?*
    A. Exercise only the joints the nurse tells you to exercise.
    B. Expose only the body part being exercised.
    C. Move the joint slowly, smoothly, and gently.
    D. Move the joint slightly beyond the point of pain.
58. You are assisting a resident with ambulation. Which is *incorrect?*
    A. The person wears nonskid shoes.
    B. Make sure the person's feet are flat on the floor.
    C. Stand on the person's weak side while he or she gains balance.
    D. Encourage the person to walk slowly and to slide his or her feet.

59. Which is *not* a safety measure for using crutches?
    A. Replace worn or torn crutch tips.
    B. Check wooden crutches for cracks.
    C. Have the person wear comfortable bedroom slippers.
    D. Keep crutches within the person's reach.
60. When using a cane to walk
    A. The cane tip is about 16 inches to the side of the foot
    B. The grip is level with the waist
    C. The cane is held on the strong side
    D. The strong leg is moved forward first
61. A walker gives more support than a cane.
    A. True
    B. False
62. To promote the person's dignity and mental comfort during exercise, you need to
    A. Provide for privacy
    B. Do as much as possible for the person
    C. Discuss the person's exercise program with the person's family
    D. Tell the person everything will be okay
63. Which is *incorrect* when considering nursing center activity programs?
    A. Activities are important for physical and mental well-being.
    B. The right to personal choice is protected.
    C. The person must participate in at least one activity each day.
    D. Listen and suggest options the person may like.

CASE STUDY

You have received the following information about a resident from the end-of-shift report and your assignment sheet.

- The person is in bed most of the day. He needs help to get out of bed. He is often unsteady when getting out of bed.
- The person needs help to walk three times a day. He uses a wheeled walker and wears a brace over his right ankle.
- The person receives active-assistive range-of-motion exercises to both knees and ankles. He is able to move up in bed and turn using a trapeze.

Answer the following questions:
1. For what complications is the person at risk?

    A. What measures can help decrease these risks?

2. What additional information do you need from the nurse and the care plan before you:
   A. Help the person with ambulation?

   B. Assist with range-of-motion exercises?

3. What safety measures are practiced when assisting the person out of bed?

4. What safety measures are practiced when helping the person with ambulation?

5. What information do you need to report and record about range-of-motion exercises?

6. When putting on and removing the person's brace, what do you need to report to the nurse at once?

7. How will you promote personal choice when providing care?

8. How will you promote the person's right to privacy when assisting with range-of-motion exercises?

ADDITIONAL LEARNING ACTIVITIES

1. Make a list of activities in your daily life that provide range-of-motion exercises.
   A. How do these activities promote your physical, social, and mental well-being?

   B. How can you use daily activities to promote ROM for patients and residents?

2. View the following video clips on the Evolve companion site to help you learn and practice the procedures:
   A. Exercising the Forearm
   B. Walking on the Weak-Side of the Person

3. Practice active range-of-motion exercises. Use the procedure checklist on pp. 323–326 as a guide. This will help you better understand the ROM of each joint.

4. Under the supervision of your instructor, practice the procedures in Chapter 27. Use the procedure checklists on pp. 323–328 as a guide.
   A. Take your turn being the patient or resident. Discuss your experience.

28 WOUND CARE

MATCHING

Match each term with the correct definition.

1. _____ To narrow
2. _____ To expand or open wider
3. _____ A break or rip in the skin; the epidermis separates from the underlying tissues
4. _____ A break in the skin or mucous membrane

A. Constrict
B. Dilate
C. Wound
D. Skin tear

FILL IN THE BLANKS

5. _____ is an accident or violent act that injures the skin, mucous membranes, bones, and organs.

6. A wound is a portal of entry for _____.

_____ is a major threat.

7. Wound care involves _____

_____

_____.

8. Before applying an elastic bandage, changing a dressing, or applying heat and cold, you need to make sure that:

A. _____

B. _____

C. _____

D. _____

E. _____

9. Skin tears are caused by:

A. _____

B. _____

C. _____

D. _____

E. _____

F. _____

G. _____

H. _____

10. An ulcer is _____

_____

_____.

11. Common sites for venous ulcers (stasis ulcers) are

_____

_____.

12. Arterial ulcers are found _____

_____

_____

_____.

13. A diabetic foot ulcer is _____

_____

_____.

14. To prevent venous ulcers:

A. _____

B. _____

C. _____

15. How do elastic stockings help prevent blood

clots? _____

_____

_____

_____

16. An embolus from a vein lodges in a lung. This

    is a _____ .

17. A pulmonary embolus can cause severe
    respiratory problems and death. You need to

    report _____
    to the nurse at once.

18. Persons at risk for thrombi include those who:

    A. _____

    B. _____

    C. _____

    D. _____

    E. _____

19. Before you apply elastic stockings, what
    information do you need from the nurse and
    the care plan?

    A. _____

    B. _____

    C. _____

    D. _____

    E. _____

    F. _____

20. Explain why elastic stockings are applied before

    the person gets out of bed. _____

    _____

    _____

    _____

21. When applying elastic stockings, why is it important
    to remove twists, creases, and wrinkles?

    _____

    _____

    _____

22. When applying elastic bandages, you need to

    start at _____

    _____ .

23. You are applying an elastic bandage to a patient's
    right leg. You should expose the person's toes

    because _____ .

24. A resident has an elastic bandage on her left arm.
    The person complains of pain and tingling in her

    fingers. What should you do? _____

    _____

    _____

25. List seven functions of wound dressings.

    A. _____

    B. _____

    C. _____

    D. _____

    E. _____

    F. _____

    G. _____

26. Tape is not applied to circle the entire body part

    because _____

    _____ .

27. A patient has a lot of pain during dressing
    changes. What measure will help promote the

    person's comfort? _____

    _____

    _____

    _____

28. Remove tape by pulling it _____

    _____ .

29. Binders are applied to the _____ ,

    _____ , or

    _____ .

30. Compression garments help to:

    A. _____

    B. _____

    C. _____

    D. _____

31. An incorrectly applied binder can cause:

    A. _____

    B. _____

    C. _____

    D. _____

32. What are the functions of heat applications?

_____

_____

_____

_____

33. When heat is applied to the skin, blood vessels in

the area _____.

34. When heat is applied to the skin, burns are a risk. What signs and symptoms do you need to report

at once? _____

_____

35. When applying heat to an area, you need to

observe for pale skin because _____

_____

_____

_____

_____

36. A hot soak involves _____

_____

37. Provide the temperature ranges in Fahrenheit and centigrade for each of the following.

A. Hot _____

B. Tepid _____

C. Cold _____

38. Cold applications are used to:

A. _____

B. _____

C. _____

D. _____

39. Explain what happens when cold is applied for a

long time. _____

_____

_____

_____

40. List eight observations you need to report and record when applying heat or cold applications.

A. _____

B. _____

C. _____

D. _____

E. _____

F. _____

G. _____

H. _____

41. You are assisting a patient with a sitz bath. How will you promote the person's safety?

_____

_____

_____

_____

_____

_____

_____

42. An aquathermia pad is placed in a flannel cover

because _____

_____

_____

MULTIPLE CHOICE

*Circle the **BEST** answer.*

43. Which measure helps prevent skin tears?
    A. Wearing rings with large stones
    B. Restricting fluids
    C. Dressing the person as quickly as possible
    D. Keeping your fingernails short and smoothly filed

44. Open sores on the lower legs and feet caused by poor blood flow through the veins are
    A. Arterial ulcers
    B. Pressure ulcers
    C. Epidermal ulcers
    D. Stasis ulcers

45. Which action will *not* help prevent circulatory ulcers?
    A. Having the person use elastic garters to hold socks in place
    B. Keeping linens clean, dry, and wrinkle-free
    C. Keeping pressure off the heels
    D. Reporting changes in skin color
46. Which measure helps prevent circulatory ulcers?
    A. Having the person sit with the legs crossed
    B. Dressing the person in tight clothes
    C. Making sure shoes fit well
    D. Massaging pressure points
47. When applying elastic stockings, the opening in the toe area is over the top of the toes.
    A. True
    B. False
48. After applying an elastic bandage to a patient's right leg, you need to check the color and temperature of the leg
    A. Every 15 minutes
    B. Every hour
    C. Every 2 hours
    D. Every shift
49. When applying a nonsterile dressing, which action is *correct*?
    A. Telling the person how you feel about the wound
    B. Removing the dressing so that the person can see the soiled side
    C. Telling the person to look at the wound
    D. Touching only the outer edges of the old and new dressings
50. When applying tape to secure a dressing, which is *correct*?
    A. Tape is applied to secure the top and bottom of the dressing.
    B. Tape is applied to secure the top, middle, and bottom of the dressing.
    C. Tape should encircle the entire body part whenever possible.
    D. The tape extends 1 inch on each side of the dressing.
51. Montgomery ties are used to secure a dressing. Which is *incorrect*?
    A. The adhesive strips are removed with each dressing change.
    B. Cloth ties are secured over the dressing.
    C. The cloth ties are undone for dressing changes.
    D. The adhesive strips are removed when soiled.

52. Heat is *not* applied to a joint replacement site.
    A. True
    B. False
53. Moist heat has greater and faster effects than dry heat.
    A. True
    B. False
54. Which is a moist cold application?
    A. Ice bag
    B. Ice collar
    C. Ice glove
    D. Cold compress
55. The prolonged application of cold has the same effects as heat applications.
    A. True
    B. False
56. You have applied an ice pack to a resident's left knee. How often do you need to check the skin at the application site?
    A. Frequently
    B. Every 5 minutes
    C. Every 10 minutes
    D. Every 15 minutes
57. Heat and cold are applied for no longer than
    A. 1 hour
    B. 30 minutes
    C. 15 to 20 minutes
    D. 5 to 10 minutes
58. To correctly and safely apply an aquathermia pad
    A. Keep the heating unit below the pad and connecting hoses
    B. Make sure hoses are free of kinks and bubbles
    C. Place the pad under the person
    D. Secure the pad with pins
59. Cold applications are used for the following *except* to
    A. Reduce pain
    B. Reduce bleeding
    C. Increase circulation to an area
    D. Prevent swelling
60. What is the correct abbreviation for centigrade?
    A. Cent
    B. CE
    C. Ct
    D. C

CASE STUDY

A 50-year-old patient at Valley View Hospital has red hair and fair skin. Her doctor has ordered sitz baths following rectal surgery. The doctor has also ordered elastic bandages to both legs. The RN has assigned you to apply the elastic bandages and to assist with the person's sitz bath.

Answer the following questions:
1. What additional information do you need before you apply the elastic bandages?

2. What safety measures are needed when applying elastic bandages?

3. After applying the elastic bandages, what observations do you need to report and record?

4. For what complications from the sitz bath is the person at risk?

A. What measures can help prevent these complications?

B. To promote the person's comfort and safety, what questions might you ask?

ADDITIONAL LEARNING ACTIVITIES

1. If available, handle the various types of dressings commonly used for wound care. Practice opening packages and applying various types of dressings. Practice applying and removing various types of tape. The greater your skill, the better care you can provide.
2. If available, handle the various types of heat and cold applications commonly used in health care agencies. Practice opening packages and applying various types of applications. The greater your skill, the better care you can provide.
3. View the video clips on the Evolve companion site to help you learn and practice the procedures:
   A. Turn Stocking Inside Out to Heel
   B. Washing Area with Soap and Water
   C. Removing Soiled Dressing
   D. Providing for Comfort
   E. Preparing Disposable Equipment
   F. Removing Application and Assessing Area
   G. Placing and Securing the Ice Bag
   H. Securing the Warm Pad
4. Under the supervision of your instructor, practice the procedures in this chapter. Use the procedure checklists on pp. 329–338 as a guide. Take your turn being the patient or resident.
   A. Discuss ways to promote the person's safety, comfort, and dignity when performing each procedure.

29 PRESSURE INJURIES

MATCHING

Match each term with the correct definition.

1. _____ Thick, leathery dead tissue that may be loose or adhered to the skin
2. _____ An area where the bone sticks out or projects from the flat surface of the body
3. _____ Dead tissue that is shed from the skin
4. _____ Normal skin and skin layers without damage or breaks
5. _____ When layers of the skin rub against each other
6. _____ A localized injury to the skin and/or underlying tissue, usually over a bony prominence, resulting from pressure or pressure in combination with shear

A. Bony prominence
B. Shear
C. Pressure injury
D. Eschar
E. Slough
F. Intact skin

FILL IN THE BLANKS

7. A bony prominence is _____

_____

_____

_____ .

8. Shearing is caused by _____

_____

_____

_____

_____ .

9. Pressure injuries result from _____

_____ .

10. Possibly painful, a pressure injury may involve

_____ or

_____ .

11. List five risk factors for pressure injury.

A. _____

B. _____

C. _____

D. _____

E. _____

12. Persons at risk for pressure injuries are those who:

A. _____

B. _____

C. _____

D. _____

E. _____

F. _____

G. _____

H. _____

I. _____

J. _____

K. _____

L. _____

13. In persons with light skin, the first sign of a

pressure injury is _____ .

In persons with dark skin, skin color may _____

_____

_____ .

14. List five common sites for pressure injury from skin-to-skin contact.

    A. _____

    B. _____

    C. _____

    D. _____

    E. _____

15. Reposition bedfast persons at least every

    _____ hours. Reposition chairfast

    persons every _____.

16. Explain how these devices help prevent or treat pressure injuries.

    A. Bed cradle _____

    _____

    _____

    _____

    B. Heel and foot elevators _____

    _____

    _____

    _____

17. Colonized refers to _____

    _____

    _____.

    _____

18. If you are interviewed by CMS staff about pressure injuries, what might you be asked about?

    A. _____

    B. _____

    C. _____

    D. _____

    E. _____

MULTIPLE CHOICE

*Circle the **BEST** answer.*

19. Any injury that results from pressure or pressure in combination with shear is
    A. A skin tear
    B. A pressure injury
    C. An intentional wound
    D. A chronic wound

20. Mr. Jones keeps sliding down in bed. The nurse tells you to raise the head of the bed no more than 30 degrees. This position will prevent tissue damage caused by
    A. Pressure over hard surfaces
    B. Shearing
    C. Poor body mechanics
    D. Poor fluid balance

21. Which measure helps prevent pressure injuries?
    A. Repositioning the person every 4 hours
    B. Raising the head of the bed 45 to 60 degrees when the person is in bed
    C. Positioning the person in the 30-degree lateral position
    D. Vigorously rubbing the skin dry after bathing

22. Remind persons sitting in chairs to shift their positions
    A. Whenever they think about it
    B. Before and after meals
    C. Every hour
    D. Every 15 minutes

23. The most common site for a pressure injury is the
    A. Elbow
    B. Sacrum
    C. Thighs
    D. Ears

24. A frame placed on the bed and over the person to keep top linens off the feet is a
    A. Bed cradle
    B. Heel elevator
    C. Flotation pad
    D. Trochanter roll

LABELING

25. Place an X on the pressure points for each position.

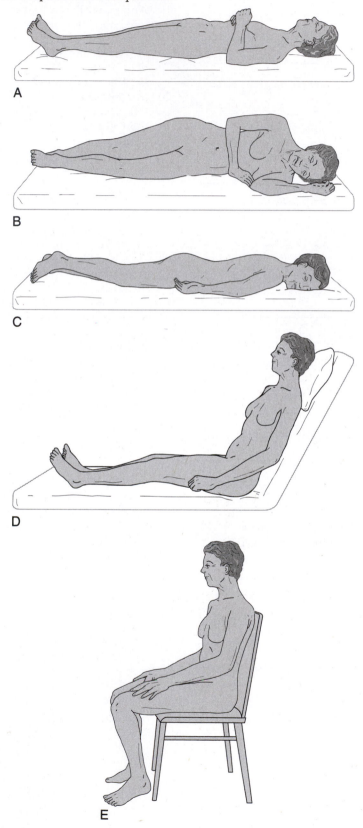

CASE STUDY

A 90-year-old patient at Valley View Hospital is currently bedfast. She is unable to turn and reposition herself. She has a reddened area on her coccyx. The nurse has delegated to you the task of turning and repositioning, as well as skin care.

Answer the following questions:

1. What additional information do you need before caring for this patient?

2. What safety measures are needed when turning and repositioning?

3. After turning and repositioning, what observations do you need to report and record?

4. For which complications may the person be at risk?

   A. What measures can help prevent these complications?

   B. To promote the person's comfort and safety, what questions might you ask?

ADDITIONAL LEARNING ACTIVITIES

1. If available, handle the various types of protective devices used for pressure injuries. Practice applying the various types of devices.

2. If available, practice turning and repositioning. The greater your skill, the better care you can provide.

3. View the following video clip on the Evolve companion site to help you learn and practice the procedures:
   A. Keep Linens Dry

30 OXYGEN NEEDS

MATCHING

Match each term with the correct definition.

1. _____ A tasteless, odorless, and colorless gas required for life
2. _____ The amount (percent) of hemoglobin containing oxygen
3. _____ Difficult, labored, or painful breathing
4. _____ Bluish color to the skin, mucous membranes, and nail beds
5. _____ Slow breathing; respirations are fewer than 12 per minute

A. Bradypnea
B. Oxygen
C. Oxygen concentration
D. Dyspnea
E. Cyanosis

FILL IN THE BLANKS

6. Early signs of low levels of oxygen (O_2) are

   _____ ,

   _____ , and

   _____ .

7. Describe normal respirations. _____

   _____

   _____

   _____

8. Describe Cheyne-Stokes respirations.

   _____

   _____

   _____

   _____

9. Kussmaul respirations are _____

   _____

   _____ .

10. Breathing is usually easier in these positions.

    A. _____

    B. _____

11. A patient has difficulty breathing. The person prefers sitting up and leaning over a table to breathe.

    This position is called _____

    _____ .

    What can you do to increase the person's comfort?

    _____

    _____

12. How do deep-breathing and coughing exercises help persons with respiratory problems?

    A. _____

    B. _____

13. How often are deep-breathing and coughing exercises usually done? _____

    _____

14. The nurse delegates deep-breathing and coughing exercises to you. What information do you need from the nurse and the care plan?

    A. _____

    B. _____

    C. _____

    D. _____

    E. _____

15. If the person has a productive cough,

    _____ and

    _____ are

    needed.

16. Oxygen is treated as a _____ .

17. Pulse oximetry measures _____

    _____

    _____ .

18. _____ is the amount (percent) of hemoglobin containing oxygen.

19. List and briefly describe four ways that oxygen is supplied.

   A. _____

   _____

   _____

   B. _____

   _____

   _____

   C. _____

   _____

   _____

   D. _____

   _____

   _____

20. Describe the following devices used to give oxygen.

   A. Nasal cannula _____

   _____

   _____

   _____

   B. Simple face mask _____

   _____

   _____

   _____

21. List two complications that can occur when using a nasal cannula.

   A. _____

   B. _____

22. The oxygen flow rate is measured in

   _____.

23. Which health team members are responsible for

   setting the oxygen flow rate? _____

   _____

24. Write the meaning of each of the following abbreviations.

   A. L/min _____

   B. O_2 _____

MULTIPLE CHOICE

Circle the BEST answer.

25. Oxygen is a gas. It has no taste, odor, or color.
   A. True
   B. False

26. In healthy adults, how often do normal respirations occur?
   A. 12 to 20 times per minute
   B. 20 to 30 times per minute
   C. 5 to 10 times per minute
   D. 35 times per minute

27. A bluish color to the skin, lips, mucous membranes, and nail beds is
   A. Dyspnea
   B. Cannula
   C. Cyanosis
   D. Oxygen concentration

28. To promote oxygenation, position changes are needed
   A. When the person complains of difficulty breathing
   B. When the person requests a position change
   C. At least every 2 hours
   D. As often as you have time

29. Respiratory hygiene and cough etiquette include the following *except*
   A. Covering the nose and mouth when coughing and sneezing
   B. Using tissues to contain respiratory secretions
   C. Disposing of tissues in the nearest waste container after use
   D. Washing the person's hands every 2 hours while awake

30. You are assisting a resident with deep-breathing and coughing exercises. Which is *incorrect*?
   A. Have the person place the hands over the rib cage.
   B. Have the person take a deep breath in through the nose.
   C. Ask the person to hold the breath for 2 to 3 seconds.
   D. Ask the person to exhale slowly through the nose.

31. Which is *not* a rule for oxygen safety?
    A. Remove the oxygen device when assisting the person with ambulation.
    B. Make sure the oxygen device is secure but not tight.
    C. Check for signs of irritation from the device.
    D. Make sure there are no kinks in the tubing.
32. The nurse tells you that a patient's oxygen flow rate needs to be at 2 L/min. When getting the person up to sit in the chair, you note that the flow rate is at 4 L/min. What should you do?
    A. Remind the person not to change the flow rate.
    B. Tell the nurse at once.
    C. Change the oxygen flow rate to 2 L/min.
    D. Check the care plan as soon as you have time.
33. The normal range for oxygen concentration is
    A. 80% to 100%
    B. 85% to 100%
    C. 90% to 100%
    D. 95% to 100%

34. Which is *not* a sensor site for pulse oximetry?
    A. The earlobes
    B. The fingers
    C. The abdomen
    D. The toes
35. Liquid oxygen is very cold. It can freeze the skin.
    A. True
    B. False
36. Smoking is allowed when a person uses oxygen, as long as the person smokes in the designated smoking area.
    A. True
    B. False
37. Always check the oxygen level when you are with or near persons using oxygen tanks or liquid oxygen systems.
    A. True
    B. False

CASE STUDY

A patient with pneumonia is in a private room. The person has difficult and painful breathing (dyspnea). The person's doctor has ordered:
- Humidified oxygen by nasal cannula at 3 liters per minute
- Position changes every 2 hours while awake
- Deep-breathing and coughing exercises every 2 hours while awake

You have been assigned to care for the person today.

Answer the following questions:

1. After assisting with deep-breathing and coughing exercises, what observations do you need to report and record?

2. How will you promote the person's comfort?

3. The person has a productive cough. What precautions are needed? How can you explain the needed precautions to the person?

4. What observations do you need to report to the nurse about the person's oxygen therapy?

5. How will you protect the person's right to privacy?

ADDITIONAL LEARNING ACTIVITIES

1. If available, handle the various types of oxygen administration devices. Place each device on yourself and observe how each feels and your comfort level.

2. Position yourself in the orthopneic position and note how it feels.

3. Review the following.
   A. The safety measures for fire and the use of oxygen in Chapter 10 in the textbook.
   B. The rules for oxygen safety listed in Chapter 30 in the textbook.
   Knowing and following these rules is needed to provide safe and effective care.

4. Under the supervision of your instructor, practice the procedures in this chapter. Use the procedure checklists on pp. 339–341 as a guide. Take your turn being the patient or resident.
   A. Discuss ways to promote the person's safety, comfort, and dignity when performing the procedures.

5. View the following video clips on the Evolve companion site to help you learn and practice the procedures:
   A. Applying Sensor
   B. Using an Incentive Spirometer

CROSSWORD

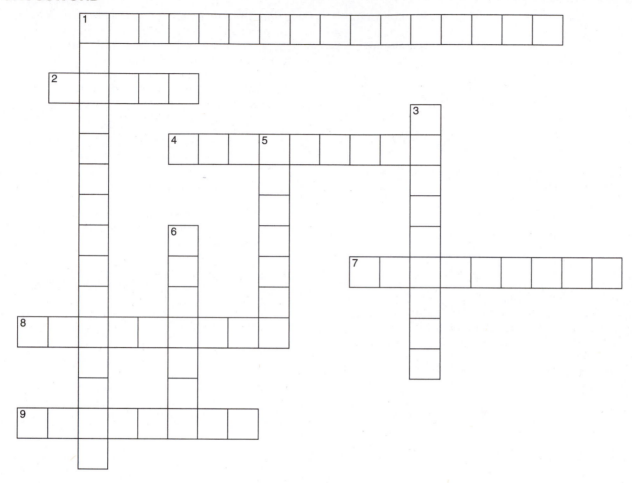

Across

1. Respirations are rapid and deeper than normal
2. Lack or absence of breathing
4. Breathing deeply and comfortably only when sitting
7. The amount of oxygen in the blood is less than normal
8. Slow breathing; respirations are fewer than 12 per minute
9. The amount of oxygen given

Down

1. Respirations are slow, shallow, and sometimes irregular
3. Rapid breathing; respirations are more than 20 per minute
5. Cells do not have enough oxygen
6. Difficult, labored, or painful breathing

31 REHABILITATION NEEDS

MATCHING

Match each term with the correct definition.

1. _____ Activities usually done during normal day in person's life
2. _____ The process of restoring the person to his or her highest possible level of physical, psychological, social, and economic function
3. _____ An artificial replacement for a missing body part
4. _____ Any lost, absent, or impaired physical or mental function
5. _____ Care that helps persons regain health, strength, and independence
6. _____ A nursing assistant with special training in restorative nursing and rehabilitation skills

A. Prosthesis
B. Restorative nursing care
C. Activities of daily living (ADL)
D. Rehabilitation
E. Disability
F. Restorative aide

FILL IN THE BLANKS

7. The goals of rehabilitation are

   A. _____

   B. _____

   C. _____.

8. Restorative nursing programs do the following.

   A. _____

   B. _____

9. Restorative nursing programs may involve measures that promote:

   A. _____

   B. _____

   C. _____

   D. _____

   E. _____

   F. _____

10. The person with a disability needs to adjust

   _____,

   _____,

   _____, and

   _____.

11. Explain why rehabilitation usually takes longer in older persons than in other age groups.

   _____

   _____

   _____

   _____

   _____

   _____

12. List three complications rehabilitation prevents.

   A. _____

   B. _____

   C. _____

13. If not used, muscles will _____.

14. The health team evaluates the person's ability to perform activities of daily living (ADL).

   Sometimes _____ are needed for self-care.

15. Some persons need bladder training. The method depends on _____

   _____.

16. A patient is learning how to use an artificial left arm. The goal is for the prosthesis to _____

_____

_____.

17. Rehabilitation is a team effort. _____ is the key team member.

18. All members of the rehabilitation team help the person regain _____

and _____.

19. Explain why family members are important.

_____

_____

20. You promote the person's _____

_____

21. Successful rehabilitation and restorative care improve the person's quality of life. To promote the person's quality of life:

A. _____

B. _____

C. _____

D. _____

E. _____

F. _____

G. _____

22. Protecting the person's privacy protects

_____ and promotes

_____.

23. You want to become a restorative aide. What qualities are required?

_____

_____

_____

_____

_____

24. Independence to the extent possible is a goal of rehabilitation and restorative care. List seven measures that promote independence.

A. _____

B. _____

C. _____

D. _____

E. _____

F. _____

G. _____

25. You need to assist a resident to apply a leg brace. Why should you practice applying the brace on yourself first? _____

_____

26. The abbreviation ADL means

_____.

MULTIPLE CHOICE

Circle the BEST answer.

27. Restorative nursing and rehabilitation both focus on
    A. The person's strengths
    B. Promoting independence
    C. Regaining physical abilities
    D. The whole person
28. When does rehabilitation start?
    A. When the person enters a rehabilitation hospital
    B. When the person goes home with home care
    C. When the person seeks health care
    D. When it is ordered by the doctor
29. Which measure will *not* help prevent complications?
    A. Good alignment
    B. Maintaining the same position for 4 hours
    C. Range-of-motion exercises
    D. Good skin care
30. Successful rehabilitation depends on the person's attitude.
    A. True
    B. False
31. You promote a person's rehabilitation by
    A. Doing as much as possible for the person
    B. Helping the person focus on remaining abilities
    C. Telling the person to work harder
    D. Focusing on what the person cannot do
32. A patient is feeling discouraged with his slow progress. Which action is *incorrect*?
    A. Remind the person of even small progress.
    B. Give support and encouragement.
    C. Give the person sympathy.
    D. Stress the person's strengths and abilities.

33. A resident is receiving physical therapy. You hear a caregiver shouting at the person in an angry voice. What should you do?
    A. Report what you heard to the nurse at once.
    B. Tell the caregiver to stop shouting.
    C. Tell the person's family what you heard.
    D. Do nothing. It is none of your business.

34. A patient wants to skip her exercises scheduled for 2:00 PM because she is tired. What should you do?
    A. Let the person take a nap.
    B. Allow the person to do only half the amount required.
    C. Check the person's care plan.
    D. Report the problem to the nurse.

35. A patient is making slow progress learning how to use a transfer board. The person tells you that he is tired and is not going to work today. You feel yourself getting impatient. What should you do?
    A. Tell the person that he will never get better if he does not keep trying.
    B. Ask a co-worker to work with the person today.
    C. Leave the room and come back when you are less impatient.
    D. Discuss your feelings with the nurse.

36. Nursing teamwork involves providing emotional support to each other.
    A. True
    B. False

CASE STUDY

A 60-year-old widow works as a secretary for a lawyer. As the result of a stroke, the person's right side is paralyzed. She has facial drooping and her speech is affected. She has trouble expressing herself. The person needs assistance with all ADLs. She is currently receiving rehabilitation in a skilled nursing center. Her goal is to learn to walk and care for herself so that she can go home. She worries that she will not be able to work as a secretary again.

The person works hard with the rehabilitation team. She tells you that she is embarrassed by her appearance. She wants to eat in her room because she is "messy." She told the nurse that she does not want visitors until she is doing better.

Answer the following questions:

1. How does the person's stroke affect her physically, psychologically, socially, and financially?

2. What effect does the stroke have on the person's self-image?

3. How can the health team protect the person's right to:
   A. Privacy?

   B. Personal choice?

   C. Be free from abuse and mistreatment?

4. How can the health team help the person deal with her emotions?

ADDITIONAL LEARNING ACTIVITIES

1. If available, handle various self-help devices used in the rehabilitation process. Becoming familiar with these devices will help you provide effective and safe care.

2. Visit a medical supply business and look at the self-help devices and other rehabilitation equipment available.

32 HEARING, SPEECH, AND VISION PROBLEMS

MATCHING

Match each term with the correct definition.

1. _____ The absence of sight
2. _____ Not being able to hear the range of sounds associated with normal hearing
3. _____ The total or partial loss of the ability to use or understand language
4. _____ Dizziness
5. _____ Hearing loss in which it is impossible for the person to understand speech through hearing alone
6. _____ A ringing, roaring, hissing, or buzzing sound in the ears or head

A. Vertigo
B. Hearing loss
C. Aphasia
D. Blindness
E. Tinnitus
F. Deafness

FILL IN THE BLANKS

7. Symptoms of Meniere's disease include

   A. _____

   B. _____

   C. _____

   D. _____

8. Hearing loss is

   _____

   _____.

   Deafness is _____

   _____

   _____.

9. List five signs of hearing loss.

   A. _____

   B. _____

   C. _____

   D. _____

   E. _____

10. List four simple measures to try when a hearing aid does not seem to be working properly.

    A. _____

    B. _____

    C. _____

    D. _____

11. The person with apraxia of speech cannot use

    _____ for understand-able speech.

12. Expressive aphasia relates to _____

    _____.

13. Receptive aphasia is _____.

14. With a _____, the lens of the eye becomes cloudy.

15. _____ is the only treatment for cataract.

16. Age-related macular degeneration causes

    _____.

17. Briefly describe what occurs with glaucoma.

    _____

    _____

    _____

    _____.

18. Treatment for glaucoma involves _____

_____.

19. _____ is a touch reading and writing system that uses raised dots.

20. What two aids are used worldwide to assist blind persons to move about safely?

    A. _____

    B. _____

21. How can you protect a person's eyeglasses from breakage or other damage? _____

_____

_____

_____

22. Contact lenses are cleaned, removed, and stored according to _____.

MULTIPLE CHOICE

*Circle the **BEST** answer.*

23. You are caring for a person with Meniere's disease. To promote safety you
   A. Have the person walk with a cane
   B. Turn on the bright overhead light
   C. Stand to the side of the person while speaking
   D. Have the person lie down

24. A person who wears a hearing aid hears better because
   A. The hearing problem is cured
   B. Background noise is decreased
   C. The person's ability to hear improves
   D. The hearing aid makes sounds louder

25. To care for a hearing aid properly, do the following *except*
   A. Follow the manufacturer's instructions
   B. Wash the mold in soapy water every day
   C. Remove the battery at night
   D. When not in use, turn the hearing aid off

26. To communicate with a hearing-impaired person, do which of the following?
   A. Shout loudly.
   B. Approach the person from behind.
   C. Speak clearly, distinctly, and slowly.
   D. Stand or sit in dim light.

27. The person with expressive aphasia has difficulty understanding language
   A. True
   B. False

28. Which is *not* a symptom of cataract?
   A. Severe eye pain
   B. Cloudy vision
   C. Sensitivity to light
   D. Poor vision at night

29. Age-related macular degeneration (AMD)
   A. Is a complication of diabetes
   B. Affects peripheral vision
   C. Blurs central vision
   D. Causes halos around lights and double vision

30. When caring for a blind person, you must avoid using the words *see*, *look*, or *read*.
   A. True
   B. False

31. When caring for a blind person, which action will *not* promote safety?
   A. Provide lighting as the person prefers.
   B. Orient the person to the room.
   C. Keep doors partly open.
   D. Tell the person when you are leaving the room.

32. When assisting a blind person to walk, which action is *correct*?
   A. Tell the person which arm is offered.
   B. Walk slightly behind the person.
   C. Guide the person in front of you.
   D. Walk very slowly.

33. A touch reading and writing system that uses raised dots is
   A. Retinopathy
   B. Glaucoma
   C. Aphasia
   D. Braille

CASE STUDY

A 60-year-old female hospital patient is legally blind. The person is alert and can assist with her daily care. She is continent and able to toilet herself with assistance. The person is not able to walk without minimal assistance.

Answer the following questions:
1. How do you provide effective communication?

2. How do you promote safety in the person's room?

3. Describe the process to assist with walking.

ADDITIONAL LEARNING ACTIVITIES

1. Discuss with your classmates how you can effectively communicate with a person with expressive aphasia.

2. View the following video clip on the Evolve companion site to help you learn and practice the procedures:
   A. Caring for Eyeglasses

3. Under the supervision of your instructor, practice the procedure in Chapter 32. Use the procedure checklist on p. 342 as a guide.

33 COMMON HEALTH PROBLEMS

MATCHING

Match each term with the correct definition.

1. _____ The surgical replacement of a joint
2. _____ A tumor that does not spread to other body parts
3. _____ Paralysis on one side of the body
4. _____ Joint inflammation
5. _____ The food and fluids expelled from the stomach through the mouth
6. _____ Malignant tumor
7. _____ Paralysis in the legs, lower trunk, and pelvic organs
8. _____ Paralysis in the arms, legs, trunk, and pelvic organs
9. _____ Inflammation and infection of lung tissue
10. _____ A new growth of abnormal cells that is benign or malignant

A. Pneumonia
B. Quadriplegia
C. Paraplegia
D. Hemiplegia
E. Vomitus
F. Arthritis
G. Tumor
H. Benign tumor
I. Arthroplasty
J. Cancer

FILL IN THE BLANKS

11. _____ tumors do not spread to other body parts.

12. List the 10 cancer risk factors described by the National Cancer Institute.

    A. _____

    B. _____

    C. _____

    D. _____

    E. _____

    F. _____

    G. _____

    H. _____

    I. _____

    J. _____

13. List and briefly describe three common cancer treatments.

    A. _____

    _____

    B. _____

    _____

    C. _____

    _____

14. List and briefly describe the two types of arthritis.

    A. _____

    _____

    _____

    _____

    _____

    B. _____

    _____

    _____

    _____

15. Treatment for osteoarthritis involves:

    A. _____

    B. _____

    C. _____

    D. _____

    E. _____

    F. _____

    G. _____

    H. _____

    I. _____

16. Arthritis risk factors include:

    A. _____

    B. _____

    C. _____

    D. _____

    E. _____

17. A person has rheumatoid arthritis. Why is weight control important? _____

    _____

    _____

18. With _____,
    the bone becomes porous and brittle. Bones are fragile and break easily.

19. List seven risk factors for osteoporosis.

    A. _____

    B. _____

    C. _____

    D. _____

    E. _____

    F. _____

    G. _____

20. Describe these types of fractures.

    A. Closed fracture _____

    _____

    B. Open fracture _____

    _____

    _____

21. The signs and symptoms of a fracture include:

    A. _____

    B. _____

    C. _____

    D. _____

    E. _____

    F. _____

    G. _____

22. Reduction means _____,
    and fixation means _____

    _____

    _____.

23. A new cast is applied to a person's right leg. You must not cover the cast with blankets or other material because _____

    _____

    _____.

24. A patient with a cast on his left arm complains of numbness in his fingers. This signals _____

    _____

    _____.

25. A patient requires a total hip replacement to repair a fractured hip. After surgery, the following hip movements are avoided:

    A. _____

    B. _____

    C. _____

    D. _____

26. A patient requires surgery to repair a fractured right hip. List three life-threatening problems that can occur after surgery.

    A. _____

    B. _____

    C. _____

27. _____ is
    the removal of all or part of an extremity.

28. A stroke or CVA occurs when

    A. _____

    B. _____.

29. Stroke is the leading cause of

    A. _____

    B. _____

30. List five warning signs of stroke.

    A. _____

    _____

    _____

    B. _____

    _____

    _____

    C. _____

    _____

    _____

    D. _____

    _____

    _____

    E. _____

    _____

    _____

31. Briefly describe Parkinson's disease. _____

    _____

    _____

    _____

32. Signs and symptoms of Parkinson's disease include:

    A. _____

    B. _____

    C. _____

    D. _____

33. _____ is a chronic disease in which the myelin in the brain and spinal cord is destroyed.

34. _____ attacks the nerve cells that control voluntary muscles. It is commonly called Lou Gehrig's disease.

35. _____ occurs from violent injury to the brain.

36. Disabilities from traumatic brain injury depend

    on _____

    _____.

37. Common causes of spinal cord injuries are:

    A. _____

    B. _____

    C. _____

    D. _____

    E. _____

    F. _____

38. With hypertension, the _____

    _____ is too high.

39. Prehypertension is _____

    _____

    _____.

40. List four risk factors for hypertension you *cannot* change.

    A. _____

    B. _____

    C. _____

    D. _____

41. The _____ supply the heart with blood.

42. The most common cause of coronary artery

    disease is _____.

43. The major complications of coronary artery disease

    (CAD) are _____,

    _____,

    _____,

    and _____.

44. Coronary artery disease (CAD) can be treated. The goals of treatment are to:

    A. _____

    B. _____

    C. _____

    D. _____

    E. _____

45. Angina is chest pain from _____.

    It is described as _____

    _____

    _____.

46. With _____,
blood flow to the heart muscle is suddenly
blocked. Part of the heart muscle dies.

47. _____ occurs
when the heart is weakened and cannot pump
blood normally. Blood backs up, and tissue
congestion occurs.

48. When the left side of the heart cannot pump blood

normally, blood backs up into the _____.

The person has _____

_____

_____.

49. A result of heart failure is _____,

_____. This is an emergency.

50. List the two disorders grouped under chronic
obstructive pulmonary disease (COPD).

A. _____

B. _____

51. _____ is
the greatest risk factor for COPD.

52. Bronchitis means _____

_____.

53. In emphysema, the _____
enlarge and become less elastic.

54. A person with emphysema develops a _____
as a result of air trapped in the lungs.

55. With _____, the airways
become inflamed and narrow. Extra mucus is
produced.

56. Pneumonia is _____

_____

It is caused by _____

_____.

57. Tuberculosis (TB) is spread by _____

_____

with coughing, sneezing, speaking, singing, or
laughing.

58. List seven signs and symptoms of TB.

A. _____

B. _____

C. _____

D. _____

E. _____

F. _____

G. _____

59. TB is detected by _____

and _____.

60. Vomitus is _____

_____.

61. A resident is vomiting. You turn the person's head

well to one side to prevent _____ .

62. Vomitus that looks like coffee grounds contains

_____.

63. Many people have small pouches in the colon.

Each pouch is called a _____.

64. The condition of having pouches in the colon is

called _____.

The pouches can become infected or inflamed.

This is called _____ .

65. _____ is an inflammation
of the liver.

66. Hepatitis A is spread by _____.

67. The hepatitis B virus is present in _____

_____

_____.

68. The hepatitis B virus is spread by:

A. _____

B. _____

C. _____

D. _____

E. _____

69. List six common causes of urinary tract infections.

    A. _____

    B. _____

    C. _____

    D. _____

    E. _____

    F. _____

70. Cystitis is _____

    _____.

71. _____

    _____

    _____ are
    signs and symptoms of cystitis.

72. _____ is
    inflammation of the kidney pelvis.

73. Cystitis and pyelonephritis are treated with

    _____ and

    _____.

74. The prostate enlarges as men get older. This is

    called _____

    _____.

75. The enlarged prostate presses against the

    _____. This causes

    _____.

76. A sexually transmitted disease (STD) is spread

    by _____

    _____.

77. Using _____ helps prevent
    the spread of STDs, especially HIV and AIDS.

78. _____ is the most common
    endocrine disorder.

79. List and briefly describe the three types of
    diabetes.

    A. _____

    _____

    _____

    _____

    B. _____

    _____

    _____

    _____

    C. _____

    _____

    _____

    _____

80. Type 1 diabetes is treated with

    _____

    _____,

    and _____.

81. Causes of hypoglycemia include:

    A. _____

    B. _____

    C. _____

    D. _____

    E. _____

    F. _____

    G. _____

82. AIDS is caused by a virus. The virus is called the

    _____.

83. The AIDS virus is transmitted mainly by:

    A. _____

    _____

    B. _____

    _____

84. Write the meaning of each of the following abbreviations:

A. AIDS _____

B. ALS _____

C. BPH _____

D. CAD _____

E. COPD _____

F. MI _____

G. MS _____

H. TIA _____

I. UTI _____

MULTIPLE CHOICE

*Circle the **BEST** answer.*

85. Which measure will *not* help prevent osteoporosis?
    A. Bedrest
    B. Calcium and vitamin supplements
    C. Exercising weight-bearing joints
    D. Not smoking

86. When caring for a person in traction, do the following *except*
    A. Keep the person in good alignment
    B. Remove the traction when making the person's bed
    C. Keep the weights off the floor
    D. Give skin care as directed

87. Care of a person following surgery to repair a fractured right hip includes the following *except*
    A. Keeping the operated leg adducted at all times
    B. Giving good skin care
    C. Preventing external rotation of the right hip
    D. Applying elastic stockings as directed

88. With which condition is there death of tissue?
    A. Amputation
    B. Gangrene
    C. Aphasia
    D. Emesis

89. A patient's right foot is amputated. The person complains of pain in his right foot. This is
    A. A delusion
    B. Sclerosis
    C. Phantom limb pain
    D. Radiating pain

90. All strokelike symptoms signal the need for emergency care.
    A. True
    B. False

91. When caring for a person with a stroke, do the following *except*
    A. Perform range-of-motion exercises to prevent contractures
    B. Approach the person from the strong side.
    C. Keep the bed in the flat position to promote breathing
    D. Encourage deep breathing and coughing

92. In the United States, the leading cause of disability in adults is
    A. Cancer
    B. Heart attack
    C. Stroke
    D. Parkinson's disease

93. When caring for a person with a stroke, which is *correct*?
    A. Keep the bed in the flat position.
    B. Turn and reposition the person every 4 hours.
    C. Do all ADLs for the person.
    D. Assist with range-of-motion exercises as directed.

94. A person has Parkinson's disease. It is important to do everything for the person.
    A. True
    B. False

95. A person has multiple sclerosis. Which is *incorrect*?
    A. There is no cure.
    B. Muscle weakness and difficulty with balance occur.
    C. Symptoms usually start after age 50.
    D. The person's condition worsens over time.

96. Which statement about ALS is *correct*?
    A. It is rapidly progressive and fatal.
    B. Symptoms usually start after age 65.
    C. The mind and memory are usually affected.
    D. The disease usually causes bowel and bladder incontinence.

97. Which statement about ALS is *incorrect*?
    A. ALS has no cure.
    B. Some drugs slow the progression of the disease.
    C. Damage cannot be reversed.
    D. Bedrest is recommended.

98. With spinal cord injuries, the higher the level of injury, the fewer functions lost.
    A. True
    B. False

99. The leading causes of death in the United States are
    A. Infections
    B. Pulmonary diseases
    C. Cardiovascular disorders
    D. Cancers

100. Which is *not* a risk factor for hypertension?
    A. Tobacco use
    B. A high-salt diet
    C. Regular exercise
    D. Being overweight
101. Angina is relieved by
    A. Exercise and fresh air
    B. Food and fluids
    C. Continuous oxygen
    D. Rest and nitroglycerin
102. Which is *not* a sign or symptom of myocardial infarction?
    A. Sudden, severe chest pain
    B. Indigestion and nausea
    C. Warm, dry, flushed skin
    D. Fear, apprehension, and a feeling of doom
103. This occurs when the right side of the heart cannot pump blood normally.
    A. Blood backs up into the lungs.
    B. The feet and ankles swell.
    C. A high-sodium diet is ordered.
    D. The dorsal recumbent position is preferred.
104. Heart failure cannot be treated.
    A. True
    B. False
105. Not smoking is the best way to prevent COPD.
    A. True
    B. False
106. This condition is usually triggered by allergies.
    A. Emphysema
    B. Chronic bronchitis
    C. Asthma
    D. Pneumonia
107. Vomitus is measured as output.
    A. True
    B. False
108. With hepatitis C, the person always has symptoms.
    A. True
    B. False
109. Which occurs only in people infected with hepatitis B?
    A. Hepatitis A
    B. Hepatitis C
    C. Hepatitis D
    D. Hepatitis E
110. Hepatitis C is spread by
    A. Blood contaminated with the hepatitis C virus
    B. Food contaminated with feces
    C. Poor hygiene
    D. Water contaminated with feces

111. Calculi are
    A. Particles in the urine
    B. Kidney stones
    C. Waste products
    D. Pus in the urine
112. Which statement about kidney failure is *incorrect?*
    A. The person has urinary frequency and urgency.
    B. The person's kidneys do not function or are severely impaired.
    C. Waste products are not removed from the blood.
    D. The body retains fluid.
113. A patient has diabetes. Which statement is *correct?*
    A. The person's body cannot produce or use insulin properly.
    B. The person is obese.
    C. The person cannot eat a balanced diet.
    D. The person needs a diet low in protein.
114. Which is a cause of hyperglycemia?
    A. Vomiting
    B. Too much insulin
    C. Eating too much food
    D. Increased exercise
115. The immune system can cause diseases by attacking the body's own normal cells, tissues, and organs.
    A. True
    B. False
116. The AIDS virus is spread through
    A. Sneezing and coughing
    B. Holding hands and hugging
    C. Insect bites
    D. Blood, semen, vaginal secretions, and breast milk
117. All persons infected with HIV have symptoms.
    A. True
    B. False
118. A resident infected with the AIDS virus does not have symptoms. The person cannot spread the disease.
    A. True
    B. False
119. Persons over age 50 do not spread HIV.
    A. True
    B. False

CASE STUDY

A 55-year-old male patient is being treated for colon cancer. He had surgery to remove a tumor and is now receiving radiation therapy. He is married and has two teenage children. He is a teacher at the high school. His wife works part time as a check-out clerk at the local grocery store.

Answer the following questions:
1. How might the person feel about having cancer?

2. What measures by the health team are helpful?

3. What are the side effects of radiation therapy?

Following hip replacement surgery, a 75-year-old woman is receiving rehabilitation at a skilled nursing center. The person fell in her driveway and fractured her right hip. She is a retired nurse. She lives alone in her home. She does volunteer work at the hospital 2 days a week.

Answer the following questions:
1. What complications is the person at risk for?

2. What care measures are needed after hip replacement surgery?

ADDITIONAL LEARNING ACTIVITIES

1. Review each of the common health problems discussed in this chapter.
   A. Identify how each problem affects the person's physical, psychological, social, and spiritual needs.

   B. List the risk factors for each of the health problems discussed in this chapter.

   (1) Identify the risk factors that can be controlled and the risk factors that cannot be controlled.

   (2) List any lifestyle changes you can make to decrease your risks for any of the common health problems discussed in this chapter.

CROSSWORD

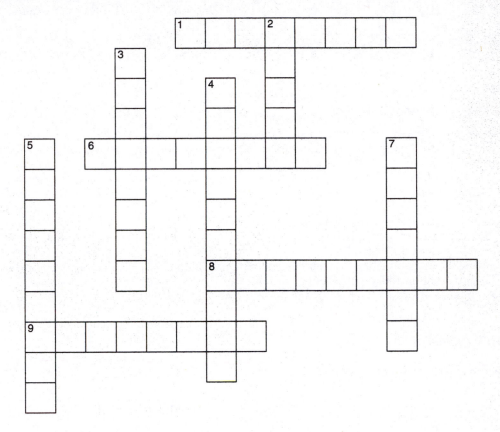

Across
1. A bladder infection
6. A broken bone
8. Joint inflammation
9. Hair loss

Down
2. A new growth of abnormal cells
3. Loss of appetite
4. The spread of cancer to other body parts
5. A tumor that grows fast and invades and destroys other tissues
7. The food and fluids expelled from the stomach through the mouth; emesis

34 MENTAL HEALTH DISORDERS

MATCHING

Match each term with the correct definition.

1. _____ A frequent, upsetting thought, idea, or image
2. _____ Reliving a trauma in thoughts during the day and in nightmares during sleep
3. _____ An intense fear
4. _____ To kill oneself
5. _____ A false belief
6. _____ Repeating an act over and over again
7. _____ The response or change in the body caused by any emotional, physical, social, or economic factor
8. _____ Seeing, hearing, smelling, or feeling something that is not real
9. _____ A vague, uneasy feeling in response to stress
10. _____ An intense or sudden feeling of fear, anxiety, terror, or dread

A. Delusion
B. Flashback
C. Stress
D. Anxiety
E. Compulsion
F. Hallucination
G. Panic
H. Obsession
I. Phobia
J. Suicide

FILL IN THE BLANKS

11. Mental health and mental illness involve

_____ .

12. Define the following terms.

   A. Mental _____

   _____

   _____

   B. Mental health _____

   _____

   _____

   C. Mental health disorder _____

   _____

   _____

13. List seven causes of mental health disorders.

   A. _____

   B. _____

   C. _____

   D. _____

   E. _____

   F. _____

   G. _____

14. _____ and

_____

are used to relieve anxiety.

15. Defense mechanisms are _____

_____

_____ .

16. Name these common phobias.

   A. _____ means fear of being in an open, crowded, or public space.

   B. _____ means fear of water.

17. A compulsion is _____ .

18. _____

occurs after a terrifying ordeal. It involves physical harm or the threat of physical harm.

19. A flashback is _____

_____

_____ .

20. Define the following terms.

    A. Delusion of grandeur _____

    _____

    _____

    B. Delusion of persecution _____

    _____

    _____

21. Persons with schizophrenia may have movement disorders. These include:

    A. _____

    B. _____

    C. _____

22. To regress means _____

    _____

23. A person hallucinates. For good communication:

    A. Remember to _____

    _____

    B. Do not _____

    _____

    _____

    C. Do not _____

    _____

24. Mood changes are called _____.

25. The person with bipolar disorder has

    _____

    _____

    _____

26. _____ involves the body, mood, and thoughts.

27. Why might depression in an older person *not* be treated? _____

    _____

    _____

    _____

28. Personality disorders involve _____

    _____

29. Maladaptive means _____

    _____.

30. Describe antisocial personality disorder.

    _____

    _____

    _____

    _____

    _____

31. _____ involves a pattern of unstable moods, behaviors, self-image, and functioning. The person is impulsive and has unstable relationships.

32. _____ is when the use of alcohol or another substance leads to health issues or problems at work, school, or home.

33. Alcoholism includes these symptoms.

    A. _____

    B. _____

    C. _____

    D. _____

34. List the reasons older persons are at risk for a substance abuse disorder:

    A. _____

    B. _____

    C. _____

    D. _____

    E. _____

    F. _____

35. Drug addiction is _____

    _____

    _____.

36. Addiction is _____

    _____.

37. A person has tolerance to a substance. This means:

    A. _____

    _____

    B. _____

    _____

38. _____
is the physical and mental response after stopping or severely reducing the use of a substance that was used regularly.

39. Name the three types of eating disorders.

    A. _____

    B. _____

    C. _____

40. If a person mentions or talks about suicide, you need to:

    A. _____

    B. _____

    C. _____

41. Define suicide contagion. _____

    _____

    _____

    _____

42. Treatment of mental health disorders involves

    _____

    _____.

    This is done through _____

    _____

    _____

    _____.

43. When interacting with persons with mental health disorders, nonverbal communication is important. You should do the following.

    A. _____

    B. _____

    C. _____

    D. _____

    E. _____

    F. _____

44. The abbreviation PTSD means

    _____

MULTIPLE CHOICE

*Circle the **BEST** answer.*

45. Which statement about anxiety is *incorrect?*
    A. Anxiety is an abnormal response to stress.
    B. Often anxiety occurs when a person's needs are not met.
    C. Signs and symptoms depend on the degree of anxiety.
    D. Defense mechanisms are used to relieve anxiety.

46. A man has a disagreement with his boss. When he gets home, he shouts at his son. Which defense mechanism is he using?
    A. Projection
    B. Displacement
    C. Regression
    D. Denial

47. A woman does not want to visit her mother. She complains of a stomachache. Which defense mechanism is she using?
    A. Compensation
    B. Conversion
    C. Projection
    D. Regression

48. A man always checks every door in his house exactly five times before leaving. He becomes very anxious if he is unable to do so. This is
    A. Compulsion
    B. Phobia
    C. Paranoia
    D. Flashback

49. A woman believes that she is the mother of Christ. This is
    A. A hallucination
    B. Paranoia
    C. A phobia
    D. A delusion

50. People with schizophrenia tend to be violent.
    A. True
    B. False

51. Which statement about bipolar disorder is *incorrect?*
    A. The disorder is also called manic-depressive illness.
    B. The disorder tends to run in families.
    C. The disorder usually develops in early childhood.
    D. The disorder requires lifelong management.

52. Depression is common in older people.
    A. True
    B. False

53. Alcoholism can be treated but not cured.
    A. True
    B. False
54. Which statement about alcohol is *incorrect*?
    A. It affects alertness and reaction time.
    B. Over time, heavy drinking damages the heart and blood vessels.
    C. It speeds up brain activity.
    D. It can cause forgetfulness and confusion.

55. Which statement about substance abuse and addiction is *incorrect*?
    A. Social and mental functions are affected.
    B. They are linked to crimes and violence.
    C. They are linked to motor vehicle crashes.
    D. Only illegal drugs are abused.
56. A person with anorexia nervosa eats large amounts of food and then purges.
    A. True
    B. False

CASE STUDY

A person you are caring for suddenly becomes angry. The person shows signs of increased anxiety.

   She is pacing back and forth in front of you. She begins to raise her voice and speak rapidly.

Answer the following question:
1. What should you do to protect yourself?

ADDITIONAL LEARNING ACTIVITIES

1. Many communities offer support groups for families and friends of persons with mental health disorders. Find out what programs and services are available in your community. The phone book yellow pages and the Internet are resources.

   B. Whom should you contact?

   C. What support resources are available in your community?

2. A friend or family member thinking of suicide may confide in you. The person may ask you not to tell anyone about his or her thoughts.
   A. What should you do?

35 CONFUSION AND DEMENTIA

MATCHING

Match each term with the correct definition.

1. _____ A false belief
2. _____ The loss of cognitive function that interferes with routine personal, social, and occupational activities
3. _____ Signs, symptoms, and behaviors of Alzheimer's disease (AD) increase during hours of darkness
4. _____ Seeing, hearing, smelling, or feeling something that is not real
5. _____ False beliefs and suspicion about a person or situation
6. _____ A state of sudden, severe confusion and rapid changes in brain function

A. Paranoia
B. Dementia
C. Delirium
D. Sundowning
E. Hallucination
F. Delusion

FILL IN THE BLANKS

7. Cognitive function involves:

A. _____

B. _____

C. _____

D. _____

E. _____

F. _____

8. The treatment of confusion is aimed at

_____.

9. List seven early warning signs of dementia.

A. _____

B. _____

C. _____

D. _____

E. _____

F. _____

G. _____

10. Treatable causes of dementia include:

A. _____

B. _____

C. _____

D. _____

E. _____

F. _____

G. _____

H. _____

I. _____

J. _____

11. _____ is the most common type of permanent dementia.

12. _____ is the most common mental health problem in older persons.

13. Depression is often overlooked in older persons

because _____

_____

_____.

14. The classic sign of AD is

   _____

   _____.

15. Describes the three stages of AD.

   Mild AD

   A. _____

   B. _____

   C. _____

   D. _____

   E. _____

   F. _____

   G. _____

   Moderate AD

   A. _____

   B. _____

   C. _____

   D. _____

   E. _____

   F. _____

   G. _____

   Severe AD

   A. _____

   B. _____

   C. _____

   D. _____

   E. _____

   F. _____

   G. _____

   H. _____

   I. _____

   J. _____

16. What is the purpose of *MedicAlert + Alzheimer's Association Safe Return*? _____

   _____

   _____

17. List 10 common behaviors in persons with AD.

   A. _____

   B. _____

   C. _____

   D. _____

   E. _____

   F. _____

   G. _____

   H. _____

   I. _____

   J. _____

18. Briefly describe catastrophic reactions.

   _____

   _____

   _____

   _____

19. Explain how caregivers can cause agitation and restlessness when caring for a person with AD.

   _____

   _____

   _____

20. Aggressive and combative behaviors include

   _____

   _____

   _____.

21. Persons with AD scream to communicate. Possible causes include:

   A. _____

   B. _____

   C. _____

   D. _____

   E. _____

   F. _____

   G. _____

   H. _____

   I. _____

22. Sexual behaviors are labeled abnormal because of

_____ .

23. Persons with AD are not oriented to person, place, and time. Therefore, sexual behaviors may involve

_____

_____ .

24. What are some nonsexual reasons a person with dementia may touch or rub the genitals?

A. _____

_____

B. _____

_____

C. _____

_____

25. A resident at Valley View Nursing Center has AD. Why is it important to report any changes in the person's usual behavior to the nurse?

_____

_____

_____

_____ .

26. Impaired communication is a common problem among persons with AD and other dementias. To promote communication, you need to avoid the following:

A. _____

B. _____

C. _____

D. _____

E. _____

F. _____

27. Some nursing centers have special secured units for persons with AD and other dementias. What is the purpose of these units?

_____

_____

_____

28. Many adult children are in the *sandwich generation.* This means _____

_____

_____ .

29. Many caregivers join AD support groups. What is the purpose of these groups?

_____

_____

_____

_____

30. Maintaining the day-night cycle is important when caring for confused persons. List measures that might help maintain the day-night cycle.

A. _____

B. _____

C. _____

31. Write the definition of each abbreviation.

A. AD _____

B. ADL _____

C. OBRA _____

MULTIPLE CHOICE

*Circle the **BEST** answer.*

32. Cognitive relates to
    A. Beliefs
    B. Changes in the brain
    C. Social function
    D. Knowledge
33. Which is *not* a change in the nervous system from aging?
    A. Reaction times are slower.
    B. Delirium occurs.
    C. Taste and smell decrease.
    D. Sleep patterns change.
34. Which statement about acute confusion is *incorrect?*
    A. Treatment is aimed at the cause.
    B. It occurs suddenly.
    C. It is usually permanent.
    D. It can occur from infection.
35. Dementia is a normal part of aging.
    A. True
    B. False
36. Delirium is an emergency.
    A. True
    B. False

37. Which statement about delirium is *incorrect*?
    A. It is common in older persons with acute or chronic illnesses.
    B. Hypoglycemia is a cause.
    C. It signals physical illness in persons with dementia.
    D. It usually lasts longer than 6 months.
38. Which statement about AD is *correct*?
    A. It is usually diagnosed before age 60.
    B. The disease is sudden in onset.
    C. The cause is unknown.
    D. It is a normal part of aging.
39. AD is often described in terms of three stages. A person in stage 1 (mild AD)
    A. Is disoriented to time and place
    B. Has fecal and urinary incontinence
    C. Has problems with movement and gait
    D. Cannot swallow
40. A person is confused. Which of the following measures is *not* helpful?
    A. Provide care in a calm, relaxed manner.
    B. Explain everything in great detail.
    C. Use touch to communicate.
    D. Tell the person the date and time each morning.
41. A person is confused. Which of the following measures is *not* helpful?
    A. Change the person's routine for staff convenience.
    B. Encourage the person to take part in self-care.
    C. Discuss current events with the person.
    D. Explain what you are going to do and why.
42. A resident has AD. You promote the person's safety by
    A. Restraining the person
    B. Explaining safety rules to the person
    C. Changing the person's room frequently
    D. Placing safety plugs in electric outlets
43. You are caring for a person with AD. Which action causes increased agitation?
    A. Rushing the person
    B. Keeping noise levels low
    C. Speaking in a calm, gentle voice
    D. Using touch to calm the person
44. A resident with AD is screaming in the dining room. You can help by
    A. Firmly asking the person to stop
    B. Taking the person to her room and closing the door
    C. Turning on loud music
    D. Having a favorite caregiver comfort and calm the person
45. When caring for a person with hallucinations, which measure is *not* helpful?
    A. Make sure the person is wearing eyeglasses and hearing aids as needed.
    B. Distract the person with some item or activity.
    C. Use touch to calm and reassure the person.
    D. Calmly explain that the hallucinations are not real.

46. A patient resists your efforts to help him into the bathtub. The person starts to scream. Which action might be helpful?
    A. Explain to the person why a bath is needed.
    B. Get help from two co-workers to force the person into the tub.
    C. Try bathing the person later, when he is calm.
    D. To show the person that there is nothing to be afraid of, step into the tub yourself.
47. Repetitive behaviors are usually harmless.
    A. True
    B. False
48. The person with AD
    A. Chooses to be incontinent
    B. Needs your support and understanding
    C. Has control over his or her actions
    D. Can understand and follow instructions
49. Catastrophic reactions are common from
    A. Wanting to go home
    B. Too many stimuli
    C. Being hungry
    D. Elimination needs
50. Validation therapy may be part of the person's care plan. Which is *not* a principle of validation therapy?
    A. All behaviors have meaning.
    B. A person may return to the past to resolve issues and emotions.
    C. Caregivers need to listen and provide empathy.
    D. Attempts are made to bring the person back to reality.
51. Proper use of validation therapy requires special training.
    A. True
    B. False
52. The right to privacy and confidentiality is *not* important for persons with dementia.
    A. True
    B. False
53. Restraints can make confusion and demented behaviors worse.
    A. True
    B. False
54. According to OBRA, secured nursing units are physical restraints.
    A. True
    B. False

CASE STUDY

A resident on the secured nursing unit was diagnosed with AD 3 years ago. Before coming to the nursing center, she lived with her daughter. The person was admitted to the nursing center after her daughter found her wandering three blocks from home at 9 o'clock at night. The person's daughter lives a few blocks from the nursing center. She visits at least three times a week. She often brings her 3-year-old son along. She has left a picture album with family pictures for her mother.

The person frequently gets up at night and wanders about the unit. She tells you that she is looking for her baby. She repeats the question "Where is my baby?" over and over. Sometimes she wanders into other resident rooms looking for her baby.

Answer the following questions:

1. What measures might be part of the person's care plan to:
   A. Promote safety?

   B. Promote dignity?

2. What measures might be used to deal with the wandering?

3. What can you do to protect the person's right to confidentiality and privacy?

4. What feelings might the person's daughter have about her mother's illness?

5. How might the person's daughter be involved in her mother's care?

ADDITIONAL LEARNING ACTIVITIES

1. Compare the signs and symptoms of delirium, depression, and early AD.
   A. How are the signs and symptoms similar?

   B. Why is a correct diagnosis needed?

2. View the following video clips on the Evolve companion site to help you learn and practice the procedures:
   A. Gentle Reminders and Hearing/Vision Aids
   B. Offering Choices With Dressing

36 EMERGENCY CARE

MATCHING

Match each term with the correct definition.

1. _____ The heart stops suddenly and without warning
2. _____ The excessive loss of blood in a short time
3. _____ The sudden loss of consciousness from an inadequate blood supply to the brain
4. _____ A life-threatening sensitivity to an antigen
5. _____ Breathing stops but heart action continues for several minutes
6. _____ Violent and sudden contractions or tremors of muscle groups
7. _____ Results when tissues and organs do not get enough blood

A. Hemorrhage
B. Respiratory arrest
C. Sudden cardiac arrest
D. Fainting
E. Shock
F. Seizure (convulsion)
G. Anaphylaxis

FILL IN THE BLANKS

8. First aid is _____

   _____

   _____.

9. The goals of first aid are to:

   A. _____

   B. _____

10. In an emergency, the _____

    _____
    is activated. To activate the Emergency Medical Services (EMS) system, do one of the following:

    A. _____

    B. _____

    C. _____

11. You have activated the EMS system. What information do you need to give the operator?

    A. _____

    B. _____

    C. _____

    D. _____

    E. _____

    F. _____

12. In the hospital, a Rapid Response Team (RRT) is called to the bedside when the person shows warning signs of a life-threatening condition.

    The RRT's goal is _____

    _____.

13. When the heart and breathing stop, the person is

    _____.

14. The American Heart Association's (AHA's) Basic Life Support courses teach the adult *Chain of Survival*. Chain of Survival actions for the adult are:

    A. _____

    B. _____

    C. _____

    D. _____

    E. _____

15. What are the three major signs of sudden cardiac arrest (SCA)?

    A. _____

    B. _____

    C. _____

16. A person is in respiratory arrest. If breathing is not restored, _____ occurs.

17. _____
    must be started at once when a person has
    sudden cardiac arrest.

18. What are the four parts involved in cardiopulmo-
    nary resuscitation (CPR)?

    A. _____

    B. _____

    C. _____

    D. _____

19. CPR procedures require

    _____ ,

    _____ , and

    _____ .

20. During CPR, _____
    force blood through the circulatory system.

21. Before starting chest compressions, check for

    _____ .

22. To give chest compressions, how should your

    hands and arms be positioned? _____

    _____

    _____

    _____

    _____

    _____

23. How far is the sternum depressed when doing
    chest compressions on an adult?

    _____

24. When giving chest compressions, the American
    Heart Association recommends that you:

    A. _____

    B. _____

25. The head tilt–chin lift method opens the airway.
    Describe how to perform the head tilt–chin lift
    method.

    A. _____

    _____

    _____

    B. _____

    _____

    _____

    C. _____

    _____

    _____

    D. _____

    _____

    _____

    E. _____

    _____

    _____

26. When you start CPR, give _____ breaths

    first. Then _____ breaths are

    given after every _____ chest
    compressions.

27. When giving mouth-to-mouth breathing, you
    need to pinch the person's nostrils shut. Why is

    this done? _____

    _____

    _____

28. What is the purpose of the barrier device used in
    mouth-to-barrier device rescue breathing?

    _____

    _____

    _____

29. The abbreviations for ventricular fibrillation are

    _____ or _____ .

30. What occurs with ventricular fibrillation?

_____

_____

_____

_____

_____

31. When a person is in V-fib, _____
    is used to deliver a shock to the heart.

32. Where will you learn about using an automated

    external defibrillator? _____

    _____

    _____

33. CPR is done if the person _____

    _____

    _____

    _____.

34. Before staring CPR in an adult, check to see if the

    person is responding by _____

    _____

    _____

    _____.

35. The recovery position is used when _____

    _____

    _____.

36. Do not use the recovery position if the person

    _____

    _____.

37. List six signs and symptoms of internal hemorrhage.

    A. _____

    B. _____

    C. _____

    D. _____

    E. _____

    F. _____

38. Bleeding from an _____
    occurs in spurts. There is a steady flow of blood

    from a _____.

39. If direct pressure over the bleeding site does not
    control external bleeding, what should you do?

    _____

    _____

40. _____,

    _____, and

    _____
    are warning signals for fainting.

41. Signs and symptoms of shock include:

    A. _____

    B. _____

    C. _____

    D. _____

    E. _____

    F. _____

    G. _____

    H. _____

42. When a person has signs and symptoms of shock,
    the following measures are needed.

    A. Keep the person _____.

    B. Maintain an open _____.

    C. Control _____.

    D. Begin _____
       if cardiac arrest occurs.

43. Signs and symptoms of anaphylaxis include:

    A. _____

    B. _____

    C. _____

    D. _____

    E. _____

    F. _____

    G. _____

    H. _____

    I. _____

    J. _____

    K. _____

44. Stroke occurs when _____
   _____
   _____ .

45. A stroke may be caused by:
   A. _____
   B. _____
   C. _____

46. Signs of stroke depend on _____
   _____ .

47. Emergency care for a stroke includes:
   A. Positioning the person _____
      _____
      _____ .
   B. Raising the _____
      without flexing the _____ .

48. List and briefly describe the three major types of seizures.
   A. _____
      _____
      _____
   B. _____
      _____
      _____
   C. _____
      _____
      _____

49. Describe the two phases of a generalized tonic-clonic seizure (grand mal seizure).
   A. _____
      _____
      _____
   B. _____
      _____
      _____

50. Common causes of burns and fires are:
   A. _____
   B. _____
   C. _____
   D. _____
   E. _____
   F. _____
   G. _____
   H. _____
   I. _____
   J. _____

51. During an emergency, your main concern is
   _____
   _____ .

52. Write the meaning of each abbreviation:
   A. BLS _____
   B. CPR _____
   C. EMS _____
   D. RRT _____
   E. AED _____
   F. SCA _____

MULTIPLE CHOICE

*Circle the **BEST** answer.*

53. When providing emergency care, it is important to do the following *except*
   A. Check for signs of life-threatening problems
   B. Move the person to a comfortable position
   C. Call for help
   D. Keep the person warm

54. For CPR, the airway is opened by
   A. Turning the head to the side
   B. Lifting the head up and tilting it forward
   C. Sitting the person up
   D. The head tilt–chin lift method

55. Which artery is used to check for a pulse before starting chest compressions?
   A. The radial artery
   B. The brachial artery
   C. The carotid artery
   D. The femoral artery

56. For chest compressions to be effective, the person
    A. Must be in a sitting position
    B. Must be supine and on a hard, flat surface
    C. Must be flat and on a soft surface
    D. Is positioned with pillows
57. A patient is in ventricular fibrillation. Defibrillation as soon as possible increases the person's chance of survival.
    A. True
    B. False
58. Hands-only CPR is used to educate
    A. Persons not trained in Basic Life Support
    B. Doctors
    C. RNs
    D. All health care professionals
59. During two-person CPR, Rescuer 2 gives
    A. 1 breath after every 5 chest compressions
    B. 1 breath after every 10 chest compressions
    C. 2 breaths after every 30 chest compressions
    D. 1 breath at the same rate as chest compressions
60. For internal hemorrhage, do the following *except*
    A. Keep the person warm until help arrives
    B. Keep the person flat
    C. Keep the person quiet until help arrives
    D. Give the person fluids
61. To control external hemorrhage, do the following *except*
    A. Elevate the affected part
    B. Remove any objects that have pierced or stabbed the person
    C. Place a sterile dressing directly over the wound
    D. Apply pressure with your hand directly over the bleeding site

62. To prevent or treat shock, do the following *except*
    A. Maintain an open airway
    B. Control bleeding
    C. Keep the person warm
    D. Keep the person in Fowler's position
63. Which action will protect the person from injury during a generalized tonic-clonic seizure?
    A. Lower the person to the floor.
    B. Turn the person onto his or her back.
    C. Restrain body movements during the seizure.
    D. Put your fingers or an object between the person's teeth.
64. Emergency care for fainting includes the following *except*
    A. Have the person sit or lie down
    B. Loosen tight clothing
    C. If the person is lying down, raise the legs
    D. Give the person sips of cool water
65. Emergency care for severe burns includes
    A. Applying warm water until pain is relieved
    B. Removing the burned clothing
    C. Breaking the blisters
    D. Removing the person from the fire or burn source
66. There is no need to protect the person's right to privacy during an emergency.
    A. True
    B. False

CASE STUDY

While a resident is eating lunch in the dining room, you notice that the left side of the person's face is drooping and he is leaning to the left. The person is having difficulty swallowing and has slurred speech.

Answer the following questions:
1. What is the person having signs of?

2. What are some possible causes?

3. What does emergency care involve?

4. How would you protect the person's right to privacy?

ADDITIONAL LEARNING ACTIVITIES

1. Identify the EMS system in your community.
   A. Check the phone book yellow pages or the Internet.

   B. Do you know how to activate the EMS system in an emergency?

2. Are you and your family prepared to respond to emergency situations in your home?
   A. Are emergency phone numbers easily found?

   B. Do members of your family know what information to give the operator in an emergency?

   C. Do you and your family know Basic Life Support procedures?

3. Do you know which agencies in your community offer classes in Basic Life Support procedures and first aid? Check the following agencies in your community.
   A. Hospitals
   B. Nursing centers
   C. Community colleges
   D. The American Heart Association
   E. The American Red Cross
   F. The National Safety Council

4. If possible, enroll in a Basic Life Support class. Your instructor can help you with this process.

5. Under the supervision of your instructor, practice the procedures in Chapter 36. Use the procedure checklists on pp. 343–344 as a guide.

37 END-OF-LIFE CARE

MATCHING

Match each term with the correct definition.

1. _____ Care that focuses on the physical, emotional, social, and spiritual needs of dying persons and their families
2. _____ Care of the body after death
3. _____ The belief that the spirit or soul is reborn in another human body or in another form of life
4. _____ The examination of the body after death
5. _____ A document about measures that support or maintain life when death is likely
6. _____ The stiffness or rigidity of skeletal muscles that occurs after death
7. _____ An illness or injury from which the person will not likely recover
8. _____ A document stating a person's wishes about health care when that person cannot make his or her own decisions
9. _____ Gives the power to make health care decisions to another person

A. Postmortem care
B. Rigor mortis
C. Hospice care
D. Durable power of attorney for health care
E. Living will
F. Advance directive
G. Terminal illness
H. Reincarnation
I. Autopsy

FILL IN THE BLANKS

10. Explain why it is important for you to understand the dying process. _____

_____

_____

_____

_____

_____

11. Palliative care involves _____

_____

_____

_____

12. The goal of hospice care is to _____

_____ .

13. A patient you are caring for is dying. Your religious beliefs about death differ from those of your patient. Effective communication with the person involves

_____

_____

_____

_____ .

14. List four fears adults may have when facing death.

A. _____

B. _____

C. _____

D. _____

15. Adults often resent death because it affects

_____ , _____ ,

_____ , and _____ .

16. Why might some older persons welcome death?

_____

_____

_____

17. List the five stages of dying described by Dr. Elisabeth Kübler-Ross.

A. _____

B. _____

C. _____

D. _____

E. _____

18. How can you use listening and touch to help meet the dying person's psychological, social, and spiritual needs?

    A. Listening _____

    _____

    _____

    _____

    B. Touch _____

    _____

    _____

    _____

19. When a patient or resident asks to visit with a

    spiritual leader, you need to _____

    _____

    _____ .

20. _____ is one of the last
    functions lost. Always assume that the person

    can _____ .

21. Which position is usually best for breathing

    problems? _____

22. List eight measures that promote the dying person's physical comfort.

    A. _____

    B. _____

    C. _____

    D. _____

    E. _____

    F. _____

    G. _____

23. _____ and

    _____ give
    persons the right to accept or refuse medical
    treatment and to make advance directives.

24. A living will may instruct doctors:

    A. _____

    B. _____

25. The doctor wrote a "Do Not Resuscitate" (DNR) order for a resident. What does this mean?

    _____

    _____

    _____

26. List six signs that signal death is near.

    A. _____

    _____

    _____

    B. _____

    _____

    _____

    C. _____

    _____

    _____

    D. _____

    _____

    _____

    E. _____

    _____

    _____

    F. _____

    _____

    _____

27. The signs of death include:

    A. _____

    B. _____

28. Which health team member determines that death

    has occurred? _____

29. When does postmortem care begin?

    _____

    _____

30. Postmortem care is done to _____

    _____ .

31. What is the purpose of an autopsy?

    _____

    _____

32. When assisting with postmortem care, what information do you need from the nurse?

   A. _____

   B. _____

   C. _____

   D. _____

   E. _____

33. A patient you are caring for has an advance directive that is against your religious values. What should you do?

   _____

   _____

   _____

34. List the dying person's rights under OBRA.

   A. _____

   B. _____

   C. _____

   D. _____

   E. _____

   F. _____

35. Write the meaning of each of the following abbreviations.

   A. CPR _____

   B. DNR _____

MULTIPLE CHOICE

*Circle the **BEST** answer.*

36. Attitudes and beliefs about death usually stay the same throughout a person's life.
   A. True
   B. False

37. Infants and toddlers do not understand the nature or meaning of death.
   A. True
   B. False

38. Children between the ages of 2 and 6 years
   A. Know that death is final
   B. Often think they will die
   C. Often blame themselves when someone dies
   D. Are not curious about death

39. The person in the bargaining stage of dying
   A. Is very sad
   B. Makes promises in exchange for more time
   C. Is calm and at peace
   D. Feels anger and rage

40. The person in the stage of acceptance
   A. Refuses to believe that he or she is dying
   B. Bargains for more time
   C. Is very sad
   D. Is calm and at peace

41. A resident is dying. The person asks you to stay and talk in the middle of the night. Which is *correct*?
   A. Tell the person to go back to sleep.
   B. Call the person's family.
   C. Call a pastor to talk with the person.
   D. Let the person express feelings and emotions.

42. A person's pastor is visiting at 11:00 PM. You need to
   A. Stay in the room while the pastor visits
   B. Provide for privacy
   C. Tell the nurse at once
   D. Ask the person why the pastor is visiting so late

43. A patient is unconscious. When providing care, do the following *except*
   A. Assume that the person can hear you
   B. Speak in a whisper
   C. Offer words of comfort
   D. Avoid topics that could upset the person

44. When caring for a dying person, you promote comfort by
   A. Playing cheerful music
   B. Asking a lot of questions to keep the person talking
   C. Providing care quickly so that the person can be alone
   D. Providing good skin care and personal hygiene

45. A darkened room is comforting to the dying person.
   A. True
   B. False

46. The family goes through stages like the dying person.
   A. True
   B. False

47. When an autopsy is to be done, postmortem care is *not* done.
   A. True
   B. False

48. Postmortem care involves the following *except*
   A. Pronouncing the person dead
   B. Positioning the body in normal alignment before rigor mortis sets in
   C. Preparing the body for viewing by the family
   D. Bathing soiled areas

49. When providing postmortem care, you must practice Standard Precautions and follow the Bloodborne Pathogen Standard.
    A. True
    B. False
50. The right to confidentiality does *not* apply after death.
    A. True
    B. False

51. The dying person has the right to receive kind and respectful care before and after death.
    A. True
    B. False

CASE STUDY

You are caring for a 59-year-old male patient receiving hospice care. The person currently sleeps most of the time. His verbal communication is minimal. He occasionally opens his eyes. His wife stays with him most of the day. She has spent the past two nights at his bedside. She says prayers and talks to her husband about important events in their lives. His son who lives in another state arrived 3 days ago. The person's daughter lives in the same town and visits several times a day. She often washes his face and applies lotion to his feet. She tells him that she loves him and that she will miss him.

After his son arrived, the person told his wife that he was ready to die and that he was at peace with his family and with God. He discussed his will and his funeral arrangements with his wife and his children.

Answer the following questions:
1. According to Elisabeth Kübler-Ross's stages of dying, what stage is the person in? Explain.

2. What physical care needs does the person have?

3. What measures will help meet the person's psychological, social, and spiritual needs?

4. What measures will help meet the family's needs?

ADDITIONAL LEARNING ACTIVITIES

1. List your thoughts and feelings about death and dying.
    A. How do your religion, culture, and age affect your feelings about death?

    B. Have you had experience with the death of a family member or friend that affects your feelings about death and dying? Explain.

    C. How do you feel about advance directives?

2. If you have fears about caring for dying persons, discuss them with your instructor.

3. Under the supervision of your instructor, practice the procedure in Chapter 37. Use the procedure checklist on pp. 345–346 as a guide.

38 GETTING A JOB

MATCHING

Match each term with the correct definition.

1. _____ An agency's official form listing questions that require factual answers
2. _____ To assist or change a position or workplace to allow an employee to do his or her job despite having a disability
3. _____ Unjust treatment based on age, race, sex, and other personal qualities
4. _____ When an employer asks a job applicant questions about his or her education and career

A. Discrimination
B. Job applications
C. Job interview
D. Reasonable accommodation

FILL IN THE BLANKS

5. List nine ways to find out about agencies and jobs.

   A. _____

   B. _____

   C. _____

   D. _____

   E. _____

   F. _____

   G. _____

   H. _____

   I. _____

6. Agencies want staff who

   A. _____

   B. _____

   C. _____

   D. _____

7. Explain why it is important for you to be at work on time and when scheduled.

   _____

   _____

   _____

   _____

8. The Omnibus Budget Reconciliation Act of 1987 (OBRA) requires each state to have a nursing

   assistant _____

   _____.

9. You are completing a job application. It is

   important to follow directions because _____

   _____

   _____.

10. You are completing a job application. A question on the application does not apply to you. What

    should you do? _____

    _____

    _____

11. When completing a job application, you will be asked to supply references. How many references should you be prepared to supply?

    _____

12. What information about each reference should

    you be prepared to give? _____

    _____

    _____

13. Lying on a job application is _____

14. You are reviewing the job description during your job interview. You should advise the interviewer of any functions you cannot perform because

    of _____

    _____ .

15. List three things you need to do when you accept a job.

    A. _____

    B. _____

    C. _____

MULTIPLE CHOICE

*Circle the **BEST** answer.*

16. You are getting ready for a job interview. You should do the following *except*
    A. Bathe, brush your teeth, and wash your hair
    B. Make sure your hands and fingernails are clean
    C. Make sure your shoes are clean and in good repair
    D. Wear clean jeans and a T-shirt

17. Being on time for a job interview shows that you are
    A. Courteous
    B. Anxious
    C. Helpful
    D. Dependable

18. When you arrive for a job interview, you should
    A. Tell the receptionist your name and why you are there
    B. Spend time visiting with the receptionist until it is time for your interview
    C. Ask the receptionist how long you will have to wait
    D. Ask the receptionist questions about the job

19. You want to make a good impression for a job interview. Which is *correct?*
    A. Stand until asked to take a seat.
    B. Look down or away from the interviewer when answering questions.
    C. Give short "yes" or "no" answers.
    D. Give long answers and explanations to all questions.

20. You can ask questions at the end of the interview. Which is *not* a good question?
    A. What is the greatest challenge of this job?
    B. What are the uniform requirements?
    C. Can I have 4 days off next month?
    D. How will my performance be evaluated?

21. How soon after a job interview should you send a thank-you note?
    A. Within 24 hours
    B. Within 3 days
    C. Within 1 week
    D. Whenever you have time

22. Drug testing may be part of the application process
    A. True
    B. False

CASE STUDY

Your classmate, Linda Jones, is often 5 to 10 minutes late for class. She has difficulty completing her homework assignments and does not get along with other classmates.

Answer the following questions:

1. Linda has asked you to be a reference for her. How do you respond?

2. Does Linda's history of tardiness in school indicate how she will perform at her new job?

3. Is Linda someone you would want as a co-worker? Explain.

ADDITIONAL LEARNING ACTIVITIES

1. You are preparing for a job interview. Discuss the following:

    A. How you will make a good impression?

    B. How you will show the employer that you have what he or she is looking for in these areas?

    (1) Hygiene measures

    (2) Professional appearance

    (3) Skills and training

    (4) Values and attitude

2. You want to find the right job. Answer the following questions:

    A. What is important to you?

    B. What questions do you want to ask the employer?

    C. Are there functions you cannot perform because of training, legal, ethical, or religious reasons?

3. You have succeeded in getting the job you want. Now, it is important to keep your job. How will you make sure that:

    A. You have dependable transportation?

    B. You have childcare, if needed?

    C. You get to work on time?

    D. You are available to work at the times you are scheduled?

    E. You stay healthy so that you can function at your best?

4. Practice writing a thank-you letter following a job interview.

PROCEDURE CHECKLISTS

Relieving Choking—Adult or Child (Over 1 Year of Age)

Name: _____   Date: _____

Procedure	S	U	Comments
1. Asked the person if he or she was choking.			
a. If the person could cough or talk, took steps to handle a mild airway obstruction.	_____	_____	_____
b. If the person was unresponsive, began CPR.	_____	_____	_____
c. If the person nodded "yes" and couldn't talk, continued to step 2.	_____	_____	_____
2. Called for help.			
a. In a public area, activated the Emergency Medical Services (EMS) system by dialing 911; sent someone to get an automated external defibrillator (AED).	_____	_____	_____
b. In an agency, called the Rapid Response Team (RRT); sent someone to get the AED.	_____	_____	_____
3. Gave abdominal thrusts.			
a. Stood or knelt behind the person.	_____	_____	_____
b. Wrapped your arms around the person's waist.	_____	_____	_____
c. Made a fist with one hand.	_____	_____	_____
d. Placed the thumb side of the fist against the abdomen. The fist was slightly above the navel in the middle of the abdomen and well below the end of the sternum (breastbone).	_____	_____	_____
e. Grasped the fist with your other hand.	_____	_____	_____
f. Pressed your fist into the person's abdomen with a quick, upward thrust.	_____	_____	_____
g. Repeated thrusts until the object was expelled or the person became unresponsive.	_____	_____	_____
4. If the object was dislodged, encouraged the person to go to the hospital.	_____	_____	_____
5. If the person became unresponsive.			
a. Lowered the person to the floor or ground. Positioned the person supine.	_____	_____	_____
b. Made sure the EMS or RRT was called. (If alone, provided 5 cycles/2 minutes of cardiopulmonary resuscitation [CPR] first, then called the EMS or RRT.)	_____	_____	_____

Date of Satisfactory Completion _____   Instructor's Initials _____

Procedure—cont'd	S	U	Comments

c. Started CPR.
   (1) Did not check for a pulse. Began with compressions. Gave 30 compressions. ___ ___ ___
   (2) Used the head tilt–chin lift method to open the airway. Opened the person's mouth. Looked for an object. Removed the object with fingers. ___ ___ ___
   (3) Gave 2 breaths. ___ ___ ___
   (4) Continued cycles of 30 compressions and 2 breaths. Looked for an object every time airway was opened for rescue breaths. ___ ___ ___

d. If choking was relieved, checked for a response, breathing, and a pulse
   (1) If no response, no normal breathing, and no pulse—continued CPR. Attached an AED. ___ ___ ___
   (2) If no response and no normal breathing but there was a pulse—gave rescue breaths. For an adult, gave 1 breath every 5 to 6 seconds (10 to 12 breaths per minute). For a child, gave 1 breath every 3 to 5 seconds (12 to 20 breaths per minute). Checked for a pulse every 2 minutes. If no pulse, began CPR. ___ ___ ___
   (3) If the person had normal breathing and a pulse—placed the person in the recovery position if there is no response. Continued to check the person until help arrived. Encouraged the person to go to the hospital if the person responds. ___ ___ ___

Date of Satisfactory Completion _____ Instructor's Initials _____

Using a Fire Extinguisher

Name: _____   Date: _____

Procedure	S	U	Comments
1. Pulled the fire alarm.	_____	_____	_____
2. Got the nearest fire extinguisher.	_____	_____	_____
3. Carried it upright.	_____	_____	_____
4. Took it to the fire.	_____	_____	_____
5. Followed the word PASS.			
a. P—pulled the safety pin.	_____	_____	_____
b. A—aimed low. Directed the hose or nozzle at the base of the fire. Did not try to spray the tops of the flames.	_____	_____	_____
c. S—squeezed or pushed down on the lever, handle, or button to start the stream. Released the lever, handle, or button to stop the stream.	_____	_____	_____
d. S—swept the stream back and forth (side to side) at the base of the fire.	_____	_____	_____

Date of Satisfactory Completion _____   Instructor's Initials _____

Using a Transfer/Gait Belt

Name: _____   Date: _____

	S	U	Comments

Quality of Life

- Knocked before entering the person's room.
- Addressed the person by name.
- Introduced self by name and title.
- Explained the procedure to the person before starting and during the procedure.
- Protected the person's rights during the procedure.
- Handled the person gently during the procedure.

Procedure

1. Reviewed *Promoting Safety and Comfort: Transfer/Gait Belts.*
2. Practiced hand hygiene.
3. Obtained a transfer/gait belt of the correct type and size.
4. Identified the person. Checked the identification (ID) bracelet against the assignment sheet. Used 2 identifiers. Called the person by name.
5. Provided for privacy.
6. Assisted the person to a sitting position.
7. Applied the belt.
    a. *For a belt with a metal buckle:*
        (1) Inserted the belt's metal tip into the buckle. Passed the belt through the side with the teeth first.
        (2) Brought the belt tip across the front of the buckle. Inserted the tip through the buckle's smooth side.
    b. *For a belt with a quick-release buckle,* pushed the belt ends together to secure the buckle.
8. Tightened the belt so that it was snug. It did not cause discomfort or impair breathing. You were able to slide your open, flat hand under the belt. Asked the person about his or her discomfort.
9. Made sure that a woman's breasts were not caught under the belt.
10. Placed the buckle off-center in the front or off-center in the back for the person's comfort. (A quick release buckle was positioned at the person's back.) The buckle was not over the spine.
11. Tucked any excess strap under the belt.
12. Completed the transfer or ambulation procedure. Grasped the belt from underneath with 2 hands. Or grasped the belt by the handles.

Post-Procedure

13. Removed the belt after the procedure in step 12. The person was not left alone wearing the belt.

Date of Satisfactory Completion _____   Instructor's Initials _____

Post-Procedure—cont'd   S   U   Comments

    a. *For a belt with a metal buckle:*
      (1) Brought the belt strap back through the
         buckle's smooth side.   _____   _____   _____
      (2) Pulled the belt through the side with the
         teeth.   _____   _____   _____
    b. *For a belt with a quick-release buckle,* pushed
       inward on the quick-release buttons.
    c. Removed the belt from the person's waist.
       Avoided dragging the belt across the waist.

14. Provided for comfort.
15. Placed the call light and other needed items within   _____   _____   _____
    reach.
16. Unscreened the person.
17. Completed a safety check of the room.   _____   _____   _____
18. Returned the transfer/gait belt to its proper place.   _____   _____   _____
19. Practiced hand hygiene.   _____   _____   _____
20. Reported and recorded your observations.   _____   _____   _____

Date of Satisfactory Completion _____   Instructor's Initials _____

Helping the Falling Person

Name: _____   Date: _____

Procedure	S	U	Comments
1. Stood behind the person with feet apart. Kept back straight.	_____	_____	_____
2. Brought the person close to your body as fast as possible. Used the transfer/gait belt. Or wrapped your arms around the person's waist. If necessary, held the person under the arms.	_____	_____	_____
3. Moved your leg so that the person's buttocks rested on it. Moved the leg near the person.	_____	_____	_____
4. Lowered the person to the floor. The person slid down your leg to the floor. Bent at hips and knees as you lowered the person.	_____	_____	_____
5. Called a nurse to check the person. Stayed with the person.	_____	_____	_____
6. Helped the nurse return the person to bed. Asked other staff to help if needed.	_____	_____	_____

Post-Procedure	S	U	Comments
7. Provided for comfort as noted on the inside of the front textbook cover.	_____	_____	_____
8. Placed the call light within reach.	_____	_____	_____
9. Raised or lowered bed rails. Followed the care plan.	_____	_____	_____
10. Completed a safety check of the room as noted on the inside of the front textbook cover.	_____	_____	_____
11. Practiced hand hygiene.	_____	_____	_____
12. Reported and recorded the following.			
• How the fall occurred	_____	_____	_____
• How far the person walked	_____	_____	_____
• How activity was tolerated before the fall	_____	_____	_____
• Complaints before the fall	_____	_____	_____
• How much help the person needed while walking	_____	_____	_____
13. Completed an incident report.	_____	_____	_____

Date of Satisfactory Completion _____   Instructor's Initials _____

Applying Restraints

Name: _____   Date: _____

Quality of Life	S	U	Comments
• Knocked before entering the person's room.			
• Addressed the person by name.			
• Introduced self by name and title.			
• Explained the procedure to the person before starting and during the procedure.			
• Protected the person's rights during the procedure.			
• Handled the person gently during the procedure.			

Pre-Procedure

1. Followed *Delegation Guidelines: Applying Restraints.* Reviewed *Promoting Safety and Comfort: Applying Restraints.*
2. Collected the following as instructed.
   - Correct type and size of restraints
   - Padding for skin and bony areas
   - Bed rail pads or gap protectors (if needed)
3. Practiced hand hygiene.
4. Identified the person. Checked the ID bracelet against the assignment sheet. Used 2 identifiers. Called the person by name.
5. Provided for privacy.

Procedure

6. Made sure the person was comfortable and in good alignment.
7. Put the bed rail pads or gap protectors (if needed) on the bed if the person was in bed. Followed the manufacturer's instructions.
8. Padded bony areas according to the nurse's instructions and the care plan.
9. Read the manufacturer's instructions. Noted the front and back of the restraint.
10. *For wrist restraints:*
    a. Applied the restraint following the manufacturer's instructions. Placed the soft or foam part toward the skin.
    b. Secured the restraint so that it was snug but not tight. Made sure you could slide 1 finger under the restraint. Followed the manufacturer's instructions. Adjusted the straps if the restraint was too loose or too tight. Checked for snugness again.
    c. Secured the straps to the movable part of the bed frame out of the person's reach. Used the buckle or quick-release tie.
    d. Repeated steps 10, a–c for the other wrist.
11. *For mitt restraints:*
    a. Made sure the person's hands were clean and dry.
    b. Inserted the person's hand into the restraint with the palm down. Followed the manufacturer's instructions.

Date of Satisfactory Completion _____   Instructor's Initials _____

Procedure—cont'd	S	U	Comments
c. Wrapped the wrist strap around the smallest part of the wrist. Secured the strap with the hook-and-loop closure.	___	___	___
d. Secured the restraint to the bed if directed to do so by the nurse. Secured the straps to the movable part of the bed frame out of the person's reach. Used the buckle or quick-release tie.	___	___	___
e. Checked for snugness. Slid 1 finger between the restraint and the wrist. Followed the manufacturer's instructions. Adjusted the straps if the restraint was too loose or too tight. Checked for snugness again.	___	___	___
f. Repeated steps 11, b–e for the other hand.	___	___	___
12. *For a belt restraint:*			
a. Assisted the person to a sitting position.	___	___	___
b. Applied the restraint. Followed the manufacturer's instructions.	___	___	___
c. Removed wrinkles or creases from the front and back of the restraint.	___	___	___
d. Brought the ties through the slots in the belt.	___	___	___
e. Positioned the straps at a 45-degree angle between the wheelchair seat and sides. If in bed, helped the person lie down.	___	___	___
f. Made sure the person was comfortable and in good alignment.	___	___	___
g. Secured the straps to the movable part of the bed frame out of the person's reach or to the chair or wheelchair. Used the buckle or quick-release tie. For a wheelchair, criss-crossed and secured the straps.	___	___	___
h. Checked for snugness. Slid an open hand between the restraint and the person. Adjusted the restraint if it was too loose or too tight. Checked for snugness again.	___	___	___
13. *For a vest restraint:*			
a. Assisted the person to a sitting position. If in a wheelchair:			
(1) Positioned him or her as far back in the wheelchair as possible.	___	___	___
(2) Made sure the buttocks were against the chair back.	___	___	___
b. Applied the restraint. Followed the manufacturer's instructions. The "V" neck is in the front.	___	___	___
c. Brought the straps through the slots.	___	___	___
d. Made sure side seams were under the arms. Made sure the vest was free of wrinkles in the front and back. Closed the zipper if the device opened in the back. Or closed with hook-and-loop closures.	___	___	___
e. Positioned the straps at a 45-degree angle between the wheelchair seat and sides. Helped the person lie down if he or she was in bed.	___	___	___
f. Made sure the person was comfortable and in good alignment.	___	___	___

Date of Satisfactory Completion _____   Instructor's Initials _____

Procedure—cont'd	S	U	Comments

g. Secured the straps underneath the chair seat or to the movable part of the bed frame. Used the buckle or quick-release tie. If secured to the bed frame, the straps were secured at waist level out of the person's reach. For a wheelchair, criss-crossed and secured the straps.

h. Checked for snugness. Slid an open hand between the restraint and the person. Adjusted the restraint if it was too loose or too tight. Checked for snugness again.

14. *For a jacket restraint:*

a. Assisted the person to a sitting position.
   (1) Positioned him or her as far back in the wheelchair as possible.
   (2) Made sure the buttocks were against the chair back.

b. Applied the restraint. Followed the manufacturer's instructions. The jacket opening was in back.

c. Made sure the side seams were under the arms. Removed any wrinkles in the front and back.

d. Closed the back with zipper or hook and loop closures.

e. Positioned the straps at a 45-degree angle between the wheelchair seat and sides. Helped the person lie down if he or she was in bed.

f. Made sure the person was comfortable and in good alignment.

g. Secured the straps to the movable part of the bed frame at waist level. Used the buckle or quick-release tie. The buckle or tie is out of the person's reach. For a wheelchair, criss-crossed and secured the straps.

h. Checked for snugness. Slid an open hand between the restraint and the person. Adjusted the restraint if it was too loose or too tight. Checked for snugness again.

Post-Procedure

15. Positioned the person as the nurse directed.

16. Provided for comfort as noted on the inside of the front textbook cover.

17. Placed the call light within the person's reach.

18. Raised or lowered the bed rails. Followed the care plan and the manufacturer's instructions for the restraint.

19. Unscreened the person.

20. Completed a safety check of the room as indicated on the inside of the front textbook cover.

21. Practiced hand hygiene.

Date of Satisfactory Completion _____   Instructor's Initials _____

Post-Procedure—cont'd	S	U	Comments
22. Checked the person and the restraints at least every 15 minutes. Reported and recorded your observations.			
a. For wrist or mitt restraints—checked the pulse, color, and temperature of the restrained parts.	_____	_____	_____
b. For a vest, jacket, or belt restraint—checked the person's breathing. Called the nurse at once if the person was not breathing or was having problems breathing. Made sure the restraint was properly positioned in the front and back.	_____	_____	_____
23. Did the following at least every 2 hours for at least 10 minutes.			
a. Removed or released the restraint.	_____	_____	_____
b. Measured vital signs.	_____	_____	_____
c. Repositioned the person.	_____	_____	_____
d. Met food, fluid, hygiene, and elimination needs.	_____	_____	_____
e. Gave skin care.	_____	_____	_____
f. Performed range-of-motion exercises or helped the person walk. Followed the care plan.	_____	_____	_____
g. Provided for physical and emotional comfort as noted on the inside of the front textbook cover.	_____	_____	_____
h. Reapplied the restraints.	_____	_____	_____
24. Completed a safety check of the room as noted on the inside of the front textbook cover.	_____	_____	_____
25. Practiced hand hygiene.	_____	_____	_____
26. Reported and recorded your observations and the care given.	_____	_____	_____

Date of Satisfactory Completion _____   Instructor's Initials _____

Hand-Washing

Name: _____   Date: _____

Procedure	S	U	Comments
1. Reviewed *Promoting Safety and Comfort: Hand Hygiene.*	_____	_____	_____
2. Made sure you had soap, paper towels, an orange stick or nail file, and a wastebasket. Collected missing items.	_____	_____	_____
3. Pushed watch up your arm 4 to 5 inches. If uniform sleeves were long, pushed them up.	_____	_____	_____
4. Stood away from the sink so that clothes did not touch the sink. Stood so that the soap and faucet were easy to reach. Did not touch inside of sink at any time.	_____	_____	_____
5. Turned on and adjusted the water until it felt warm.	_____	_____	_____
6. Wet wrists and hands. Kept your hands lower than your elbows. Wet the area 3 to 4 inches above your wrists.	_____	_____	_____
7. Applied about 1 teaspoon of soap to hands.	_____	_____	_____
8. Rubbed your palms together and interlaced fingers to work up a good lather. Lathered your wrists, hands, and fingers. Kept your hands lower than your elbows. This step lasted at least 15 to 20 seconds.	_____	_____	_____
9. Washed each hand and wrist thoroughly. Cleaned backs of fingers and between the fingers well.	_____	_____	_____
10. Cleaned under the fingernails. Rubbed your fingertips against your palms.	_____	_____	_____
11. Cleaned under the fingernails with a nail file or orange stick. Did this for the first hand washing of the day and when your hands were highly soiled.	_____	_____	_____
12. Rinsed wrists, hands, and fingers well. Water flowed from above the wrists to the fingertips.	_____	_____	_____
13. Repeated steps 7 through 12, if needed.	_____	_____	_____
14. Dried your wrists and hands with a clean, dry paper towel. Patted dry starting at your fingertips.	_____	_____	_____
15. Discarded the paper towels into the wastebasket.	_____	_____	_____
16. Turned off faucets with clean, dry paper towels. Used a clean paper towel for each faucet or used knee or foot controls to turn off the faucet.	_____	_____	_____
17. Discarded paper towels into the wastebasket.	_____	_____	_____

Date of Satisfactory Completion _____   Instructor's Initials _____

Using an Alcohol-Based Hand Sanitizer

Name: _____   Date: _____

Procedure	S	U	Comments
1. Reviewed *Promoting Safety and Comfort: Hand Hygiene.*	_____	_____	_____
2. Applied a palmful of an alcohol-based hand sanitizer into a cupped hand.	_____	_____	_____
3. Rubbed your palms together.	_____	_____	_____
4. Rubbed the palm of 1 hand over the back of the other. Did the same for the other hand.	_____	_____	_____
5. Rubbed your palms together with your fingers interlaced.	_____	_____	_____
6. Interlocked your fingers. Rubbed your fingers back and forth.	_____	_____	_____
7. Rubbed the thumb of 1 hand in the palm of the other. Did the same for the other thumb.	_____	_____	_____
8. Rubbed the fingers of 1 hand into the palm of the other hand. Used a circular motion. Did the same for the fingers of the other hand.	_____	_____	_____
9. Continued rubbing your hands until they were dry.	_____	_____	_____

Date of Satisfactory Completion _____   Instructor's Initials _____

Donning and Removing PPE

Name: _____   Date: _____

Procedure	S	U	Comments
1. Followed *Delegation Guidelines: Transmission-Based Precautions*	_____	_____	_____
2. Removed watch and all jewelry.	_____	_____	_____
3. Rolled up uniform sleeves.	_____	_____	_____
4. Practiced hand hygiene.	_____	_____	_____
5. Put on a gown.			
a. Held a clean gown out in front of you.	_____	_____	_____
b. Unfolded the gown. Faced the back of the gown. Did not shake it.	_____	_____	_____
c. Put hands and arms through the sleeves.	_____	_____	_____
d. Made sure the gown covered from neck to knees and covered arms to the end of wrists.	_____	_____	_____
e. Tied the strings at the back of the neck.	_____	_____	_____
f. Overlapped the back of the gown. Made sure it covered uniform. The gown was snug, not loose.	_____	_____	_____
g. Tied the waist strings. Tied them at the back or the side. Did not tie them in front.	_____	_____	_____
6. Put on a mask or respirator.			
a. Picked up a mask by its upper ties. Did not touch the part that will cover face.	_____	_____	_____
b. Placed the mask over nose and mouth.	_____	_____	_____
c. Placed the upper strings above ears. Tied them at the back in the middle of head.	_____	_____	_____
d. Tied the lower strings at the back of neck. The lower part of the mask is under chin.	_____	_____	_____
e. Pinched the metal band around nose. The top of the mask is snug over nose. If wearing eyeglasses, the mask must be snug under the bottom of the eyeglasses.	_____	_____	_____
f. Made sure the mask was snug over face and under chin.	_____	_____	_____
7. Put on goggles or a face shield (if needed and if not part of the mask).			
a. Placed the device over face and eyes.	_____	_____	_____
b. Adjusted the device to fit.	_____	_____	_____
8. Put on gloves. Made sure the gloves covered the wrists of the gown.	_____	_____	_____
9. Provided care.	_____	_____	_____
10. Removed and discarded the PPE. Practiced hand hygiene between each step if hands became contaminated.			
a. Method 1—*Gloves, goggles or face shield, gown, mask or respirator*			
(1) Removed and discarded the gloves.			
a) Made sure that glove touches only glove.	_____	_____	_____
b) Grasped a glove at the palm. Grasp it on the outside.	_____	_____	_____
c) Pulled the glove down over your hand so that it is inside-out.	_____	_____	_____
d) Held the removed glove with the other gloved hand.	_____	_____	_____

Date of Satisfactory Completion _____   Instructor's Initials _____

Procedure—cont'd	S	U	Comments
e) Reached inside the other glove. Use the first 2 fingers of the ungloved hand.	_____	_____	_____
f) Pulled the glove down (inside-out) over your hand and the other glove.	_____	_____	_____
g) Discarded the gloves.	_____	_____	_____
(2) Removed and discarded the goggles or face shield if worn.			
a) Lifted the headband or earpieces from the back. Did not touch the front of the device.	_____	_____	_____
b) Discarded the device.	_____	_____	_____
(3) Removed and discarded the gown. Did not touch the outside of the gown.			
a) Untied the neck and then the waist strings.	_____	_____	_____
b) Pulled the gown down and away from neck and shoulders. Only touched the inside of the gown.	_____	_____	_____
c) Turned the gown inside-out as it was removed. Held it at the inside shoulder seams and brought hands together.	_____	_____	_____
d) Folded or rolled up the gown away from body. Kept it inside-out. Did not let the gown touch the floor.	_____	_____	_____
e) Discarded the gown.	_____	_____	_____
(4) Removed and discarded the mask if worn.			
a) Untied the lower strings of the mask.	_____	_____	_____
b) Untied the top strings.	_____	_____	_____
c) Held the top strings. Removed the mask without touching the front of the mask.	_____	_____	_____
d) Discarded the mask.	_____	_____	_____
b. Method 2—*Gown and gloves, goggles or face shield, mask or respirator.*			
(1) Removed and discarded the gown and gloves.			
a) Grasped the gown in front with gloved hands. Pulled away from body so that the ties break. Only touched the outside of the gown.	_____	_____	_____
b) Folded or rolled the gown inside-out into a bundle while removing the gown. Kept it inside out. Did not let the gown touch the floor.	_____	_____	_____
c) Peeled off gloves as removed the gown. Only touched the inside of the gloves and gown with bare hands.	_____	_____	_____
d) Discarded the gown and gloves.	_____	_____	_____
(2) Removed and discarded the goggles or face shield.			
a) Lifted the headband or earpieces from the back. Did not touch the front of the device.	_____	_____	_____
b) Discarded the device. If reusable, follow agency policy.	_____	_____	_____
(3) Removed and discarded the mask if worn.			
a) Untied the lower strings of the mask.	_____	_____	_____
b) Untied the top strings.	_____	_____	_____
c) Held the top strings. Removed the mask.	_____	_____	_____
d) Discarded the mask.	_____	_____	_____
11. Practiced hand hygiene after removing all PPE.	_____	_____	_____

Date of Satisfactory Completion _____   Instructor's Initials _____

Moving the Person Up in Bed

VIDEO

Name: _____   Date: _____

Quality of Life	S	U	Comments
• Knocked before entering the person's room.	_____	_____	_____
• Addressed the person by name.	_____	_____	_____
• Introduced self by name and title.	_____	_____	_____
• Explained the procedure to the person before starting and during the procedure.	_____	_____	_____
• Protected the person's rights during the procedure.	_____	_____	_____
• Handled the person gently during the procedure.	_____	_____	_____

Pre-Procedure

	S	U	Comments
1. Followed *Delegation Guidelines:* a. *Preventing Work-Related Injuries* b. *Moving Persons in Bed* Reviewed *Promoting Safety and Comfort:* a. *Assisting with Moving and Transfers* b. *Preventing Work-Related Injuries* c. *Moving the Person Up in Bed*	_____ _____	_____ _____	_____ _____
2. Asked a co-worker to help.	_____	_____	_____
3. Practiced hand hygiene.	_____	_____	_____
4. Identified the person. Checked the ID bracelet against the assignment sheet. Used 2 identifiers. Called the person by name.	_____	_____	_____
5. Provided for privacy.	_____	_____	_____
6. Locked the bed wheels.	_____	_____	_____
7. Raised the bed for body mechanics. Bed rails were up if used.	_____	_____	_____

Procedure

	S	U	Comments
8. Lowered the head of the bed to a level appropriate for the person. It was as flat as possible.	_____	_____	_____
9. Stood on one side of the bed. Your co-worker stood on the other side.	_____	_____	_____
10. Lowered the bed rails if up.	_____	_____	_____
11. Removed the pillow as directed by the nurse. Placed a pillow upright against the head-board if the person could be without it.	_____	_____	_____
12. Stood with a wide base of support. Pointed the foot near the head of the bed toward the head of the bed. Faced the head of the bed.	_____	_____	_____
13. Bent your hips and knees. Kept your back straight.	_____	_____	_____
14. Placed 1 arm under the person's shoulder and 1 arm under the thighs. Your co-worker did the same. Grasped each other's forearms.	_____	_____	_____
15. Asked the person to grasp the trapeze.	_____	_____	_____
16. Had the person flex both knees.	_____	_____	_____
17. Explained the following. a. You will count "1, 2, 3." b. The move will be on "3." c. On "3," the person pushes against the bed with the feet if able and pulls up with the trapeze.	_____ _____ _____	_____ _____ _____	_____ _____ _____

Date of Satisfactory Completion _____   Instructor's Initials _____

Procedure—cont'd	**S**	**U**	**Comments**
18. Moved the person to the head of the bed on the count of "3." Shifted your weight from your rear leg to your front leg. Your co-worker did the same.	_____	_____	_____
19. Repeated steps 12 through 18 if necessary.	_____	_____	_____
Post-Procedure			
20. Put the pillow under the person's head and shoulders. Straightened linens.	_____	_____	_____
21. Positioned the person in good alignment. Raised the head of the bed to a level appropriate for the person.	_____	_____	_____
22. Provided for comfort as noted on the inside of the front textbook cover.	_____	_____	_____
23. Placed the call light and other needed items within reach.	_____	_____	_____
24. Lowered the bed to a safe and comfortable level appropriate for the person. Followed the care plan.	_____	_____	_____
25. Raised or lowered bed rails. Followed the care plan.	_____	_____	_____
26. Unscreened the person.	_____	_____	_____
27. Completed a safety check of the room as noted on the inside of the front textbook cover.	_____	_____	_____
28. Practiced hand hygiene.	_____	_____	_____
29. Reported and recorded your observations.	_____	_____	_____

Date of Satisfactory Completion _____   Instructor's Initials _____

Moving the Person Up in Bed with an Assist Device

Name: _____   Date: _____

Quality of Life	S	U	Comments

Quality of Life
- Knocked before entering the person's room.
- Addressed the person by name.
- Introduced self by name and title.
- Explained the procedure to the person before starting and during the procedure.
- Protected the person's rights during the procedure.
- Handled the person gently during the procedure.

Pre-Procedure
1. Followed *Delegation Guidelines:*
   a. *Preventing Work-Related Injuries*
   b. *Moving Persons in Bed*
   Reviewed *Promoting Safety and Comfort:*
   a. *Assisting with Moving and Transfers*
   b. *Preventing Work-Related Injuries*
   c. *Moving the Person Up in Bed*
   d. *Moving the Person Up in Bed with an Assist Device*
2. Asked a co-worker to help.
3. Obtained the needed assist device
4. Practiced hand hygiene.
5. Identified the person. Checked the ID bracelet against the assignment sheet. Called the person by name.
6. Provided for privacy.
7. Locked the bed wheels.
8. Raised the bed for body mechanics. Bed rails were up if used.

Procedure
9. Lowered the head of the bed to a level appropriate for the person. It was as flat as possible.
10. Stood on one side of the bed. Your co-worker stood on the other side.
11. Lowered the bed rails if up.
12. Removed pillows as directed by the nurse. Placed a pillow upright against the head-board if the person could be without it.
13. Positioned the assist device.
14. Stood with a broad base of support. Pointed the foot near the head of the bed toward the head of the bed. Faced that direction.
15. Rolled the sides of the assist device up close to the person. (Omitted this step if device had handles.)
16. Grasped the rolled-up assist device firmly near the person's shoulders and hips. Grasped it by handles if present. Supported the head.
17. Bent hips and knees.

Date of Satisfactory Completion _____   Instructor's Initials _____

Procedure—cont'd	S	U	Comments
18. Moved the person up in bed on the count of "3." Shifted your weight from your rear leg to your front leg.	_____	_____	_____
19. Repeated steps 14 through 18 if necessary.	_____	_____	_____
20. Unrolled the assist device. (Omitted this step if device had handles.) Turned the person to remove the slide sheet if used.	_____	_____	_____

Post-Procedure

	S	U	Comments
21. Put the pillow under the person's head and shoulders.	_____	_____	_____
22. Positioned the person in good alignment.	_____	_____	_____
23. Provided for comfort as noted on the inside of the front textbook cover.	_____	_____	_____
24. Placed the call light and other items within reach.	_____	_____	_____
25. Lowered the bed to a safe and comfortable level appropriate for the person. Followed the care plan.	_____	_____	_____
26. Raised or lowered bed rails. Followed the care plan.	_____	_____	_____
27. Unscreened the person.	_____	_____	_____
28. Completed a safety check of the room as noted on the inside of the front textbook cover.	_____	_____	_____
29. Practiced hand hygiene.	_____	_____	_____
30. Reported and recorded your observations.	_____	_____	_____

Date of Satisfactory Completion _____   Instructor's Initials _____

Moving the Person to the Side of the Bed

Name: _____   Date: _____

Quality of Life	S	U	Comments
• Knocked before entering the person's room.	_____	_____	_____
• Addressed the person by name.	_____	_____	_____
• Introduced yourself by name and title.	_____	_____	_____
• Explained the procedure to the person before starting and during the procedure.	_____	_____	_____
• Protected the person's rights during the procedure.	_____	_____	_____
• Handled the person gently during the procedure.	_____	_____	_____

Pre-Procedure

	S	U	Comments
1. Followed *Delegation Guidelines:* 　a. *Preventing Work-Related Injuries* 　b. *Moving Persons in Bed*	_____	_____	_____
Reviewed *Promoting Safety and Comfort:* 　a. *Assisting with Moving and Transfers* 　b. *Preventing Work-Related Injuries* 　c. *Moving the Person to the Side of the Bed*	_____	_____	_____
2. Asked 1 or 2 co-workers to help if using an assist device.	_____	_____	_____
3. Obtained a drawsheet.	_____	_____	_____
4. Practiced hand hygiene.	_____	_____	_____
5. Identified the person. Checked the ID bracelet against the assignment sheet. Used 2 Identifiers. Called the person by name.	_____	_____	_____
6. Provided for privacy.	_____	_____	_____
7. Locked the bed wheels.	_____	_____	_____
8. Raised the bed for body mechanics. Bed rails were up if used.	_____	_____	_____

Procedure

	S	U	Comments
9. Lowered the head of the bed to a level appropriate for the person. It was as flat as possible.	_____	_____	_____
10. Stood on the side of the bed to which you would move the person.	_____	_____	_____
11. Lowered the bed rail near you if bed rails were used. (Both bed rails were lowered for step 16.)	_____	_____	_____
12. Removed pillows as directed by the nurse.	_____	_____	_____
13. Crossed the person's arms over the person's chest.	_____	_____	_____
14. Stood with your feet about 12 inches apart. One foot was in front of the other. Flexed your knees.	_____	_____	_____
15. *Method 1—Moving the person in segments:* 　a. Placed your arm under the person's neck and shoulders. Grasped the far shoulder.	_____	_____	_____
b. Placed your other arm under the mid-back.	_____	_____	_____
c. Moved the upper part of the person's body toward you. Rocked backward and shifted your weight to your rear leg.	_____	_____	_____
d. Placed 1 arm under the person's waist and 1 under the thighs.	_____	_____	_____
e. Rocked backward to move the lower part of the person toward you.	_____	_____	_____
f. Repeated the procedure for the legs and feet. Your arms were under the person's thighs and calves.	_____	_____	_____

Date of Satisfactory Completion _____   Instructor's Initials _____

Procedure—cont'd	S	U	Comments
16. *Method 2—Moving the person with a drawsheet:*			
a. Positioned the drawsheet.	_____	_____	_____
b. Rolled up the drawsheet close to the person.	_____	_____	_____
c. Grasped the rolled-up drawsheet near the person's shoulders and hips. Your co-worker did the same. Supported the person's head.	_____	_____	_____
d. Rocked backward on the count of "3," moving the person toward you. Your co-worker rocked backward slightly and then forward toward you while keeping the arms straight.	_____	_____	_____
e. Unrolled the drawsheet. Removed any wrinkles.	_____	_____	_____
Post-Procedure			
17. Put the pillow under the person's head and shoulders.			
18. Positioned the person in good alignment.	_____	_____	_____
19. Provided for comfort as noted on the inside of the front textbook cover.	_____	_____	_____
20. Placed the call light and other needed items within reach.	_____	_____	_____
21. Lowered the bed to a safe and comfortable level appropriate for the person. Followed the care plan.	_____	_____	_____
22. Raised or lowered bed rails. Followed the care plan.	_____	_____	_____
23. Unscreened the person.	_____	_____	_____
24. Completed a safety check of the room as noted on the inside of the front textbook cover.	_____	_____	_____
25. Practiced hand hygiene.	_____	_____	_____
26. Reported and recorded your observations.	_____	_____	_____

Date of Satisfactory Completion _____   Instructor's Initials _____

Turning and Repositioning the Person

Name: _____   Date: _____

Quality of Life	S	U	Comments
• Knocked before entering the person's room.	_____	_____	_____
• Addressed the person by name.	_____	_____	_____
• Introduced yourself by name and title.	_____	_____	_____
• Explained the procedure to the person before starting and during the procedure.	_____	_____	_____
• Protected the person's rights during the procedure.	_____	_____	_____
• Handled the person gently during the procedure.	_____	_____	_____

Pre-Procedure

1. Followed *Delegation Guidelines:*
   a. *Preventing Work-Related Injuries*
   b. *Moving Persons in Bed*
   c. *Turning Persons*
   Reviewed *Promoting Safety and Comfort:*
   a. *Assisting with Moving and Transfers*
   b. *Preventing Work-Related Injuries*
   c. *Moving the Person to the Side of the Bed*
   d. *Turning Persons*
2. Practiced hand hygiene.
3. Identified the person. Checked the ID bracelet against the assignment sheet. Used 2 Identifiers. Called the person by name.
4. Provided for privacy.
5. Locked the bed wheels.
6. Raised the bed for body mechanics. Bed rails were up.

Procedure

7. Lowered the head of the bed to a level appropriate for the person. It was as flat as possible.
8. Stood on the side of the bed opposite to where you would turn the person.
9. Lowered the bed rail.
10. Moved the person to the side near you. (Followed the procedure: *Moving the Person to the Side of the Bed.*)
11. Crossed the person's arms over the person's chest. Crossed the leg near you over the far leg.
12. *Turning the person away from you:*
    a. Stood with a wide base of support. Flexed the knees.
    b. Placed 1 hand on the person's shoulder. Placed the other on the hip near you.
    c. Rolled the person gently away from you toward the raised bed rail.
    d. Shifted your weight from your rear leg to your front leg.
13. *Turning the person toward you:*
    a. Raised the bed rail.
    b. Went to the other side. Lowered the bed rail.
    c. Stood with a wide base of support. Flexed your knees.

Date of Satisfactory Completion _____   Instructor's Initials _____

Procedure—cont'd	S	U	Comments
d. Placed 1 hand on the person's far shoulder. Placed the other on the far hip.	_____	_____	_____
e. Rolled the person toward you gently.	_____	_____	_____
14. Positioned the person. Followed the nurse's directions and the care plan. The following is common.			
a. Placed a pillow under the head and neck.	_____	_____	_____
b. Adjusted the shoulder. The person did not lie on an arm.	_____	_____	_____
c. Placed a small pillow under the upper hand and arm.	_____	_____	_____
d. Positioned a pillow against the back.	_____	_____	_____
e. Flexed the upper knee. Positioned the upper leg in front of the lower leg.	_____	_____	_____
f. Supported the upper leg and thigh on pillows. Made sure the ankle was supported.	_____	_____	_____
Post-Procedure			
15. Provided for comfort as noted on the inside of the front textbook cover.	_____	_____	_____
16. Placed the call light and other needed items within reach.	_____	_____	_____
17. Lowered the bed to a safe and comfortable level appropriate for the person. Followed the care plan.	_____	_____	_____
18. Raised or lowered bed rails. Followed the care plan.	_____	_____	_____
19. Unscreened the person.	_____	_____	_____
20. Completed a safety check of the room as noted on the inside of the front textbook cover.	_____	_____	_____
21. Practiced hand hygiene.	_____	_____	_____
22. Reported and recorded your observations.	_____	_____	_____

Date of Satisfactory Completion _____   Instructor's Initials _____

Logrolling the Person

Name: _____   Date: _____

Quality of Life	S	U	Comments
• Knocked before entering the person's room.	_____	_____	_____
• Addressed the person by name.	_____	_____	_____
• Introduced yourself by name and title.	_____	_____	_____
• Explained the procedure to the person before starting and during the procedure.	_____	_____	_____
• Protected the person's rights during the procedure.	_____	_____	_____
• Handled the person gently during the procedure.	_____	_____	_____

Pre-Procedure

	S	U	Comments

1. Followed *Delegation Guidelines:*
  a. *Preventing Work-Related Injuries*
  b. *Moving Persons in Bed*
  c. *Turning Persons*
Reviewed *Promoting Safety and Comfort:*
  a. *Assisting with Moving and Transfers*
  b. *Preventing Work-Related Injuries*
  c. *Turning Persons*
  d. *Logrolling*
	_____
	
	_____
		_____
		
		_____
			_____
			
			_____

2. Asked a co-worker to help.	_____	_____	_____
3. Obtained the needed assist device	_____	_____	_____
4. Practiced hand hygiene.	_____	_____	_____
5. Identified the person. Checked the ID bracelet against the assignment sheet. Used 2 Identifiers. Called the person by name.	_____	_____	_____
6. Provided for privacy.	_____	_____	_____
7. Locked the bed wheels.	_____	_____	_____
8. Raised the bed for body mechanics. Bed rails were up if used.	_____	_____	_____

Procedure

	S	U	Comments
9. Made sure the bed was flat.	_____	_____	_____
10. Stood on the side opposite to which you would turn the person. Your co-worker stood on the other side.	_____	_____	_____
11. Lowered the bed rails if used.	_____	_____	_____
12. Positioned the assist device	_____	_____	_____
13. Moved the person as a unit to the side of the bed near you. Used the assist device. (If the person had a spinal cord injury, assisted the nurse as directed.)	_____	_____	_____
14. Placed the person's arms across the chest. Placed a pillow between the knees.	_____	_____	_____
15. Raised the bed rail if used.	_____	_____	_____
16. Went to the other side.	_____	_____	_____
17. Stood near the shoulders and chest. Your co-worker stood near the hips and thighs.	_____	_____	_____
18. Stood with a broad base of support. One foot was in front of the other.	_____	_____	_____
19. Asked the person to hold his or her body rigid.	_____	_____	_____
20. Rolled the person toward you or used the assist device. Turned the person as a unit.	_____	_____	_____
21. Removed the slide sheet if used.	_____	_____	_____

Date of Satisfactory Completion _____   Instructor's Initials _____

Procedure—cont'd	S	U	Comments
22. Positioned the person in good alignment. Used pillows as directed by the nurse and care plan. The following is common unless the spinal cord is involved.			
a. Placed a pillow under the head and neck if allowed.	_____	_____	_____
b. Adjusted the shoulder. The person was not on an arm.	_____	_____	_____
c. Placed a small pillow under the upper hand and arm.	_____	_____	_____
d. Positioned a pillow against the back.	_____	_____	_____
e. Flexed the upper knee. Positioned the upper leg in front of the lower leg.	_____	_____	_____
f. Supported the upper leg and thigh on pillows. Made sure the ankle was supported.	_____	_____	_____

Post-Procedure

	S	U	Comments
23. Provided for comfort as noted on the inside of the front textbook cover.	_____	_____	_____
24. Placed the call light and other needed items within reach.	_____	_____	_____
25. Lowered the bed to a safe and comfortable level appropriate for the person. Followed the care plan.	_____	_____	_____
26. Raised or lowered bed rails. Followed the care plan.	_____	_____	_____
27. Unscreened the person.	_____	_____	_____
28. Completed a safety check of the room as noted on the inside of the front textbook cover.	_____	_____	_____
29. Practiced hand hygiene.	_____	_____	_____
30. Reported and recorded your observations.	_____	_____	_____

Date of Satisfactory Completion _____   Instructor's Initials _____

Sitting on the Side of the Bed (Dangling)

Name: _____   Date: _____

Quality of Life	S	U	Comments
• Knocked before entering the person's room.	_____	_____	_____
• Addressed the person by name.	_____	_____	_____
• Introduced yourself by name and title.	_____	_____	_____
• Explained the procedure to the person before starting and during the procedure.	_____	_____	_____
• Protected the person's rights during the procedure.	_____	_____	_____
• Handled the person gently during the procedure.	_____	_____	_____

Pre-Procedure

1. Followed *Delegation Guidelines:*
   a. *Preventing Work-Related Injuries*
   b. *Dangling*
   Reviewed *Promoting Safety and Comfort:*
   a. *Assisting with Moving and Transfers*
   b. *Preventing Work-Related Injuries*
   c. *Dangling*
2. Asked a co-worker to help you.
3. Practiced hand hygiene.
4. Identified the person. Checked the ID bracelet against the assignment sheet. Used 2 Identifiers. Called the person by name.
5. Provided for privacy.
6. Decided what side of the bed to use.
7. Moved furniture to provide moving space.
8. Locked the bed wheels.
9. Raised the bed for body mechanics. Bed rails were up if used.

Procedure

10. Lowered the bed rail if up.
11. Positioned the person in a side-lying position facing you. The person lay on the strong side.
12. Raised the head of the bed to a sitting position.
13. Stood by the person's hips. Faced the foot of the bed.
14. Stood with your feet apart. The foot near the head of the bed was in front of the other foot.
15. Slid 1 arm under the person's neck and shoulders. Grasped the far shoulder. Placed your other hand over the thighs near the knees.
16. Pivoted toward the foot of the bed while moving the person's legs and feet over the side of the bed. As the legs went over the edge of the mattress, the trunk was upright.
17. Asked the person to hold on to the edge of the mattress. This supported the person in the sitting position. If possible, raised a half-length bed rail for the person to grasp. Raised the bed rail on the person's strong side. Your co-worker supported the person at all times.

Date of Satisfactory Completion _____   Instructor's Initials _____

Procedure—cont'd	S	U	Comments

18. Checked the person's condition:
    a. Asked how the person felt. Asked if the person felt dizzy or light-headed.
    b. Checked the pulse and respirations.
    c. Checked for difficulty breathing.
    d. Noted if the skin was pale or bluish in color (cyanosis).
19. Reversed the procedure to return the person to bed. (Or prepared the person to walk or for a transfer to a chair or wheelchair. Lowered the bed to a safe and comfortable level. The person's feet were flat on the floor.
20. Lowered the head of the bed after the person returned to bed. Helped him or her move to the center of the bed.
21. Positioned the person in good alignment.

Post-Procedure

22. Provided for comfort as noted on the inside of the front textbook cover.
23. Placed the call light and other needed items within reach.
24. Lowered the bed to a safe and comfortable level appropriate for the person. Followed the care plan.
25. Raised or lowered bed rails. Followed the care plan.
26. Returned furniture to its proper place.
27. Unscreened the person.
28. Completed a safety check of the room as noted on the inside of the front textbook cover.
29. Practiced hand hygiene.
30. Reported and recorded your observations.

Date of Satisfactory Completion _____   Instructor's Initials _____

Transferring the Person to a Chair or Wheelchair

Name: _____   Date: _____

Quality of Life	S	U	Comments
• Knocked before entering the person's room.	___	___	___
• Addressed the person by name.	___	___	___
• Introduced yourself by name and title.	___	___	___
• Explained the procedure to the person before starting and during the procedure.	___	___	___
• Protected the person's rights during the procedure.	___	___	___
• Handled the person gently during the procedure.	___	___	___

Pre-Procedure

1. Followed *Delegation Guidelines:*   ___   ___   ___
   a. *Transferring the Person*
   b. *Stand and Pivot Transfers*
   Reviewed *Promoting Safety and Comfort:* ___   ___   ___
   a. *Transfer Belts*
   b. *Transferring the Person*
   c. *Stand and Pivot Transfers*
   d. *Bed to Chair or Wheelchair Transfers*
2. Collected:
   a. Wheelchair or armchair   ___   ___   ___
   b. Bath blanket   ___   ___   ___
   c. Lap blanket   ___   ___   ___
   d. Robe and non-skid footwear ___   ___   ___
   e. Paper or sheet   ___   ___   ___
   f. Transfer belt if needed   ___   ___   ___
   g. Seat cushion if needed   ___   ___   ___
3. Practiced hand hygiene.   ___   ___   ___
4. Identified the person. Checked the ID bracelet against the assignment sheet. Used 2 Identifiers. Called the person by name.   ___   ___   ___
5. Provided for privacy.   ___   ___   ___
6. Decided which side of the bed to use. Moved furniture for a safe transfer.   ___   ___   ___

Procedure

7. Raised the wheelchair footplates. Removed or swung front rigging out of the way if possible. Positioned the chair or wheelchair near the bed on the person's strong side.
   a. If at the head of the bed, it faced the foot of the bed.   ___   ___   ___
   b. If at the foot of the bed, it faced the head of the bed.   ___   ___   ___
   c. The armrest almost touched the bed.   ___   ___   ___
8. Placed a folded bath blanket or cushion on the seat if needed.   ___   ___   ___
9. Locked wheelchair wheels.   ___   ___   ___
10. Fan-folded top linens to the foot of the bed.   ___   ___   ___
11. Placed the paper or sheet under the person's feet. Put footwear on the person.   ___   ___   ___
12. Lowered the bed to a safe and comfortable level. The person's feet were flat on the floor. Locked the bed wheels.   ___   ___   ___

Date of Satisfactory Completion _____   Instructor's Initials _____

Procedure—cont'd	S	U	Comments
13. Helped the person sit on the side of the bed. His or her feet touched the floor.	_____	_____	_____
14. Helped the person put on a robe.	_____	_____	_____
15. Applied the transfer belt if needed. It was applied at the waist over clothing.	_____	_____	_____
16. *Method 1—Using a transfer belt:*			
a. Stood in front of the person.	_____	_____	_____
b. Had the person hold on to the mattress.	_____	_____	_____
c. Made sure the person's feet were flat on the floor.	_____	_____	_____
d. Had the person lean forward.	_____	_____	_____
e. Grasped the transfer belt at each side. Grasped the handles or grasped the belt from underneath.	_____	_____	_____
f. Prevented the person from sliding or falling by doing one of the following.			
(1) Braced your knees against the person's knees. Blocked the person's feet with your feet.	_____	_____	_____
(2) Used the knee and foot of one leg to block the person's weak leg or foot. Placed your other foot slightly behind you for balance.	_____	_____	_____
(3) Straddled your legs around the person's weak leg.	_____	_____	_____
g. Explained the following.			
(1) You will count "1, 2, 3."	_____	_____	_____
(2) The move will be on "3."	_____	_____	_____
(3) On "3" the person will push down on the mattress and stand.	_____	_____	_____
h. Asked the person to push down on the mattress and to stand on the count of "3." Pulled the person into a standing position as you straightened your knees.	_____	_____	_____
17. *Method 2—No transfer belt (This method was used only if directed by the nurse and the care plan.):*			
a. Followed steps 16, a–c.	_____	_____	_____
b. Placed your hands under the person's arms. Your hands were around the person's shoulder blades.	_____	_____	_____
c. Had the person lean forward.	_____	_____	_____
d. Prevented the person from sliding or falling by doing one of the following.			
(1) Braced your knees against the person's knees. Blocked the person's feet with your feet.	_____	_____	_____
(2) Used the knee and foot of one leg to block the person's weak leg or foot. Placed your other foot slightly behind you for balance.	_____	_____	_____
(3) Straddled your legs around the person's weak leg.	_____	_____	_____
e. Explained the count of "3" as in step 16, g.	_____	_____	_____
f. Asked the person to push down on the mattress and to stand on the count of "3." Pulled the person up into a standing position as you straightened your knees.	_____	_____	_____
18. Supported the person in the standing position. Held the transfer belt or kept your hands around the person's shoulder blades. Continued to prevent the person from sliding or falling.	_____	_____	_____

Date of Satisfactory Completion _____   Instructor's Initials _____

Procedure—cont'd	S	U	Comments
19. Helped the person turn so that he or she could grasp the far arm of the chair or wheelchair. The legs touched the edge of the seat.	_____	_____	_____
20. Continued to help the person turn until the other armrest was grasped.	_____	_____	_____
21. Lowered the person into the chair or wheelchair as you bent your hips and knees. The person assisted by leaning forward and bending the elbows and knees.	_____	_____	_____
22. Made sure the hips were to the back of the seat. Positioned the person in good alignment.	_____	_____	_____
23. Attached the wheelchair front rigging. Positioned the person's feet on the wheelchair footplates.	_____	_____	_____
24. Covered the person's lap and legs with a lap blanket. Kept the blanket off the floor and the wheels.	_____	_____	_____
25. Removed the transfer belt if used.	_____	_____	_____
26. Positioned the chair as the person preferred. Locked the wheelchair wheels according to the care plan.	_____	_____	_____
Post-Procedure			
27. Provided for comfort as noted on the inside of the front textbook cover.	_____	_____	_____
28. Placed the call light and other needed items within reach.	_____	_____	_____
29. Unscreened the person.	_____	_____	_____
30. Completed a safety check of the room as noted on the inside of the front textbook cover.	_____	_____	_____
31. Practiced hand hygiene.	_____	_____	_____
32. Reported and recorded your observations.	_____	_____	_____
33. Followed the procedure: *Transferring the Person from a Chair or Wheelchair to Bed* to return the person to bed.	_____	_____	_____

Date of Satisfactory Completion _____   Instructor's Initials _____

Transferring the Person from a Chair or Wheelchair to Bed

NATCEP™

Name: _____   Date: _____

Quality of Life	S	U	Comments
• Knocked before entering the person's room.	_____	_____	_____
• Addressed the person by name.	_____	_____	_____
• Introduced yourself by name and title.	_____	_____	_____
• Explained the procedure to the person before starting and during the procedure.	_____	_____	_____
• Protected the person's rights during the procedure.	_____	_____	_____
• Handled the person gently during the procedure.	_____	_____	_____

Pre-Procedure

	S	U	Comments
1. Followed *Delegation Guidelines:*	_____	_____	_____
a. *Transferring the Person*			
b. *Stand and Pivot Transfers*			
Reviewed *Promoting Safety and Comfort:*	_____	_____	_____
a. *Transfer/Gait Belts*			
b. *Transferring the Person*			
c. *Stand and Pivot Transfers*			
d. *Bed to Chair or Wheelchair Transfers*			
2. Collected a transfer belt if needed.	_____	_____	_____
3. Practiced hand hygiene.	_____	_____	_____
4. Identified the person. Checked the ID bracelet against the assignment sheet. Called the person by name.	_____	_____	_____
5. Provided for privacy.	_____	_____	_____

Procedure

	S	U	Comments
6. Moved furniture for moving space.	_____	_____	_____
7. Raised the head of the bed to a sitting position. Lowered the bed to a safe and comfortable level. The person's feet were flat on the floor.	_____	_____	_____
8. Moved the call light so that it was on the strong side when the person was in bed.	_____	_____	_____
9. Positioned the chair or wheelchair so that the person's strong side was next to the bed. Had a co-worker help if necessary.	_____	_____	_____
10. Locked the wheelchair and bed wheels.	_____	_____	_____
11. Removed and folded the lap blanket.	_____	_____	_____
12. Removed the person's feet from the footplates. Raised the footplates. Removed or swung the front rigging out of the way. (The person had on non-skid footwear.)	_____	_____	_____
13. Applied the transfer belt if needed.	_____	_____	_____
14. Made sure the person's feet were flat on the floor.	_____	_____	_____
15. Stood in front of the person.	_____	_____	_____
16. Asked the person to hold on to the armrests. (If the nurse directed you to do so, placed your arms under the person's arms. Your hands were around the shoulder blades.)	_____	_____	_____
17. Had the person lean forward.	_____	_____	_____

Date of Satisfactory Completion _____   Instructor's Initials _____

Procedure—cont'd	S	U	Comments
18. Grasped the transfer belt on each side if using it. Grasped the handles or grasped the belt from underneath.	_____	_____	_____
19. Prevented the person from sliding or falling by doing one of the following.			
a. Braced your knees against the person's knees. Blocked the person's feet with your feet.	_____	_____	_____
b. Used the knee and foot of one leg to block the person's weak leg or foot. Placed your other foot slightly behind you for balance.	_____	_____	_____
c. Straddled your legs around the person's weak leg.	_____	_____	_____
20. Explained the count of "3" as in procedure: *Transferring the Person to a Chair or Wheelchair.*	_____	_____	_____
21. Asked the person to push down on the armrests on the count of "3." Pulled the person into a standing position as you straightened your knees.	_____	_____	_____
22. Supported the person in the standing position. Held the transfer belt or kept your hands around the person's shoulder blades. Continued to prevent the person from sliding or falling.	_____	_____	_____
23. Turned the person so that he or she could reach the edge of the mattress. The person's legs touched the mattress.	_____	_____	_____
24. Continued to turn the person until he or she could reach the mattress with both hands.	_____	_____	_____
25. Lowered the person onto the bed as you bent your hips and knees. The person assisted by leaning forward and bending the elbows and knees.	_____	_____	_____
26. Removed the transfer belt.	_____	_____	_____
27. Removed the robe and footwear.	_____	_____	_____
28. Helped the person lie down.	_____	_____	_____
Post-Procedure			
29. Provided for comfort as noted on the inside of the front textbook cover.	_____	_____	_____
30. Placed the call light and other needed items within reach.	_____	_____	_____
31. Raised or lowered bed rails. Followed the care plan.	_____	_____	_____
32. Arranged furniture to meet the person's needs.	_____	_____	_____
33. Unscreened the person.	_____	_____	_____
34. Completed a safety check of the room as noted on the inside of the front textbook cover.	_____	_____	_____
35. Practiced hand hygiene.	_____	_____	_____
36. Reported and recorded your observations.	_____	_____	_____

Date of Satisfactory Completion _____ Instructor's Initials _____

Transferring the Person to and from the Toilet

Name: _____   Date: _____

Quality of Life	S	U	Comments
• Knocked before entering the person's room.	___	___	___
• Addressed the person by name.	___	___	___
• Introduced yourself by name and title.	___	___	___
• Explained the procedure to the person before starting and during the procedure.	___	___	___
• Protected the person's rights during the procedure.	___	___	___
• Handled the person gently during the procedure.	___	___	___

Pre-Procedure

1. Followed *Delegation Guidelines:*
   a. *Transferring the Person*
   b. *Stand and Pivot Transfers*   ___ ___ ___

   Reviewed *Promoting Safety and Comfort:*
   a. *Transfer/Gait Belts*
   b. *Transferring the Person*   ___ ___ ___
   c. *Stand and Pivot Transfers*
   d. *Bed to Chair or Wheelchair Transfers*
   e. *Transferring the Person to and from the Toilet*

2. Practiced hand hygiene.   ___ ___ ___

Procedure

3. Had the person wear non-skid footwear.   ___ ___ ___
4. Positioned the wheelchair next to the toilet if there was enough room. If not, positioned the wheelchair at a right angle (90-degree angle) to the toilet. (If possible, the person's strong side was near the toilet.)   ___ ___ ___
5. Locked the wheelchair wheels.   ___ ___ ___
6. Raised the footplates. Removed or swung front rigging out of the way.   ___ ___ ___
7. Applied the transfer belt.   ___ ___ ___
8. Helped the person unfasten clothing.   ___ ___ ___
9. Used the transfer belt to help the person stand and to turn to the toilet. (See procedure: *Transferring the Person From Chair or Wheelchair to Bed.*) The person used the grab bars to turn to the toilet.   ___ ___ ___
10. Supported the person with the transfer belt while he or she lowered clothing or had the person hold on to the grab bars for support. Lowered the person's pants and undergarments.   ___ ___ ___
11. Used the transfer belt to lower the person onto the toilet seat. Checked for proper positioning on the toilet.   ___ ___ ___
12. Removed the transfer belt.   ___ ___ ___
13. Told the person you would stay nearby. Reminded the person to use the call light or call for help when needed. Stayed with the person if required by the care plan.   ___ ___ ___
14. Closed the bathroom door to provide for privacy.   ___ ___ ___
15. Stayed near the bathroom. Completed other tasks in the person's room. Checked on the person every 5 minutes.   ___ ___ ___

Date of Satisfactory Completion _____   Instructor's Initials _____

Procedure—cont'd	S	U	Comments
16. Knocked on the bathroom door when the person called.	_____	_____	_____
17. Helped with wiping, perineal care, flushing, and hand washing as needed. Wore gloves and practiced hand hygiene after removing gloves.	_____	_____	_____
18. Applied the transfer belt.	_____	_____	_____
19. Used the transfer belt to help the person stand.	_____	_____	_____
20. Helped the person raise and secure clothing.	_____	_____	_____
21. Used the transfer belt to transfer the person to the wheelchair. (See procedure: *Transferring the Person to a Chair or Wheelchair.*)	_____	_____	_____
22. Made sure the person's buttocks were to the back of the seat. Positioned the person in good alignment.	_____	_____	_____
23. Positioned the person's feet on the footplates.	_____	_____	_____
24. Removed the transfer belt.	_____	_____	_____
25. Covered the person's lap and legs with a lap blanket. Kept the blanket off the floor and wheels.	_____	_____	_____
26. Positioned the chair as the person preferred. Locked the wheelchair wheels according to the care plan.	_____	_____	_____

Post-Procedure

	S	U	Comments
27. Provided for comfort as noted on the inside of the front textbook cover.	_____	_____	_____
28. Placed the call light and other needed items within the person's reach.	_____	_____	_____
29. Unscreened the person.	_____	_____	_____
30. Completed a safety check of the room as noted on the inside of the front textbook cover.	_____	_____	_____
31. Practiced hand hygiene.	_____	_____	_____
32. Reported and recorded your observations.	_____	_____	_____

Date of Satisfactory Completion _____   Instructor's Initials _____

Transferring the Person Using a Stand-Assist Mechanical Lift

Name: _____   Date: _____

	S	U	Comments
Quality of Life			
• Knocked before entering the person's room.	___	___	___
• Addressed the person by name.	___	___	___
• Introduced self by name and title.	___	___	___
• Explained the procedure to the person before starting and during the procedure.	___	___	___
• Protected the person's rights during the procedure.	___	___	___
• Handled the person gently during the procedure.	___	___	___
Pre-Procedure			
1. Followed *Delegation Guidelines:*	___	___	___
a. *Transferring the Person*			
b. *Using a Mechanical Lift*			
See *Promoting Safety and Comfort:*	___	___	___
a. *Transferring the Person*			
b. *Using a Mechanical Lift*			
2. Asked a co-worker to help (if needed).	___	___	___
3. Collected the following.			
• Mechanical lift and sling	___	___	___
• Arm chair or wheelchair	___	___	___
• Footwear	___	___	___
• Bath blanket or cushion	___	___	___
• Lap blanket (if used)	___	___	___
4. Practiced hand hygiene.	___	___	___
5. Identified the person. Checked the ID bracelet against the assignment sheet. Used 2 identifiers. Also called the person by name.	___	___	___
6. Provided for privacy.	___	___	___
Procedure			
7. Placed the chair (wheelchair) at the head of the bed. It was even with the head-board and about 1 foot away from the bed. Locked (brake) the wheelchair wheels. Placed a folded bath blanket or cushion in the seat if needed.	___	___	___
8. Assisted the person to a seated position on the side of the bed. See procedure: *Sitting on the Side of the Bed (Dangling)* in Chapter 15. The person's feet were flat on the floor. Bed wheels are locked.	___	___	___
9. Put footwear on the person.	___	___	___
10. Applied the sling.			
a. Positioned the sling at the lower back.	___	___	___
b. Brought the straps around to the front of the chest. The straps are positioned under the arms.	___	___	___
c. Secured the waist belt around the person's waist. Adjusted the belt so that it was snug but not tight.	___	___	___
11. Positioned the lift in front of the person.	___	___	___
12. Widen the lift's base.	___	___	___
13. Locked (brake) the lift's wheels.	___	___	___

Date of Satisfactory Completion _____   Instructor's Initials _____

Procedure—cont'd   S   U   Comments

14. Had the person place the feet on the foot plate and
    the knees against the knee pad. Assisted as needed.
    If the lift has a knee strap, secured the strap around
    the legs. Adjusted the strap so that it was snug but
    not tight.
15. Attached the sling to the sling hooks.
16. Had the person grasp the lift's hand grips.
17. Unlocked the lift's wheels. (released the brakes)
18. Raised the person slightly off the bed. Checked that
    the sling is secure, the feet were on the footplate,
    and the knees were against the knee pad. If not,
    lowered the person and corrected the problem.
19. Raised the lift until the person was cleared of the
    bed. Or raised the person to a standing position.
    Followed the care plan.
20. Adjusted the base's width to move from the bed to
    the chair (wheelchair) if needed. Kept the base in
    the wide or open position as much as possible.
21. Moved the lift to the chair (wheelchair). The person's
    back was toward the seat.
22. Lowered the person into the chair (wheelchair).
    Guided the person into the seat.
23. Locked (brake) the lift's wheels.
24. Unhooked the sling from the sling hooks.
25. Unbuckled the waist belt. Remove the sling.
26. Unlocked the lift's wheels. (released the brakes)
27. Had the person lift the feet off of the footplate.
    Assisted as needed. Moved the lift. Positioned the
    person's feet flat on the floor or on the wheelchair
    footplates.
28. Covered the lap and legs with a lap blanket (if
    used). Kept it off the floor.

Post-Procedure
29. Provided for comfort.
30. Placed the call light and other needed items within
    reach.
31. Unscreened the person.
32. Completed a safety check of the room.
33. Practiced hand hygiene.
34. Reported and recorded your observations.
35. Reversed the procedure to return the person to bed.

Date of Satisfactory Completion _____   Instructor's Initials _____

Transferring the Person Using a Full-Sling Mechanical Lift

Name: _____   Date: _____

	S	U	Comments

Quality of Life

- Knocked before entering the person's room.
- Addressed the person by name.
- Introduced self by name and title.
- Explained the procedure to the person before starting and during the procedure.
- Protected the person's rights during the procedure.
- Handled the person gently during the procedure.

Pre-Procedure

1. Followed *Delegation Guidelines:*
   a. *Transferring the Person,*
   b. *Using a Mechanical Lift,*
   See *Promoting Safety and Comfort:*
   a. *Transferring the Person,*
   b. *Using a Mechanical Lift,*
2. Asked a co-worker to help.
3. Collected the following.
   - Full-sling mechanical lift and sling
   - Arm chair or wheelchair
   - Footwear
   - Bath blanket or cushion
   - Lap blanket (if used)
4. Practiced hand hygiene.
5. Identified the person. Checked the ID bracelet against the assignment sheet. Used 2 identifiers. Also called the person by name.
6. Provided for privacy.
7. Raised the bed for body mechanics. Bed rails are up if used.

Procedure

8. Lowered the head of the bed to a level appropriate for the person. It is as flat as possible.
9. Stood on one side of the bed. Co-worker stood on the other side.
10. Lowered the bed rails if up. Locked (brake) the bed wheels.
11. Centered the sling under the person. To position the sling, turned the person from side to side (Chapter 15). Follow the manufacturer's instructions to position the sling.
12. Positioned the person in the semi-Fowler's position.
13. Placed the chair (wheelchair) at the head of the bed. It was even with the headboard and about 1 foot away from the bed. Placed a folded bath blanket or cushion in the seat if needed. Locked (brake) the wheelchair wheels.
14. Lowered the bed so that it was level with the chair.
15. Raised the lift to position it over the person.
16. Positioned the lift over the person.

Date of Satisfactory Completion _____   Instructor's Initials _____

Procedure—cont'd	S	U	Comments
17. Widened the lift's base. Locked (brake) the lift wheels.	___	___	___
18. Attached the sling to the sling hooks.	___	___	___
19. Raised the head of the bed to a comfortable level for the person.	___	___	___
20. Crossed the person's arms over the chest.	___	___	___
21. Unlocked the lift's wheels. (released the brakes)	___	___	___
22. Raised the person slightly from the bed. Checked that the sling is secure. If not, lowered the person and corrected the problem.	___	___	___
23. Raised the lift until the person and sling were free of the bed.	___	___	___
24. Had co-worker support the person's legs as you moved the lift and the person away from the bed.	___	___	___
25. Adjusted the base's width to move from the bed to the chair (wheelchair) if needed. Kept the base in the wide or open position as much as possible.	___	___	___
26. Positioned the lift so that the person's back was toward the chair (wheelchair).	___	___	___
27. Adjusted the position of the chair (wheelchair) as needed to lower the person into it. Locked the wheelchair wheels.	___	___	___
28. Lowered the person into the chair (wheelchair). Guided the person into the seat.	___	___	___
29. Locked the lift wheels.	___	___	___
30. Unhooked the sling. Unlocked the lift's wheels (released the brakes). Moved the lift. Removed the sling from under the person unless otherwise indicated.	___	___	___
31. Put footwear on the person. Positioned the feet flat on the floor or on the wheelchair footplates.	___		___
32. Covered the lap and legs with a lap blanket (if used). Kept it off the floor and wheels.	___		___
33. Positioned the chair (wheelchair) as the person prefers. Locked the wheelchair wheels according to the care plan.	___		___
Post-Procedure			
34. Provided for comfort.			
35. Placed the call light and other needed items within reach.	___	___	___
36. Unscreened the person.	___	___	___
37. Completed a safety check of the room as noted on the inside front cover of the textbook.	___	___	___
38. Practiced hand hygiene.	___	___	___
39. Reported and recorded your observations.	___	___	___
40. Reversed the procedure to return the person to bed.	___	___	___

Date of Satisfactory Completion _____   Instructor's Initials _____

Making a Closed Bed

Name: _____ Date: _____

	S	U	Comments
Quality of Life			
• Knocked before entering the person's room.	___	___	___
• Addressed the person by name.	___	___	___
• Introduced yourself by name and title.	___	___	___
• Explained the procedure to the person before starting and during the procedure.	___	___	___
• Protected the person's rights during the procedure.	___	___	___
• Handled the person gently during the procedure.	___	___	___

Pre-Procedure

1. Followed *Delegation Guidelines: Making Beds.* Reviewed *Promoting Safety and Comfort: Making Beds.* ___ ___ ___
2. Practiced hand hygiene. ___ ___ ___
3. Collected clean linen.
   - Mattress pad (if needed) ___ ___ ___
   - Bottom sheet (flat sheet or fitted sheet) ___ ___ ___
   - Waterproof under-pad (if needed) ___ ___ ___
   - Cotton drawsheet or padded waterproof draw-sheet (if needed) ___ ___ ___
   - Top sheet ___ ___ ___
   - Blanket ___ ___ ___
   - Bedspread ___ ___ ___
   - A pillowcase for each pillow ___ ___ ___
   - Bath towel ___ ___ ___
   - Hand towel ___ ___ ___
   - Washcloth ___ ___ ___
   - Gown or pajamas ___ ___ ___
   - Bath blanket ___ ___ ___
   - Gloves ___ ___ ___
   - Laundry bag ___ ___ ___
   - Paper towels (if required as a barrier for clean linens) ___ ___ ___
4. Placed linen on a clean surface. Used paper towels as a barrier between the clean surface and clean linen if required by agency policy. ___ ___ ___
5. Raised the bed for body mechanics. Bed rails were down. ___ ___ ___

Procedure

6. Put on the gloves. ___ ___ ___
7. Removed linen. Rolled each piece away from you. Placed each piece in a laundry bag. Discarded incontinence products or disposable bed protectors in the trash. Did not put them in the laundry bag. ___ ___ ___
8. Cleaned the bed frame and mattress if this is part of your job. ___ ___ ___
9. Removed and discarded gloves. Practiced hand hygiene. ___ ___ ___
10. Moved the mattress to the head of the bed. ___ ___ ___
11. Put the mattress pad on the mattress. It was even with the top of the mattress. ___ ___ ___

Date of Satisfactory Completion _____ Instructor's Initials _____

Procedure—cont'd   S   U   Comments

12. Placed the bottom sheet on the mattress pad.
    Unfolded it lengthwise. Placed the center crease in
    the middle of the bed (if using a flat sheet).
    a. Positioned the lower edge even with the bottom   _____   _____   _____
       of the mattress.
    b. Placed the large hem at the top and the small   _____   _____   _____
       hem at the bottom.
    c. Faced hem-stitching downward, away from the   _____   _____   _____
       person.
13. Opened the sheet. Fanfolded it to the other side of   _____   _____   _____
    the bed.
14. Tucked the corners of a fitted sheet over the mattress _____   _____   _____
    at the top and then foot of the bed. For a flat sheet,
    tucked the top of the sheet under the mattress. The
    sheet was tight and smooth.
15. Made a mitered corner if using a flat sheet.   _____   _____   _____
16. Placed the cotton drawsheet or padded waterproof
    drawsheet on the bed. It was in the middle of the
    mattress.
    a. Opened the drawsheet. Fanfolded it to the other   _____   _____   _____
       side of the bed.
    b. Tucked the drawsheet under the mattress.   _____   _____   _____
17. Went to the other side of the bed.   _____   _____   _____
18. Mitered the top corner of the flat bottom sheet.   _____   _____   _____
19. Pulled the bottom sheet tight so there were no   _____   _____   _____
    wrinkles. Tucked in the sheet.
20. Pulled the drawsheets tight so that there were no   _____   _____   _____
    wrinkles. Tucked in the drawsheets.
21. *If using a waterproof under-pad:* Placed the waterproof _____   _____   _____
    pad on the bed. It was in the middle of the mattress.
22. Went to the other side of the bed.   _____   _____   _____
23. Put the top sheet on the bed.
    a. Unfolded it lengthwise. Placed the center crease   _____   _____   _____
       in the middle
    b. Placed the large hem even with the top of the   _____   _____   _____
       mattress.
    c. Opened the sheet. Fanfolded it to the other side. _____   _____   _____
    d. Faced hem-stitching outward, away from the   _____   _____   _____
       person.
    e. Did not tuck the bottom in yet.   _____   _____   _____
    f. Did not tuck top linens in on the sides.   _____   _____   _____
24. Placed the blanket on the bed.
    a. Unfolded it so that the center crease was in the   _____   _____   _____
       middle.
    b. Put the upper hem about 6 to 8 inches from the   _____   _____   _____
       top of the mattress.
    c. Opened the blanket. Fanfolded it to the other side. _____   _____   _____
    d. If steps 30 and 31 were not done, turned the top   _____   _____   _____
       sheet down over the blanket. Hem-stitching was
       down, away from the person.

Date of Satisfactory Completion _____   Instructor's Initials _____

Procedure—cont'd	S	U	Comments
25. Placed the bedspread on the bed.			
a. Unfolded it so that the center crease was in the middle.	_____	_____	_____
b. Placed the upper hem even with the top of the mattress.	_____	_____	_____
c. Opened and fanfolded the bedspread to the other side.	_____	_____	_____
d. Made sure the bedspread facing the door was even. It covered all top linens.	_____	_____	_____
26. Tucked in top linens together at the foot of the bed. They were smooth and tight. Made a mitered corner. Left the side of the top linens untucked.	_____	_____	_____
27. Went to the other side.	_____	_____	_____
28. Straightened all top linen. Worked from the head of the bed to the foot.	_____	_____	_____
29. Tucked in the top linens together at the foot of the bed. Made a mitered corner. Left the side of the top linens untucked.	_____	_____	_____
30. Turned the top hem of the bedspread under the blanket to make a cuff.	_____	_____	_____
31. Turned the top sheet down over the bedspread. Hem-stitching was down. (If steps 30 and 31 were not done, the bedspread covered the pillow and was tucked under the pillow.)	_____	_____	_____
32. Put the pillowcase on the pillow. Folded extra material under the pillow at the seam end of the pillowcase.	_____	_____	_____
33. Placed the pillow on the bed. The open end of the pillowcase was away from the door. The seam was toward the head of the bed.	_____	_____	_____
Post-Procedure			
34. Provided for comfort as noted on the inside of the front textbook cover. (Omitted this step if bed was prepared for a new patient or resident.)	_____	_____	_____
35. Attached the call light to the bed or placed it within the person's reach.	_____	_____	_____
36. Lowered the bed to a safe and comfortable level appropriate for the person. Followed the care plan. Locked the bed wheels.	_____	_____	_____
37. Put towels, washcloth, gown or pajamas, and bath blanket in the bedside stand.	_____	_____	_____
38. Completed a safety check of the room as noted on the inside of the front textbook cover.	_____	_____	_____
39. Followed agency policy for dirty linen.	_____	_____	_____
40. Practiced hand hygiene.	_____	_____	_____

Date of Satisfactory Completion _____   Instructor's Initials _____

Making an Occupied Bed

Name: _____ Date: _____

	S	U	Comments

Quality of Life
- Knocked before entering the person's room.
- Addressed the person by name.
- Introduced yourself by name and title.
- Explained the procedure to the person before starting and during the procedure.
- Protected the person's rights during the procedure.
- Handled the person gently during the procedure.

Pre-Procedure
1. Followed *Delegation Guidelines: Making Beds.* Reviewed *Promoting Safety and Comfort:*
   a. *Making Beds*
   b. *The Occupied Bed*
2. Practiced hand hygiene.
3. Collected the following.
   - Gloves
   - Laundry bag
   - Clean linen
   - Paper towels (if required as a barrier for clean linen)
4. Placed linen on a clean surface. Used paper towels as a barrier between the clean surface and clean linen if required by agency policy.
5. Identified the person. Checked the ID bracelet against the assignment sheet. Used 2 identifiers. Called the person by name.
6. Provided for privacy.
7. Removed the call light.
8. Raised the bed for body mechanics. Bed rails were up if used. Bed wheels were locked.
9. Lowered the head of the bed. It was as flat as possible.

Procedure
10. Practiced hand hygiene. Put on gloves.
11. Loosened top linens at the foot of the bed.
12. Lowered the bed rail near you if up.
13. Folded and removed the bedspread. Then removed the blanket. Placed each over the chair.
14. Covered the person with a bath blanket. Used the blanket in the bedside stand.
    a. Unfolded a bath blanket over the top sheet.
    b. Asked the person to hold on to the bath blanket. If the person could not, tucked the top part under the person's shoulders.
    c. Grasped the top sheet under the bath blanket at the shoulders. Brought the sheet down to the foot of the bed. Removed the sheet from under the blanket.
15. Positioned the person on the side of the bed away from you. Adjusted the pillow for comfort.

Date of Satisfactory Completion _____   Instructor's Initials _____

Procedure—cont'd	S	U	Comments
16. Loosened bottom linens from the head to the foot of the bed.	_____	_____	_____
17. Fanfolded bottom linens 1 at a time toward the person. Started with the item on top. (If reusing the mattress pad, did not fanfold it.)	_____	_____	_____
18. Removed and discarded the gloves. Practiced hand hygiene. Put on clean gloves.	_____	_____	_____
19. Placed a clean mattress pad on the bed. Unfolded it lengthwise. The center crease was in the middle. Fanfolded the top part toward the person. (If reusing the mattress pad, straightened and smoothed any wrinkles.)	_____	_____	_____
20. Placed the bottom sheet on the mattress pad. Hem-stitching was away from the person. Unfolded the sheet so that the crease was in the middle. The small hem was even with the bottom of the mattress. Fanfolded the top part toward the person.	_____	_____	_____
21. Tucked the corners of a fitted sheet over the mattress. If using a flat sheet, made a mitered corner at the head of the bed. Tucked the sheet under the mattress from the head to the foot.	_____	_____	_____
22. *If using a cotton drawsheet:*			
a. Placed the drawsheet on the bed. It was in the middle of the mattress.	_____	_____	_____
b. Opened the drawsheet.	_____	_____	_____
c. Fanfolded it toward the person.	_____	_____	_____
d. Tucked in excess fabric.	_____	_____	_____
23. *If using a waterproof pad:*			
a. Placed the waterproof pad on the bed. It was in the middle of the mattress.	_____	_____	_____
b. Fanfolded it toward the person.	_____	_____	_____
24. Explained to the person that he or she would roll over a bump. Assured the person that he or she would not fall.	_____	_____	_____
25. Helped the person turn to the other side. Adjusted the pillow for comfort.	_____	_____	_____
26. Raised the bed rail. Went to the other side and lowered the bed rail.	_____	_____	_____
27. Loosened bottom linens. Removed one piece at a time. Placed each piece in the laundry bag. Discarded disposable bed protectors and incontinence products in the trash. (Did not put them in the laundry bag.)	_____	_____	_____
28. Removed and discarded the gloves. Practiced hand hygiene.	_____	_____	_____
29. Straightened and smoothed the mattress pad.	_____	_____	_____
30. Pulled the clean bottom sheet toward you. Tucked the corners of a fitted sheet over the mattress. If using a flat sheet, made a mitered corner at the top. Tucked the sheet under the mattress from the head to the foot of the bed.	_____	_____	_____
31. Pulled the drawsheets tightly toward you. Tucked both under together or separately.	_____	_____	_____

Date of Satisfactory Completion _____   Instructor's Initials _____

Procedure—cont'd	S	U	Comments
32. Positioned the person supine in the center of the bed. Adjusted the pillow for comfort.	___	___	___
33. Put the top sheet on the bed. Unfolded it lengthwise. The crease was in the middle. The large hem was even with the top of the mattress. Hem-stitching was on the outside.	___	___	___
34. Asked the person to hold on to the top sheet so that you could remove the bath blanket or tucked the top sheet under the person's shoulders. Removed the bath blanket. Placed it in the laundry bag.	___	___	___
35. Placed the blanket on the bed. Unfolded it so that the crease was in the middle and it covered the person. The upper hem was 6 to 8 inches from the top of the mattress.	___	___	___
36. Placed the bedspread on the bed. Unfolded it so that the center crease was in the middle and it covered the person. The top hem was even with the mattress top.	___	___	___
37. Turned the top hem of the bedspread under the blanket to make a cuff.	___	___	___
38. Brought the top sheet down over the bedspread to form a cuff.	___	___	___
39. Went to the foot of the bed.	___	___	___
40. Made a 2-inch toe pleat across the foot of the bed. It was 6 to 8 inches from the foot of the bed.	___	___	___
41. Lifted the mattress corner with 1 arm. Tucked all top linens under the mattress. Made a mitered corner.	___	___	___
42. Raised the bed rail. Went to the other side and lowered the bed rail.	___	___	___
43. Straightened and smoothed top linens.	___	___	___
44. Tucked all top linens under the mattress. Made a mitered corner. Left the side of the top linens untucked.	___	___	___
45. Changed the pillowcase(s).	___	___	___
Post-Procedure			
46. Provided for comfort as noted on the inside of the front textbook cover.	___	___	___
47. Placed the call light within reach.	___	___	___
48. Lowered the bed to a safe and comfortable level appropriate for the person. Followed the care plan. Locked the bed wheels.	___	___	___
49. Raised or lowered bed rails. Followed the care plan.	___	___	___
50. Put the towels, washcloth, gown or pajamas, and bath blanket in the bedside stand.	___	___	___
51. Unscreened the person.	___	___	___
52. Completed a safety check of the room as noted on the inside of the front textbook cover.	___	___	___
53. Followed agency policy for dirty linen.	___	___	___
54. Practiced hand hygiene.	___	___	___

Date of Satisfactory Completion _____   Instructor's Initials _____

Making a Surgical Bed

Name: _____   Date: _____

	S	U	Comments
Pre-Procedure			
1. Followed *Delegation Guidelines: Making Beds.*	_____	_____	_____
Reviewed *Promoting Safety and Comfort:*	_____	_____	_____
a. *Making Beds*			
b. *The Surgical Bed*			
2. Practiced hand hygiene.	_____	_____	_____
3. Collected the following.			
• Clean linen as for procedure: *Making a Closed Bed*	_____	_____	_____
• Gloves	_____	_____	_____
• Laundry bag	_____	_____	_____
• Equipment requested by the nurse	_____	_____	_____
• Paper towels (if required as a barrier for clean linens)	_____	_____	_____
4. Placed linen on a clean surface. Used paper towels as a barrier between the clean surface and clean linen if required by agency policy.	_____	_____	_____
5. Removed the call light.	_____	_____	_____
6. Raised the bed for body mechanics.	_____	_____	_____
Procedure			
7. Removed all linen from the bed and placed in laundry bag. Wore gloves. Practiced hand hygiene after removing gloves and discarding them.	_____	_____	_____
8. Made a closed bed. (Reviewed procedure: *Making a Closed Bed.*) Did not tuck the top linens under the mattress.	_____	_____	_____
9. Folded all top linens at the foot of the bed back onto the bed. The fold was even with the edge of the mattress.	_____	_____	_____
10. Knew on which side of the bed the stretcher was placed. Fanfolded linen lengthwise to the other side of the bed.	_____	_____	_____
11. Put the pillowcase(s) on the pillow(s).	_____	_____	_____
12. Placed the pillow(s) on a clean surface.	_____	_____	_____
Post-Procedure			
13. Left the bed in its highest position.	_____	_____	_____
14. Left both bed rails down.	_____	_____	_____
15. Put the towels, washcloth, gown or pajamas, and bath blanket in the bedside stand.	_____	_____	_____
16. Moved furniture away from the bed. Allowed room for the stretcher and for the staff.	_____	_____	_____
17. Did not attach the call light to the bed.	_____	_____	_____
18. Completed a safety check of the room as noted on the inside of the front textbook cover.	_____	_____	_____
19. Followed agency policy for soiled linen.	_____	_____	_____
20. Practiced hand hygiene.	_____	_____	_____

Date of Satisfactory Completion _____   Instructor's Initials _____

Giving a Back Massage

Name:_____   Date:_____

	S	U	Comments

Quality of Life
- Knocked before entering the person's room.
- Addressed the person by name.
- Introduced yourself by name and title.
- Explained the procedure to the person before starting and during the procedure.
- Protected the person's rights during the procedure.
- Handled the person gently during the procedure.

Pre-Procedure
1. Followed *Delegation Guidelines: The Back Massage.* Reviewed *Promoting Safety and Comfort: The Back Massage.*
2. Practiced hand hygiene.
3. Identified the person. Checked the ID bracelet against the assignment sheet. Used 2 identifiers. Called the person by name.
4. Collected the following.
   - Bath blanket
   - Bath towel
   - Lotion
5. Provided for privacy.
6. Raised the bed for body mechanics. Bed rails were up if used.

Procedure
7. Lowered the bed rail near you if up.
8. Positioned the person in the prone or side-lying position with the back toward you.
9. Exposed the back, shoulders, upper arms. Covered the rest of the body with the bath blanket.
10. Laid the towel on the bed along the back (if the person was in a side-lying position).
11. Warmed the lotion.
12. Explained that the lotion may feel cool and wet.
13. Applied lotion to the lower back area.
14. Stroked up from the lower back to the shoulders. Then stroked down over the upper arms. Stroked up the upper arms, across the shoulders, and down the back using firm strokes. Kept your hands in contact with the person's skin.
15. Repeated step 14 for at least 3 minutes.
16. Kneaded the back.
    a. Grasped the skin between your thumb and fingers.
    b. Kneaded half of the back. Started at the buttocks and moved up to the shoulder. Then kneaded down from the shoulder to the lower back.
    c. Repeated on the other half of the back.

Date of Satisfactory Completion _____   Instructor's Initials _____

Procedure—cont'd	S	U	Comments
18. Flossed the person's teeth (optional).			
a. Broke off an 18-inch piece of floss from the dispenser.	_____	_____	_____
b. Held the floss between the middle fingers of each hand.	_____	_____	_____
c. Stretched the floss with your thumbs.	_____	_____	_____
d. Started at the upper back tooth on the right side. Worked around to the left side.	_____	_____	_____
e. Moved the floss gently up and down between the teeth. Moved floss up and down against the sides of each tooth. Worked from the top of the crown to the gum line.	_____	_____	_____
f. Moved to a new section of floss after every second tooth.	_____	_____	_____
g. Flossed the lower teeth. Used up and down motions as for the upper teeth. Started on the right side. Worked around to the left side.	_____	_____	_____
19. Let the person use mouthwash or other solution. Held the kidney basin under the chin.	_____	_____	_____
20. Wiped the person's mouth and removed the towel.	_____	_____	_____
21. Removed and discarded the gloves. Practiced hand hygiene.	_____	_____	_____
Post-Procedure			
22. Provided for comfort as noted on the inside of the front textbook cover.	_____	_____	_____
23. Placed the call light within reach.	_____	_____	_____
24. Lowered the bed to a safe and comfortable level appropriate for the person. Followed the care plan.	_____	_____	_____
25. Raised or lowered bed rails. Followed the care plan.	_____	_____	_____
26. Rinsed the toothbrush. Cleaned, rinsed, and dried equipment. Returned the toothbrush and equipment to their proper place. Wore gloves.	_____	_____	_____
27. Wiped off the over-bed table with the paper towels. Discarded the paper towels.	_____	_____	_____
28. Unscreened the person.	_____	_____	_____
29. Completed a safety check of the room as noted on the inside of the front textbook cover.	_____	_____	_____
30. Followed agency policy for dirty linen.	_____	_____	_____
31. Removed the gloves. Practiced hand hygiene.	_____	_____	_____
32. Reported and recorded your observations.	_____	_____	_____

Date of Satisfactory Completion _____   Instructor's Initials _____

Providing Mouth Care for the Unconscious Person

Name: _____   Date: _____

Quality of Life	S	U	Comments
• Knocked before entering the person's room.	_____	_____	_____
• Addressed the person by name.	_____	_____	_____
• Introduced yourself by name and title.	_____	_____	_____
• Explained the procedure to the person before starting and during the procedure.	_____	_____	_____
• Protected the person's rights during the procedure.	_____	_____	_____
• Handled the person gently during the procedure.	_____	_____	_____

Pre-Procedure

	S	U	Comments
1. Followed *Delegation Guidelines: Oral Hygiene.* Reviewed *Promoting Safety and Comfort:*	_____	_____	_____
a. *Oral Hygiene*			
b. *Hygiene Needs*			
c. *Mouth Care for the Unconscious Person*			
2. Practiced hand hygiene.	_____	_____	_____
3. Collected the following.			
• Cleaning agent according to the care plan	_____	_____	_____
• Sponge swabs	_____	_____	_____
• Plastic tongue depressor	_____	_____	_____
• Water cup with cool water	_____	_____	_____
• Hand towel	_____	_____	_____
• Kidney basin	_____	_____	_____
• Lip lubricant	_____	_____	_____
• Paper towels	_____	_____	_____
• Gloves	_____	_____	_____
4. Placed the paper towels on the over-bed table. Arranged items on top of them.	_____	_____	_____
5. Identified the person. Checked the ID bracelet against the assignment sheet. Used 2 identifiers. Called the person by name.	_____	_____	_____
6. Provided for privacy.	_____	_____	_____
7. Raised the bed for body mechanics. Bed rails were up if used.	_____	_____	_____

Procedure

	S	U	Comments
8. Lowered the bed rail near you if up.	_____	_____	_____
9. Positioned the person in a side-lying position near you. Turned the person's head well to the side.	_____	_____	_____
10. Placed the towel under the person's face.	_____	_____	_____
11. Put on the gloves.	_____	_____	_____
12. Placed the kidney basin under the chin.	_____	_____	_____
13. Separated the upper and lower teeth. Used the plastic tongue depressor. Was gentle. Never used force. Asked the nurse for help as needed.	_____	_____	_____
14. Moistened the sponge swabs with the cleaning agent. Squeezed out excess cleaning agent.	_____	_____	_____

Date of Satisfactory Completion _____   Instructor's Initials _____

Procedure—cont'd	S	U	Comments
15. Cleaned the mouth using sponge swabs moistened with the cleaning agent.			
a. Cleaned the chewing and inner surfaces of the teeth.	_____	_____	_____
b. Cleaned the gums and outer surfaces of the teeth.	_____	_____	_____
c. Swabbed the roof of the mouth, inside of the cheeks, and the lips.	_____	_____	_____
d. Swabbed the tongue.	_____	_____	_____
e. Moistened and squeezed out a clean swab with water. Swabbed the mouth to rinse.	_____	_____	_____
f. Placed used swabs in the kidney basin.	_____	_____	_____
16. Removed the kidney basin and supplies.	_____	_____	_____
17. Wiped the person's mouth. Removed the towel.	_____	_____	_____
18. Applied lubricant to the lips.	_____	_____	_____
19. Removed and discarded the gloves. Practiced hand hygiene.	_____	_____	_____
Post-Procedure			
20. Provided for comfort as noted on the inside of the front textbook cover.	_____	_____	_____
21. Placed the call light within reach.	_____	_____	_____
22. Lowered the bed to a safe and comfortable level appropriate for the person. Followed the care plan.	_____	_____	_____
23. Raised or lowered bed rails. Followed the care plan.	_____	_____	_____
24. Cleaned, rinsed, dried, and returned equipment to its proper place. Used clean, dry paper towels for drying. Discarded disposable items. (Wore gloves.)	_____	_____	_____
25. Wiped off the over-bed table with paper towels. Discarded the paper towels.	_____	_____	_____
26. Unscreened the person.	_____	_____	_____
27. Completed a safety check of the room as noted on the inside of the front textbook cover.	_____	_____	_____
28. Told the person that you were leaving the room. Told him or her when you would return.	_____	_____	_____
29. Followed agency policy for dirty linen.	_____	_____	_____
30. Removed the gloves. Practiced hand hygiene.	_____	_____	_____
31. Reported and recorded your observations.	_____	_____	_____

Date of Satisfactory Completion _____   Instructor's Initials _____

Post-Procedure—cont'd   S   U   Comments

35. Placed the call light within reach.   _____   _____   _____
36. Lowered the bed to a safe and comfortable level   _____   _____   _____
    appropriate for the person. Followed the care plan.
37. Raised or lowered bed rails. Followed the care plan.   _____   _____   _____
38. Removed the towel from the sink. Drained the sink.   _____   _____   _____
39. Rinsed the brushes. Emptied and rinsed the denture   _____   _____   _____
    cup. Cleaned, rinsed, and dried equipment. Used
    clean, dry paper towels for drying. Returned the
    brushes and equipment to their proper place.
    Discarded disposable items. Wore gloves for this
    step.
40. Wiped off the over-bed table with paper towels.   _____   _____   _____
    Discarded the paper towels.
41. Unscreened the person.   _____   _____   _____
42. Completed a safety check of the room as noted on   _____   _____   _____
    the inside of the front textbook cover.
43. Followed agency policy for dirty linen.   _____   _____   _____
44. Removed gloves. Practiced hand hygiene.   _____   _____   _____
45. Reported and recorded your observations.   _____   _____   _____

Date of Satisfactory Completion _____   Instructor's Initials _____

Giving a Complete Bed Bath

Name: _____   Date: _____

	S	U	Comments
Quality of Life			
• Knocked before entering the person's room.	_____	_____	_____
• Addressed the person by name.	_____	_____	_____
• Introduced yourself by name and title.	_____	_____	_____
• Explained the procedure to the person before starting and during the procedure.	_____	_____	_____
• Protected the person's rights during the procedure.	_____	_____	_____
• Handled the person gently during the procedure.	_____	_____	_____
Pre-Procedure			
1. Followed *Delegation Guidelines: Bathing.*	_____	_____	_____
Reviewed *Promoting Safety and Comfort:*	_____	_____	_____
a. *Hygiene Needs*			
b. *Bathing*			
2. Practiced hand hygiene.	_____	_____	_____
3. Identified the person. Checked the ID bracelet against the assignment sheet. Used 2 identifiers. Called the person by name.	_____	_____	_____
4. Collected clean linen for a closed bed. (See procedure: *Making a Closed Bed* in Chapter 17.) Placed linen on a clean surface.	_____	_____	_____
5. Collected the following.			
• Wash basin	_____	_____	_____
• Soap	_____	_____	_____
• Water thermometer	_____	_____	_____
• Orangewood stick or nail file	_____	_____	_____
• Washcloth (and at least four washcloths for perineal care)	_____	_____	_____
• Two bath towels and two hand towels	_____	_____	_____
• Bath blanket	_____	_____	_____
• Clothing or sleepwear	_____	_____	_____
• Lotion	_____	_____	_____
• Powder	_____	_____	_____
• Deodorant or antiperspirant	_____	_____	_____
• Brush and comb	_____	_____	_____
• Other grooming items as requested	_____	_____	_____
• Paper towels	_____	_____	_____
• Gloves	_____	_____	_____
6. Covered the over-bed table with paper towels. Arranged items on the over-bed table. Adjusted the height as needed.	_____	_____	_____
7. Provided for privacy.	_____	_____	_____
8. Raised the bed for body mechanics. Bed rails were up if used.	_____	_____	_____
Procedure			
9. Practiced hand hygiene. Put on gloves.	_____	_____	_____
10. Removed the sleepwear. Did not expose the person. Followed agency policy for dirty sleepwear.	_____	_____	_____
11. Covered the person with a bath blanket. Removed top linens. (See procedure: *Making an Occupied Bed* in Chapter 17.)	_____	_____	_____

Date of Satisfactory Completion _____   Instructor's Initials _____

Procedure—cont'd

	S	U	Comments
12. Lowered the head of the bed. It was as flat as possible. The person had at least one pillow.	____	____	_____
13. Filled the wash basin two-thirds full with water. Raised the bed rail before leaving the bedside. Followed the care plan for water temperature. Water temperature was 110° F to 115° F [43.3° C to 46.1° C] for adults or as directed by the nurse. Measured water temperature. Used a bath thermometer or tested the water by dipping your elbow or inner wrist into the basin.	____	____	_____
14. Lowered the bed rail near you if up.	____	____	_____
15. Asked the person to check the water temperature. Adjusted temperature if too hot or too cold. Raised the bed rail before leaving the bedside. Lowered it when you returned.	____	____	_____
16. Placed the basin on the over-bed table.	____	____	_____
17. Placed a hand towel over the person's chest.	____	____	_____
18. Made a mitt with the washcloth. Used a mitt for the entire bath.	____	____	_____
19. Washed around the person's eyes with water. Did not use soap.			
a. Cleaned the far eye. Gently wiped from the inner to the outer aspect of the eye with a corner of the mitt.	____	____	_____
b. Cleaned around the near eye. Used a clean part of the washcloth for each stroke.	____	____	_____
20. Asked the person if you should use soap to wash the face.	____	____	_____
21. Washed the face, ears, and neck. Rinsed and patted dry with the towel on the chest.	____	____	_____
22. Helped the person move to the side of the bed near you.	____	____	_____
23. Exposed the far arm. Placed a bath towel lengthwise under the arm. Applied soap to the washcloth.	____	____	_____
24. Supported the arm with your palm under the person's elbow. The person's forearm rested on your forearm.	____	____	_____
25. Washed the arm, shoulder, and underarm. Used long, firm strokes. Rinsed and patted dry.	____	____	_____
26. Placed the basin on the towel. Put the person's hand into the water. Washed it well. Cleaned under the fingernails with an orangewood stick or nail file.	____	____	_____
27. Had the person exercise the hand and fingers.	____	____	_____
28. Removed the basin. Dried the hand well. Covered the arm with the bath blanket.	____	____	_____
29. Repeated steps 23 to 28 for the near arm.	____	____	_____
30. Placed a bath towel over the chest cross-wise. Held the towel in place. Pulled the bath blanket from under the towel to the waist. Applied soap to the washcloth.	____	____	_____
31. Lifted the towel slightly and washed the chest. Did not expose the person. Rinsed and patted dry, especially under breasts.	____	____	_____
32. Moved the towel lengthwise over the chest and abdomen. Did not expose the person. Pulled the bath blanket down to the pubic area. Applied soap to the washcloth.	____	____	_____

Date of Satisfactory Completion _____   Instructor's Initials _____

Procedure—cont'd	S	U	Comments
33. Lifted the towel slightly and washed the abdomen. Rinsed and patted dry.	_____	_____	_____
34. Pulled the bath blanket up to the shoulders, covering both arms. Removed the towel.	_____	_____	_____
35. Changed soapy or cool water. Measured bath water temperature as in step 13. If bed rails were used, raised the bed rail near you before leaving the bedside. Lowered it when you returned.	_____	_____	_____
36. Uncovered the far leg. Did not expose the genital area. Placed a towel lengthwise under the foot and leg. Applied soap to the washcloth.	_____	_____	_____
37. Bent the knee and supported the leg with your arm. Washed it with long, firm strokes. Rinsed and patted dry.	_____	_____	_____
38. Placed the basin on the towel near the foot.	_____	_____	_____
39. Lifted the leg slightly. Slid the basin under the foot.	_____	_____	_____
40. Placed the foot in the basin. Used an orangewood stick or nail file to clean under toenails if necessary. If the person could not bend the knees:			
a. Washed the foot. Carefully separated the toes. Rinsed and patted dry.	_____	_____	_____
b. Cleaned under the toenails with an orangewood stick or nail file if necessary.	_____	_____	_____
41. Removed the basin. Dried the leg and foot. Applied lotion to the foot if directed by the nurse and the care plan. Covered the leg with the bath blanket. Removed the towel.	_____	_____	_____
42. Repeated steps 36 to 41 for the near leg.	_____	_____	_____
43. Changed the water. Measured water temperature as in step 13. If bed rails were used, raised the bed rail near you before leaving the bedside. Lowered it when you returned.	_____	_____	_____
44. Turned the person onto the side away from you. The person was covered with the bath blanket.	_____	_____	_____
45. Uncovered the back and buttocks. Did not expose the person. Placed a towel lengthwise on the bed along the back. Applied soap to the washcloth.	_____	_____	_____
46. Washed the back. Worked from the back of the neck to the lower end of the buttocks. Used long, firm, continuous strokes. Rinsed and dried well.	_____	_____	_____
47. Turned the person onto his or her back.	_____	_____	_____
48. Changed water for perineal care. Saw step 14 in procedure: *Giving Female Perineal Care* for water temperature. (Some state competency tests also require changing gloves and hand hygiene at this time.) Raised the bed rail near you before leaving the bedside. Lowered it when you returned.	_____	_____	_____
49. Allowed the person to perform perineal care if able. Provided perineal care if the person cannot do so. At least four washcloths were used. (Practiced hand hygiene and wore gloves for perineal care.)	_____	_____	_____
50. Removed and discarded gloves. Practiced hand hygiene.	_____	_____	_____

Date of Satisfactory Completion _____   Instructor's Initials _____

Procedure—cont'd	S	U	Comments
51. Gave a back massage.			
52. Applied lotion, powder, and deodorant or antiperspirant as requested.			
53. Put clean garments on the person.			
54. Combed and brushed the hair.			
55. Made the bed.			
Post-Procedure			
56. Provided for comfort as noted on the inside of the front textbook cover.			
57. Placed the call light within reach.			
58. Lowered the bed to a safe and comfortable level appropriate for the person. Followed the care plan.			
59. Raised or lowered bed rails. Followed the care plan.			
60. Put on clean gloves.			
61. Emptied, cleaned, rinsed, and dried the wash basin. Used clean, dry paper towels for drying. Returned it and other supplies to their proper place.			
62. Wiped off the over-bed table with paper towels. Discarded the paper towels.			
63. Unscreened the person.			
64. Completed a safety check of the room as noted on the inside of the front textbook cover.			
65. Followed agency policy for dirty linen.			
66. Removed and discarded gloves. Practiced hand hygiene.			
67. Reported and recorded your observations.			

Date of Satisfactory Completion _____   Instructor's Initials _____

Assisting with the Partial Bath

Name: _____   Date: _____

Quality of Life	S	U	Comments
• Knocked before entering the person's room.	_____	_____	_____
• Addressed the person by name.	_____	_____	_____
• Introduced yourself by name and title.	_____	_____	_____
• Explained the procedure to the person before starting and during the procedure.	_____	_____	_____
• Protected the person's rights during the procedure.	_____	_____	_____
• Handled the person gently during the procedure.	_____	_____	_____

Pre-Procedure

	S	U	Comments
1. Followed *Delegation Guidelines: Bathing.* Reviewed *Promoting Safety and Comfort:*	_____	_____	_____
a. *Hygiene Needs*			
b. *Bathing*			
2. Followed steps 2 through 7 in procedure: *Giving a Complete Bed Bath.*	_____	_____	_____

Procedure

	S	U	Comments
3. Made sure the bed was in the lowest position.	_____	_____	_____
4. Practiced hand hygiene. Put on gloves.	_____	_____	_____
5. Covered the person with a bath blanket. Removed top linens.	_____	_____	_____
6. Filled the wash basin two-thirds full with water. (Water temperature was 110°F to 115°F [43.3°C to 46.1°C] or as directed by the nurse.) Measured water temperature with the bath thermometer or tested bath water by dipping your elbow or inner wrist into the basin.	_____	_____	_____
7. Asked the person to check the water temperature. Adjusted temperature if too hot or too cold.	_____	_____	_____
8. Placed the basin on the over-bed table.	_____	_____	_____
9. Positioned the person in Fowler's position or assisted the person to sit at the bedside.	_____	_____	_____
10. Adjusted the over-bed table so that the person could reach the basin and supplies.	_____	_____	_____
11. Helped the person undress. Provided for privacy and warmth with the bath blanket.	_____	_____	_____
12. Asked the person to wash easy to reach body parts. Explained that you would wash the back and areas the person could not reach.	_____	_____	_____
13. Placed the call light within reach. Asked the person to signal when help was needed or bathing was complete.	_____	_____	_____
14. Removed and discarded the gloves. Practiced hand hygiene. Then left the room.	_____	_____	_____
15. Returned when the call light was on. Knocked before entering. Practiced hand hygiene.	_____	_____	_____
16. Changed the bath water. Measured bath water temperature as in step 6.	_____	_____	_____
17. Raised the bed for body mechanics. The far bed rail was up if used.	_____	_____	_____

Date of Satisfactory Completion _____   Instructor's Initials _____

Procedure—cont'd

	S	U	Comments
18. Asked what was washed. Put on gloves. Washed and dried areas the person could not reach. Made sure that the face, hands, underarms, back, buttocks, and perineal area were washed.			
19. Removed the gloves. Practiced hand hygiene.			
20. Gave a back massage.			
21. Applied lotion, powder, and deodorant or antiperspirant as requested.			
22. Helped the person put on clean garments.			
23. Assisted with hair care and other grooming needs.			
24. Made the bed.			

Post-Procedure

	S	U	Comments
25. Provided for comfort as noted on the inside of the front textbook cover.			
26. Placed the call light within reach.			
27. Lowered the bed to a safe and comfortable level appropriate for the person. Followed the care plan.			
28. Raised or lowered bed rails. Followed the care plan.			
29. Put on clean gloves.			
30. Emptied, cleaned, and dried the bath basin. Used clean, dry paper towels for drying. Returned the basin and supplies to their proper place.			
31. Wiped off the over-bed table with the paper towels. Discarded the paper towels.			
32. Unscreened the person.			
33. Completed a safety check of the room as noted on the inside of the front textbook cover.			
34. Followed agency policy for dirty linen.			
35. Removed the gloves. Practiced hand hygiene.			
36. Reported and recorded your observations.			

Date of Satisfactory Completion _____   Instructor's Initials _____

Assisting with a Tub Bath or Shower

Name: _____   Date: _____

	S	U	Comments
Quality of Life			
• Knocked before entering the person's room.	_____	_____	_____
• Addressed the person by name.	_____	_____	_____
• Introduced yourself by name and title.	_____	_____	_____
• Explained the procedure to the person before starting and during the procedure.	_____	_____	_____
• Protected the person's rights during the procedure.	_____	_____	_____
• Handled the person gently during the procedure.	_____	_____	_____

Pre-Procedure

1. Followed *Delegation Guidelines:*
   a. *Bathing*
   b. *Tub Baths and Showers*
   Reviewed *Promoting Safety and Comfort:*
   a. *Hygiene Needs*
   b. *Bathing*
   c. *Tub Baths and Showers*
2. Reserved the bathtub or shower.
3. Practiced hand hygiene.
4. Identified the person. Checked the ID bracelet against the assignment sheet. Used 2 identifiers. Called the person by name.
5. Collected the following.
   • Washcloth and two bath towels
   • Soap
   • Water thermometer (for a tub bath)
   • Clothing or sleepwear
   • Grooming items as requested
   • Robe and non-skid footwear
   • Rubber bath mat if needed
   • Disposable bath mat
   • Gloves
   • Wheelchair, shower chair, and so on as needed

Procedure

6. Placed items in the tub or shower room. Used the space provided or a chair.
7. Cleaned, disinfected, and dried the tub or shower.
8. Placed a rubber bath mat in the tub or on the shower floor. Did not block the drain.
9. Placed the disposable bath mat on the floor in front of the tub or shower.
10. Put the occupied sign on the door.
11. Returned to the person's room. Provided for privacy. Practiced hand hygiene.
12. Helped the person sit on the side of the bed.
13. Helped the person put on a robe and non-skid footwear. (Or the person left clothing on.)
14. Assisted or transported the person to the tub or shower room.

Date of Satisfactory Completion _____   Instructor's Initials _____

Procedure—cont'd

	S	U	Comments
15. Had the person sit on a chair if he or she walked to the tub or shower room.	_____	_____	_____
16. Provided for privacy.	_____	_____	_____
17. *For a tub bath:*			
a. Filled the tub halfway with warm water (105°F; 40.5°C). Followed the care plan for water temperature.	_____	_____	_____
b. Measured water temperature with the bath thermometer or checked the digital display.	_____	_____	_____
c. Asked the person to check the water temperature. Adjusted temperature if it was too hot or too cold.	_____	_____	_____
18. *For a shower:*			
a. Turned on the shower.	_____	_____	_____
b. Adjusted water temperature and pressure. Checked the digital display. Water temperature was 105°F/40.5°C.	_____	_____	_____
c. Asked the person to check the water temperature. Adjusted water temperature if it was too hot or too cold.	_____	_____	_____
19. Helped the person undress and remove footwear.	_____	_____	_____
20. Helped the person into the tub or shower. Positioned the shower chair and locked the wheels.	_____	_____	_____
21. Assisted with washing if necessary. Wore gloves.	_____	_____	_____
22. Asked the person to use the call light when done or when help was needed. Reminded the person that a tub bath lasts no longer than 20 minutes.	_____	_____	_____
23. Placed a towel across the chair.	_____	_____	_____
24. Left the room if the person could bathe alone. If not, stayed in the room or nearby. Removed the gloves and practiced hand hygiene if you left the room.	_____	_____	_____
25. Checked the person at least every 5 minutes.	_____	_____	_____
26. Returned when the person signaled. Knocked before entering. Practiced hand hygiene.	_____	_____	_____
27. Turned off the shower or drained the tub. Covered the person while the tub drained.	_____	_____	_____
28. Helped the person out of the shower or tub and onto the chair.	_____	_____	_____
29. Helped the person dry off. Patted gently. Dried under breasts, between skin folds, in the perineal area, and between the toes.	_____	_____	_____
30. Assisted with lotion and other grooming items as needed.	_____	_____	_____
31. Helped the person dress and put on footwear.	_____	_____	_____
32. Helped the person return to the room. Provided for privacy.	_____	_____	_____
33. Assisted the person to a chair or into bed.	_____	_____	_____
34. Provided a back massage if the person returned to bed.	_____	_____	_____
35. Assisted with hair care and other grooming needs.	_____	_____	_____

Post-Procedure

	S	U	Comments
36. Provided for comfort as noted on the inside of the front textbook cover.	_____	_____	_____
37. Placed the call light within reach.	_____	_____	_____

Date of Satisfactory Completion _____   Instructor's Initials _____

Post-Procedure—cont'd	**S**	**U**	**Comments**
38. Raised or lowered bed rails. Followed the care plan.	_____	_____	_____
39. Unscreened the person.	_____	_____	_____
40. Completed a safety check of the room as noted on the inside of the front textbook cover.	_____	_____	_____
41. Cleaned, disinfected, and dried the tub or shower. Dried the tub or shower room floor. Removed soiled linen. Wore gloves.	_____	_____	_____
42. Discarded disposable items. Put the unoccupied sign on the door. Returned supplies to their proper place.	_____	_____	_____
43. Followed agency policy for dirty linen.	_____	_____	_____
44. Removed the gloves. Practiced hand hygiene.	_____	_____	_____
45. Reported and recorded your observations.	_____	_____	_____

Date of Satisfactory Completion _____   Instructor's Initials _____

Giving Female Perineal Care

Name: _____   Date: _____

Quality of Life	S	U	Comments

Quality of Life
- Knocked before entering the person's room.
- Addressed the person by name.
- Introduced yourself by name and title.
- Explained the procedure to the person before starting and during the procedure.
- Protected the person's rights during the procedure.
- Handled the person gently during the procedure.

Pre-Procedure
1. Followed *Delegation Guidelines: Perineal Care.*
   Reviewed *Promoting Safety and Comfort:*
   a. *Hygiene Needs*
   b. *Perineal Care*
2. Practiced hand hygiene.
3. Collected the following.
   - Soap or other cleaning agent as directed
   - At least four washcloths
   - Bath towel
   - Bath blanket
   - Water thermometer
   - Wash basin
   - Waterproof under-pad
   - Gloves
   - Laundry bag
   - Paper towels
4. Covered the over-bed table with paper towels. Arranged items on top of them.
5. Identified the person. Checked the ID bracelet against the assignment sheet. Used 2 identifiers. Called the person by name.
6. Provided for privacy.
7. Raised the bed for body mechanics. Bed rails were up if used.

Procedure
8. Lowered the bed rail near you if up.
9. Practiced hand hygiene. Put on gloves.
10. Covered the person with a bath blanket. Moved top linens to the foot of the bed.
11. Positioned the person on the back.
12. Draped the person.
13. Raised the bed rail if used.
14. Filled the wash basin. Followed the care plan for water temperature. Water temperature is usually 105°F to 109°F [40.5°C to 42.7°C]. Measured water temperature according to agency policy.
15. Asked the person to check the water temperature. Adjusted water temperature if too hot or too cold. Raised the bed rail before leaving the bedside. Lowered it when you returned.
16. Placed the basin on the over-bed table.
17. Lowered the bed rail if up.

Date of Satisfactory Completion _____   Instructor's Initials _____

Procedure—cont'd	S	U	Comments

Procedure—cont'd

18. Helped the person flex her knees and spread her legs. Or helped her spread her legs as much as possible with the knees straight.

19. Folded the corner of the bath blanket between her legs onto her abdomen.

20. Placed a waterproof pad under her buttocks. Removed any wet or soiled incontinence products.

21. Removed and discarded the gloves. Practiced hand hygiene. Put on clean gloves.

22. Wet the washcloths.

23. Squeezed out excess water from the washcloth. Made a mitted washcloth. Applied soap. Squeezed out water every time you changed washcloths. Did not place used washcloths back in the basin. Put used washcloths in the laundry bag.

24. Cleaned the perineum. Changed washcloths as needed.
    a. Separated the labia.
    b. Cleaned 1 side of the labia. Cleaned downward from front to back (top to bottom) with 1 stroke. Used 1 part of a washcloth.
    c. Cleaned the other side of the labia. Cleaned downward from front to back (top to bottom) with 1 stroke. Used a clean part of a washcloth.
    d. Cleaned the vaginal area. Cleaned downward from front to back (top to bottom) with 1 stroke. Used a clean part of a washcloth.

25. Rinsed the perineum with a clean washcloth. Changed washcloths as needed.
    a. Separated the labia.
    b. Rinsed 1 side of the labia. Rinsed downward from front to back (top to bottom) with 1 stroke. Used 1 part of a washcloth.
    c. Rinsed the other side of the labia. Rinsed downward from front to back (top to bottom) with 1 stroke. Used a clean part of a washcloth.
    d. Rinsed the vaginal area. Rinsed downward from front to back (top to bottom) with 1 stroke. Used a clean part of a washcloth.

26. Patted the area dry with the towel. Dried from front to back. (top to bottom)

27. Folded the blanket back between her legs.

28. Helped the person lower her legs and turn onto her side away from you.

29. Applied soap to a mitted washcloth.

30. Cleaned and rinsed the rectal area.
    a. Cleaned from the vagina to the anus with 1 stroke. Used 1 part of the washcloth.
    b. Repeated steps 29 and 30-a until the area was clean. Used a clean part of the washcloth for each stroke. Changed washcloths as needed.
    c. Rinsed the rectal area with a clean washcloth. Rinsed from the vagina to the anus. Repeated as necessary. Used a clean part of the washcloth for each stroke. Changed washcloths as needed.

Date of Satisfactory Completion _____   Instructor's Initials _____

Procedure—cont'd

	S	U	Comments
31. Patted the area dry with the towel. Dried from front to back.	_____	_____	_____
32. Removed the waterproof under-pad.	_____	_____	_____
33. Removed and discarded the gloves. Practiced hand hygiene. Put on clean gloves.	_____	_____	_____
34. Provided clean and dry linens and incontinence products as needed.	_____	_____	_____
35. Positioned the person on her back.	_____	_____	_____

Post-Procedure

	S	U	Comments
36. Covered the person. Removed the bath blanket.	_____	_____	_____
37. Provided for comfort as noted on the inside of the front textbook cover.	_____	_____	_____
38. Placed the call light and other needed items within reach.	_____	_____	_____
39. Lowered the bed to a safe and comfortable level appropriate for the person. Followed the care plan.	_____	_____	_____
40. Raised or lowered bed rails. Followed the care plan.	_____	_____	_____
41. Emptied, cleaned, rinsed, and dried the wash basin. Used a clean dry paper towel for drying.	_____	_____	_____
42. Returned the basin and supplies to their proper place.	_____	_____	_____
43. Wiped off the over-bed table with the paper towels. Discarded the paper towels.	_____	_____	_____
44. Unscreened the person.	_____	_____	_____
45. Completed a safety check of the room as noted on the inside of the front textbook cover.	_____	_____	_____
46. Followed agency policy for dirty linen.	_____	_____	_____
47. Removed and discarded the gloves. Practiced hand hygiene.	_____	_____	_____
48. Reported and recorded your observations.	_____	_____	_____

Date of Satisfactory Completion _____   Instructor's Initials _____

Giving Male Perineal Care

Name: _____   Date: _____

Quality of Life	S	U	Comments

Quality of Life
- Knocked before entering the person's room.
- Addressed the person by name.
- Introduced yourself by name and title.
- Explained the procedure to the person before starting and during the procedure.
- Protected the person's rights during the procedure.
- Handled the person gently during the procedure.

Procedure
1. Followed steps 1 through 17 in procedure: *Giving Female Perineal Care.* Draped the person.
2. Folded the corner of the bath blanket between the legs onto his abdomen.
3. Placed a waterproof pad under his buttocks. Removed any wet or soiled incontinence products.
4. Removed and discarded the gloves. Practiced hand hygiene. Put on clean gloves.
5. Wet the washcloths.
6. Squeezed out water from a washcloth. Made a mitted washcloth. Applied soap. Squeezed out water every time you changed washcloths. Did not place used washcloths back in the basin. Put used washcloths in the laundry bag.
7. Retracted the foreskin if the person was uncircumcised.
8. Grasped the penis.
9. Cleaned the tip. Used a circular motion. Started at the meatus of the urethra and worked outward. Repeated as needed. Used a clean part of the washcloth each time.
10. Rinsed the area with another washcloth. Used the same circular motion.
11. Returned the foreskin to its natural position immediately after rinsing.
12. Cleaned the shaft of the penis. Used firm downward strokes. Used a clean part of a washcloth for each stroke.
13. Rinsed the shaft. Used the same downward motion. Used a clean part of a washcloth for each stroke.
14. Helped the person flex his knees and spread his legs. Or helped him spread his legs as much as possible with his knees straight.
15. Cleaned the scrotum. Used a clean part of a washcloth.
16. Rinsed the scrotum. Rinsed well. Used a clean part of a washcloth. Observed for redness and irritation in the skin folds.
17. Patted dry the penis and scrotum with the towel.
18. Folded the bath blanket back between his legs.

Date of Satisfactory Completion _____   Instructor's Initials _____

Procedure—cont'd

	S	U	Comments
19. Helped him lower his legs and turn onto his side away from you.	_____	_____	_____
20. Cleaned the rectal area. Cleaned from the scrotum (front to top) to the anus (back to bottom). (See procedure: *Giving Female Perineal Care.*) Rinsed and dried well.	_____	_____	_____
21. Removed the waterproof pad.	_____	_____	_____
22. Removed and discarded the gloves. Practiced hand hygiene. Put on clean gloves.	_____	_____	_____
23. Provided clean and dry linens and incontinence products.	_____	_____	_____
24. Positioned the person on his back	_____	_____	_____
25. Followed steps 36 through 48 in procedure: *Giving Female Perineal Care.*	_____	_____	_____

Date of Satisfactory Completion _____   Instructor's Initials _____

Brushing and Combing Hair

Name: _____   Date: _____

Quality of Life	S	U	Comments
• Knocked before entering the person's room.	___	___	___
• Addressed the person by name.	___	___	___
• Introduced yourself by name and title.	___	___	___
• Explained the procedure to the person before starting and during the procedure.	___	___	___
• Protected the person's rights during the procedure.	___	___	___
• Handled the person gently during the procedure.	___	___	___

Pre-Procedure

	S	U	Comments
1. Followed *Delegation Guidelines: Brushing and Combing Hair.*	___	___	___
Reviewed *Promoting Safety and Comfort: Brushing and Combing Hair.*	___	___	___
2. Practiced hand hygiene.	___	___	___
3. Identified the person. Checked the ID bracelet against the assignment sheet. Used 2 identifiers. Called the person by name.	___	___	___
4. Asked the person how to style hair.	___	___	___
5. Collected the following.			
• Comb and brush	___	___	___
• Bath towel	___	___	___
• Other hair care items as requested	___	___	___
6. Arranged items on the bedside stand.	___	___	___
7. Provided for privacy.	___	___	___

Procedure

	S	U	Comments
8. Lowered the bed rail if up.	___	___	___
9. Position the person.			
a. *In a chair*—Helped the person to the chair. The person put on a robe and non-skid footwear when up.	___	___	___
b. *In bed*—Raised the bed for body mechanics. Bed rails are up if used. Lowered the bed rail near you. Assisted the person to a semi-Fowler's position if allowed.	___	___	___
10. Placed a towel across the person's back and shoulders or across the pillow.	___	___	___
11. Asked the person to remove eyeglasses. Put them in the eyeglass case. Put the case inside the bedside stand.	___	___	___
12. Brushed and combed hair that was not matted or tangled.			
a. Used the comb to part the hair.	___	___	___
(1) Parted hair down the middle into two sides.	___	___	___
(2) Divided one side into two smaller sections.	___	___	___
b. Brushed one of the small sections of hair. Started at the scalp and brushed toward the hair ends. Did the same for the other small sections of hair.	___	___	___
c. Repeated steps 12, a(2) and b for the other side.	___	___	___
13. Brushed and combed matted or tangled hair.			
a. Took a small section of hair near the ends.	___	___	___
b. Combed or brushed through to the hair ends.	___	___	___

Date of Satisfactory Completion _____   Instructor's Initials _____

Procedure—cont'd	S	U	Comments

   c. Added small sections of hair as you worked up to the scalp.

   d. Combed or brushed through each longer section to the hair ends.

14. Styled the hair as the person preferred.
15. Removed the towel.
16. Let the person put on the eyeglasses.

Post-Procedure

17. Provided for comfort as noted on the inside of the front textbook cover.
18. Placed the call light within reach.
19. Lowered the bed to a safe and comfortable level appropriate for the person. Followed the care plan.
20. Raised or lowered bed rails. Followed the care plan.
21. Removed hair from the brush or comb. Cleaned rinsed, dried, and returned hair care items to their proper place. Used clean, dry paper towels for drying. Wore gloves for this step. Removed and discarded the gloves. Practiced hand hygiene.
22. Unscreened the person.
23. Completed a safety check of the room as noted on the inside of the front textbook cover.
24. Followed agency policy for dirty linen.
25. Practiced hand hygiene.

Date of Satisfactory Completion _____ Instructor's Initials _____

Shampooing the Person's Hair

Name: _____   Date: _____

Quality of Life	S	U	Comments
• Knocked before entering the person's room.	_____	_____	_____
• Addressed the person by name.	_____	_____	_____
• Introduced yourself by name and title.	_____	_____	_____
• Explained the procedure to the person before starting and during the procedure.	_____	_____	_____
• Protected the person's rights during the procedure.	_____	_____	_____
• Handled the person gently during the procedure.	_____	_____	_____

Pre-Procedure

	S	U	Comments
1. Followed *Delegation Guidelines: Shampooing.*	_____	_____	_____
Reviewed *Promoting Safety and Comfort: Shampooing.*	_____	_____	_____
2. Practiced hand hygiene.	_____	_____	_____
3. Collected the following.			
• Two bath towels	_____	_____	_____
• Washcloth	_____	_____	_____
• Shampoo	_____	_____	_____
• Hair conditioner (if requested)	_____	_____	_____
• Water thermometer	_____	_____	_____
• Pitcher or hand-held nozzle (if needed)	_____	_____	_____
• Shampoo tray (if needed)	_____	_____	_____
• Basin or pan (if needed)	_____	_____	_____
• Waterproof pad (if needed)	_____	_____	_____
• Gloves (if needed)	_____	_____	_____
• Comb and brush	_____	_____	_____
• Hair dryer	_____	_____	_____
4. Arranged items nearby.	_____	_____	_____
5. Identified the person. Checked the ID bracelet against the assignment sheet. Used 2 identifiers. Called the person by name.	_____	_____	_____
6. Provided for privacy.	_____	_____	_____
7. Raised the bed for body mechanics for a shampoo in bed. Bed rails were up if used.	_____	_____	_____
8. Practiced hand hygiene.	_____	_____	_____

Procedure

	S	U	Comments
9. Lowered the bed rail near you if up.	_____	_____	_____
10. Covered the person's chest with a bath towel.	_____	_____	_____
11. Brushed and combed the hair to remove snarls and tangles.	_____	_____	_____
12. Positioned the person for the method used. To shampoo the person in bed:			
a. Lowered the head of the bed and removed the pillow.	_____	_____	_____
b. Placed the waterproof pad and shampoo tray under the head and shoulders.	_____	_____	_____
c. Supported the head and neck with a folded towel if necessary.	_____	_____	_____
13. Raised the bed rail if used.	_____	_____	_____

Date of Satisfactory Completion _____   Instructor's Initials _____

Procedure—cont'd   S   U   Comments

14. Obtained water. Water temperature was 105°F (40.5°C). Tested water temperature according to agency policy. Asked the person to check the water temperature. Adjusted water temperature as needed. Raised the bed rail before leaving the bedside.

15. Lowered the bed rail near you if up.

16. Put on gloves (if needed).

17. Asked the person to hold a washcloth over the eyes. It did not cover the nose and mouth. (Some agencies require a dry washcloth.)

18. Used the pitcher or nozzle to wet the hair.

19. Applied a small amount of shampoo.

20. Worked up a lather with both hands. Started at the hairline. Worked toward the back of the head.

21. Massaged the scalp with your fingertips. Did not scratch the scalp.

22. Rinsed the hair until the water ran clear.

23. Repeated steps 19 through 22.

24. Applied conditioner. Followed directions on the container.

25. Squeezed water from the person's hair.

26. Covered the hair with a bath towel.

27. Removed the shampoo tray, basin, and waterproof pad.

28. Dried the person's face with the towel. Used the towel on the person's chest.

29. Helped the person raise the head if appropriate. For the person in bed, raised the head of the bed.

30. Rubbed the hair and scalp with the towel. Used the second towel if the first was wet.

31. Combed the hair to remove snarls and tangles.

32. Dried and styled hair as quickly as possible.

33. Removed and discarded the gloves (if used). Practiced hand hygiene.

Post-Procedure

34. Provided for comfort as noted on the inside of the front textbook cover.

35. Placed the call light within reach.

36. Lowered the bed to a safe and comfortable level appropriate for the person. Followed the care plan.

37. Raised or lowered bed rails. Followed the care plan.

38. Unscreened the person.

39. Completed a safety check of the room as noted on the inside of the front textbook cover.

40. Cleaned, rinsed, dried, and returned equipment to its proper place. Cleaned the brush and comb. Used clean, dry paper towels for drying. Wore gloves for this step. Discarded disposable items. Removed and discarded gloves.

41. Followed agency policy for dirty linen.

42. Practiced hand hygiene.

43. Reported and recorded your observations.

Date of Satisfactory Completion _____   Instructor's Initials _____

Shaving the Person's Face with a Safety Razor

Name: _____   Date: _____

Quality of Life	S	U	Comments
• Knocked before entering the person's room.	___	___	_____
• Addressed the person by name.	___	___	_____
• Introduced yourself by name and title.	___	___	_____
• Explained the procedure to the person before starting and during the procedure.	___	___	_____
• Protected the person's rights during the procedure.	___	___	_____
• Handled the person gently during the procedure.	___	___	_____

Pre-Procedure

	S	U	Comments
1. Followed *Delegation Guidelines: Shaving.* Reviewed *Promoting Safety and Comfort: Shaving.*	___	___	_____
2. Practiced hand hygiene.	___	___	_____
3. Collected the following.			
• Wash basin	___	___	_____
• Bath towel	___	___	_____
• Hand towel	___	___	_____
• Washcloth	___	___	_____
• Safety razor	___	___	_____
• Mirror	___	___	_____
• Shaving cream, soap, or lotion	___	___	_____
• Shaving brush	___	___	_____
• Aftershave or lotion	___	___	_____
• Tissues or paper towels	___	___	_____
• Paper towels	___	___	_____
• Gloves	___	___	_____
4. Arranged paper towels and supplies on the over-bed table.	___	___	_____
5. Identified the person. Checked the ID bracelet against the assignment sheet. Called the person by name.	___	___	_____
6. Provided for privacy.	___	___	_____
7. Raised the bed for body mechanics. Bed rails were up if used.	___	___	_____

Procedure

	S	U	Comments
8. Filled the wash basin with warm water.	___	___	_____
9. Placed the basin on the over-bed table.	___	___	_____
10. Lowered the bed rail near you if up.	___	___	_____
11. Practiced hand hygiene. Put on gloves.	___	___	_____
12. Assisted the person to semi-Fowler's position if allowed or to the supine position.	___	___	_____
13. Adjusted lighting to clearly see the person's face.	___	___	_____
14. Placed the bath towel over the person's chest and shoulders.	___	___	_____
15. Adjusted the over-bed table for easy reach.	___	___	_____
16. Tightened the razor blade to the shaver.	___	___	_____
17. Washed the person's face. Did not dry.	___	___	_____
18. Wet the washcloth or towel. Wrung it out.	___	___	_____
19. Applied the washcloth or towel to the face for a few minutes.	___	___	_____

Date of Satisfactory Completion _____   Instructor's Initials _____

Procedure—cont'd   **S**   **U**   **Comments**

20. Applied shaving cream with your hands, or used a shaving brush to apply lather.
21. Held the skin taut with one hand.
22. Shaved in the direction of hair growth. Used shorter strokes around the chin and lips.
23. Rinsed the razor often. Wiped it with tissues or paper towels.
24. Applied direct pressure to any bleeding areas.
25. Washed off any remaining shaving cream or soap. Patted dry with a towel.
26. Applied after-shave or lotion if requested. (If there were nicks or cuts, did not apply aftershave or lotion.)
27. Removed the towel and gloves. Practiced hand hygiene.

Post-Procedure

28. Provided for comfort as noted on the inside of the front textbook cover.
29. Placed the call light within reach.
30. Lowered the bed to a safe and comfortable level appropriate for the person. Followed the care plan.
31. Raised or lowered bed rails. Followed the care plan.
32. Cleaned, rinsed, dried, and returned equipment and supplies to their proper place. Used clean, dry paper towels for drying. Discarded a razor blade or a disposable razor into the sharps container. Discarded other disposable items. Wore gloves.
33. Wiped off the over-bed table with paper towels. Discarded the paper towels.
34. Unscreened the person.
35. Completed a safety check of the room as noted on the inside of the front textbook cover.
36. Followed agency policy for dirty linen.
37. Removed the gloves. Practiced hand hygiene.
38. Reported nicks, cuts, irritation, or bleeding to the nurse at once. Reported and recorded other observations.

Date of Satisfactory Completion _____   Instructor's Initials _____

Giving Nail and Foot Care

Name: _____   Date: _____

Quality of Life	S	U	Comments
• Knocked before entering the person's room.	___	___	___
• Addressed the person by name.	___	___	___
• Introduced yourself by name and title.	___	___	___
• Explained the procedure to the person before starting and during the procedure.	___	___	___
• Protected the person's rights during the procedure.	___	___	___
• Handled the person gently during the procedure.	___	___	___

Pre-Procedure

	S	U	Comments
1. Followed *Delegation Guidelines: Nail and Foot Care.* Reviewed *Promoting Safety and Comfort: Nail and Foot Care.*	___	___	___
2. Practiced hand hygiene.	___	___	___
3. Collected the following.			
• Wash basin or whirlpool foot bath	___	___	___
• Soap	___	___	___
• Water thermometer	___	___	___
• Bath towel	___	___	___
• Hand towel	___	___	___
• Washcloth	___	___	___
• Kidney basin	___	___	___
• Nail clippers	___	___	___
• Orangewood stick	___	___	___
• Emery board or nail file	___	___	___
• Lotion for the hands	___	___	___
• Lotion or petroleum jelly for the feet	___	___	___
• Paper towels	___	___	___
• Bath mat	___	___	___
• Gloves	___	___	___
4. Arranged paper towels and other items on the over-bed table.	___	___	___
5. Identified the person. Checked the ID bracelet against the assignment sheet. Used 2 Identifiers. Called the person by name.	___	___	___
6. Provided for privacy.	___	___	___
7. Assisted the person to the bedside chair. Removed footwear and socks or stockings. Placed the call light within reach.	___	___	___

Procedure

	S	U	Comments
8. Placed the bath mat under the feet.	___	___	___
9. Filled the wash basin or whirlpool foot bath two-thirds full with water. Followed the nurse's directions for water temperature. (Measured water temperature with a bath thermometer or tested it by dipping your elbow or inner wrist into the basin. Followed agency policy.) Asked the person to check the water temperature. Adjusted water temperature as needed.	___	___	___
10. Placed the basin or foot bath on the bath mat.	___	___	___
11. Put on gloves.	___	___	___
12. Helped the person put the feet into the basin or foot bath. Made sure both feet were completely covered by water.	___	___	___

Date of Satisfactory Completion _____   Instructor's Initials _____

Procedure—cont'd	S	U	Comments
13. Adjusted the over-bed table in front of the person.	___	___	___
14. Filled the kidney basin two-thirds full with water. Measured water temperature (see step 9).	___	___	___
15. Placed the kidney basin on the over-bed table.	___	___	___
16. Placed the person's fingers into the basin. Positioned the arms for comfort.	___	___	___
17. Let the fingers soak for 5 to 10 minutes. Let the feet soak for 15 to 20 minutes. Rewarmed water as needed.	___	___	___
18. Removed the kidney basin.	___	___	___
19. Dried the hands and between the fingers thoroughly.	___	___	___
20. Cleaned under the fingernails with the orangewood stick. Used a towel to wipe the orangewood stick after each nail.	___	___	___
21. Pushed cuticles back gently with the orangewood stick or a washcloth.	___	___	___
22. Clipped fingernails straight across with the nail clippers.	___	___	___
23. Shaped nails with an emery board or nail file. Nails were smooth with no rough edges. Checked each nail for smoothness. Filed as needed.	___	___	___
24. Applied lotion to the hands. Warmed lotion before applying it.	___	___	___
25. Moved the over-bed table to the side.	___	___	___
26. Removed and discarded the gloves. Practiced hand hygiene. Put on clean gloves.	___	___	___
27. Lifted a foot out of the water. Supported the foot and ankle with one hand. With your other hand, washed the foot and between the toes with soap and a washcloth. Returned the foot to the water for rinsing. Made sure to rinse between the toes.	___	___	___
28. Repeated step 27 for the other foot.	___	___	___
29. Removed the feet from the basin or foot bath. Dried thoroughly, especially between the toes. Supported the foot and ankle as needed.	___	___	___
30. Applied lotion or petroleum jelly to the tops and soles of the feet. Did not apply between the toes. Warmed lotion or petroleum jelly before applying it. Removed excess lotion or petroleum jelly with a towel. Supported the foot and ankle as needed.	___	___	___
31. Removed and discarded the gloves. Practiced hand hygiene.	___	___	___
32. Helped the person put on non-skid footwear.	___	___	___
Post-Procedure			
33. Provided for comfort as noted on the inside of the front textbook cover.	___	___	___
34. Placed the call light within reach.	___	___	___
35. Raised or lowered bed rails. Followed the care plan.	___	___	___
36. Cleaned, dried, and returned equipment and supplies to their proper place. Used clean, dry paper towels for drying. Discarded disposable items. Wore gloves.	___	___	___
37. Unscreened the person.	___	___	___
38. Completed a safety check of the room as noted on the inside of the front textbook cover.	___	___	___
39. Followed agency policy for dirty linen.	___	___	___
40. Removed the gloves. Practiced hand hygiene.	___	___	___
41. Reported and recorded your observations.	___	___	___

Date of Satisfactory Completion _____   Instructor's Initials _____

Undressing the Person

Name: _____ Date: _____

Quality of Life	S	U	Comments
• Knocked before entering the person's room.	_____	_____	_____
• Addressed the person by name.	_____	_____	_____
• Introduced yourself by name and title.	_____	_____	_____
• Explained the procedure to the person before starting and during the procedure.	_____	_____	_____
• Protected the person's rights during the procedure.	_____	_____	_____
• Handled the person gently during the procedure.	_____	_____	_____

Pre-Procedure

	S	U	Comments
1. Followed *Delegation Guidelines: Dressing and Undressing.*	_____	_____	_____
Reviewed *Promoting Safety and Comfort: Dressing and Undressing.*	_____	_____	_____
2. Asked a co-worker to help turn and position the person if needed.	_____	_____	_____
3. Practiced hand hygiene.	_____	_____	_____
4. Collected a bath blanket and clothing requested by the person.	_____	_____	_____
5. Identified the person. Checked the ID bracelet against the assignment sheet. Used 2 identifiers. Called the person by name.	_____	_____	_____
6. Provided for privacy.	_____	_____	_____
7. Raised the bed for body mechanics. Bed rails were up if used.	_____	_____	_____
8. Lowered the bed rail on the person's weak side.	_____	_____	_____
9. Positioned the person supine.	_____	_____	_____
10. Covered the person with a bath blanket. Fanfolded linens to the foot of the bed.	_____	_____	_____

Procedure

	S	U	Comments
11. *To remove garments that opened in the back:*			
a. Raised the head and shoulders. Or turned the person onto the side away from you.	_____	_____	_____
b. Undid buttons, zippers, ties, or snaps.	_____	_____	_____
c. Brought the sides of the garment to the sides of the person. If the person was in a side-lying position, tucked the far side under the person. Folded the near side onto the chest.	_____	_____	_____
d. Positioned the person supine.	_____	_____	_____
e. Slid the garment off the shoulder on the strong side. Removed it from the arm.	_____	_____	_____
f. Removed the garment from the weak side.	_____	_____	_____
12. *To remove garments that opened in the front:*			
a. Undid buttons, zippers, ties, or snaps.	_____	_____	_____
b. Slid the garment off the shoulder and arm on the strong side.	_____	_____	_____
c. Assisted the person to sit up or raised the head and shoulders. Brought the garment over to the weak side.	_____	_____	_____
d. Lowered the head and shoulders. Removed the garment from the weak side.	_____	_____	_____

Date of Satisfactory Completion _____ Instructor's Initials _____

Procedure—cont'd	S	U	Comments
e. If you could not raise the head and shoulders:			
(1) Turned the person toward you. Tucked the removed part under the person.	___	___	___
(2) Turned the person onto the side away from you.	___	___	___
(3) Pulled the side of the garment out from under the person. Made sure he or she would not lie on it when supine.	___	___	___
(4) Returned the person to the supine position.	___	___	___
(5) Removed the garment from the weak side.	___	___	___
13. Removed pullover garments.			
a. Undid buttons, zippers, ties, or snaps.	___	___	___
b. Removed the garment from the strong side.	___	___	___
c. Raised the head and shoulders. Or turned the person onto the side away from you. Brought the garment up to the person's neck.	___	___	___
d. Removed the garment from the weak side.	___	___	___
e. Brought the garment over the person's head.	___	___	___
f. Positioned the person in the supine position.	___	___	___
14. Removed pants or slacks.			
a. Removed footwear and socks.	___	___	___
b. Positioned the person supine.	___	___	___
c. Undid buttons, zippers, ties, snaps, or buckles.	___	___	___
d. Removed the belt.	___	___	___
e. Asked the person to lift the buttocks off the bed. Slid the pants down over the hips and buttocks. Had the person lower the hips and buttocks.	___	___	___
f. If the person could not raise the hips off the bed:			
(1) Turned the person toward you.	___	___	___
(2) Slid the pants off the hip and buttock on the strong side.	___	___	___
(3) Turned the person away from you.	___	___	___
(4) Slid the pants off the hip and buttock on the weak side.	___	___	___
g. Slid the pants down the legs and over the feet.	___	___	___
15. Dressed the person. See procedure: *Dressing the Person.*	___	___	___
Post-Procedure			
16. Provided for comfort as noted on the inside of the front textbook cover.	___	___	___
17. Placed the call light within reach.	___	___	___
18. Lowered the bed to a safe and comfortable level appropriate for the person. Followed the care plan.	___	___	___
19. Raised or lowered bed rails. Followed the care plan.	___	___	___
20. Unscreened the person.	___	___	___
21. Completed a safety check of the room as noted on the inside of the front textbook cover.	___	___	___
22. Followed agency policy for removed clothing.	___	___	___
23. Practiced hand hygiene.	___	___	___
24. Reported and recorded your observations.	___	___	___

Date of Satisfactory Completion _____   Instructor's Initials _____

Dressing the Person

Name: _____   Date: _____

Quality of Life	S	U	Comments
• Knocked before entering the person's room.	_____	_____	_____
• Addressed the person by name.	_____	_____	_____
• Introduced yourself by name and title.	_____	_____	_____
• Explained the procedure to the person before starting and during the procedure.	_____	_____	_____
• Protected the person's rights during the procedure.	_____	_____	_____
• Handled the person gently during the procedure.	_____	_____	_____

Pre-Procedure

	S	U	Comments
1. Followed *Delegation Guidelines: Dressing and Undressing.*	_____	_____	_____
Reviewed *Promoting Safety and Comfort: Dressing and Undressing.*	_____	_____	_____
2. Asked a co-worker to help turn and position the person if needed.	_____	_____	_____
3. Practiced hand hygiene.	_____	_____	_____
4. Asked the person what he or she would like to wear.	_____	_____	_____
5. Got a bath blanket and clothing requested by the person.	_____	_____	_____
6. Identified the person. Checked the ID bracelet against the assignment sheet. Used 2 identifiers. Called the person by name.	_____	_____	_____
7. Provided for privacy.	_____	_____	_____
8. Raised the bed for body mechanics. Bed rails were up if used.	_____	_____	_____
9. Lowered the bed rail (if up) on the person's weak side.	_____	_____	_____
10. Positioned the person supine.	_____	_____	_____
11. Covered the person with the bath blanket. Fanfolded linens to the foot of the bed.	_____	_____	_____
12. Undressed the person. (See procedure: *Undressing the Person.*)	_____	_____	_____

Procedure

	S	U	Comments
13. Put on garments that open in the back.			
a. Slid the garment onto the arm and shoulder of the weak side.	_____	_____	_____
b. Slid the garment onto the arm and shoulder of the strong side.	_____	_____	_____
c. Raised the person's head and shoulders.	_____	_____	_____
d. Brought the sides to the back.	_____	_____	_____
e. If you could not raise the person's head and shoulders:			
(1) Turned the person toward you.	_____	_____	_____
(2) Brought one side of the garment to the person's back.	_____	_____	_____
(3) Turned the person away from you.	_____	_____	_____
(4) Brought the other side to the person's back.	_____	_____	_____
f. Fastened buttons, zippers, snaps, or other closures.	_____	_____	_____
g. Positioned the person supine.	_____	_____	_____
14. Put on garments that open in the front.			
a. Slid the garment onto the arm and shoulder on the weak side.	_____	_____	_____

Date of Satisfactory Completion _____   Instructor's Initials _____

Procedure—cont'd	S	U	Comments
b. Raised the head and shoulders. Brought the side of the garment around to the back. Lowered the person down. Slid the garment onto the arm and shoulder of the strong arm.	___	___	___
c. If the person could not raise the head and shoulders:			
(1) Turned the person away from you.	___	___	___
(2) Tucked the garment under the person.	___	___	___
(3) Turned the person toward you.	___	___	___
(4) Pulled the garment out from under him or her.	___	___	___
(5) Turned the person back to the supine position.	___	___	___
(6) Slid the garment over the arm and shoulder of the strong arm.	___	___	___
d. Fastened buttons, zippers, ties, snaps, or other closures.	___	___	___
15. Put on pullover garments.			
a. Slid the arm and shoulder of the garment onto the weak side.	___	___	___
b. Raised the person's head and shoulders.	___	___	___
c. Brought the neck of the garment over the head.	___	___	___
d. Slid the arm and shoulder of the garment onto the strong side.	___	___	___
e. If the person could not assume a semi-sitting position:			
(1) Brought the neck of the garment over the head.	___	___	___
(2) Slid the arm and shoulder of the garment onto the strong side.	___	___	___
(3) Turned the person onto the strong side.	___	___	___
(4) Pulled the garment down on the person's weak side.	___	___	___
(5) Turned the person onto the weak side.	___	___	___
(6) Pulled the garment down on the person's strong side.	___	___	___
f. Positioned the person supine.	___	___	___
16. Put on pants or slacks.			
a. Slid the pants over the feet and up the legs.	___	___	___
b. Asked the person to raise the hips and buttocks off the bed.	___	___	___
c. Brought the pants up over the buttocks and hips on the weak side.	___	___	___
d. Brought the pants up over the buttocks and hips on the strong side.	___	___	___
e. If the person could not raise the hips and buttocks:			
(1) Turned the person onto the strong side.	___	___	___
(2) Pulled the pants over the buttock and hip on the weak side.	___	___	___
(3) Turned the person onto the weak side.	___	___	___
(4) Pulled the pants over the buttock and hip on the strong side.	___	___	___
(5) Positioned the person supine.	___	___	___
f. Fastened buttons, zippers, ties, snaps, a belt buckle, or other closures.	___	___	___

Date of Satisfactory Completion _____   Instructor's Initials _____

Procedure—cont'd	S	U	Comments
17. Put socks and non-skid footwear on the person. Made sure socks were up all the way and were smooth.	_____	_____	_____
18. Helped the person get out of bed. If the person stayed in bed, covered the person. Removed the bath blanket.	_____	_____	_____

Post-Procedure

	S	U	Comments
19. Provided for comfort as noted on the inside of the front textbook cover.	_____	_____	_____
20. Placed the call light within reach.	_____	_____	_____
21. Lowered the bed to a safe and comfortable level appropriate for the person. Followed the care plan.	_____	_____	_____
22. Raised or lowered bed rails. Followed the care plan.	_____	_____	_____
23. Unscreened the person.	_____	_____	_____
24. Completed a safety check of the room as noted on the inside of the front textbook cover.	_____	_____	_____
25. Followed agency policy for removed clothing.	_____	_____	_____
26. Practiced hand hygiene.	_____	_____	_____
27. Reported and recorded your observations.	_____	_____	_____

Date of Satisfactory Completion _____ Instructor's Initials _____

Changing a Standard Patient Gown on a Person with an IV

Name: _____   Date: _____

	S	U	Comments

Quality of Life

- Knocked before entering the person's room.
- Addressed the person by name.
- Introduced yourself by name and title.
- Explained the procedure to the person before starting and during the procedure.
- Protected the person's rights during the procedure.
- Handled the person gently during the procedure.

Pre-Procedure

1. Followed *Delegation Guidelines: Changing Patient Gowns.*
   Reviewed *Promoting Safety and Comfort: Changing Patient Gowns.*
2. Practiced hand hygiene.
3. Got a clean gown and a bath blanket.
4. Identified the person. Checked the ID bracelet against the assignment sheet. Used 2 identifiers. Called the person by name.
5. Provided for privacy.
6. Raised the bed for body mechanics. Bed rails were up if used.

Procedure

7. Lowered the bed rail near you if up.
8. Covered the person with a bath blanket. Fanfolded linens to the foot of the bed.
9. Untied the gown. Freed parts that the person was lying on.
10. Removed the gown from the arm with no IV.
11. Gathered up the sleeve of the arm with the IV. Slid it over the IV site and tubing. Removed the arm and hand from the sleeve.
12. Kept the sleeve gathered. Slid your arm along the tubing to the bag.
13. Removed the bag from the pole. Slid the bag and tubing through the sleeve. Did not pull on the tubing. Kept the bag above the person.
14. Hung the IV bag on the pole.
15. Gathered the sleeve of the clean gown that would go on the arm with the IV infusion.
16. Removed the bag from the pole. Slipped the sleeve over the bag at the shoulder part of the gown. Hung the bag.
17. Slid the gathered sleeve over the tubing, hand, arm, and IV site. Then slid it onto the shoulder.
18. Put the other side of the gown on the person. Fastened the gown.
19. Covered the person. Removed the bath blanket.

Post-Procedure

20. Provided for comfort as noted on the inside of the front textbook cover.

Date of Satisfactory Completion _____   Instructor's Initials _____

Post-Procedure—cont'd	**S**	**U**	**Comments**
21. Placed the call light within reach.	_____	_____	_____
22. Lowered the bed to a safe and comfortable level appropriate for the person. Followed the care plan.	_____	_____	_____
23. Raised or lowered bed rails. Followed the care plan.	_____	_____	_____
24. Unscreened the person.	_____	_____	_____
25. Completed a safety check of the room as noted on the inside of the front textbook cover.	_____	_____	_____
26. Followed agency policy for dirty linen.	_____	_____	_____
27. Practiced hand hygiene.	_____	_____	_____
28. Asked the nurse to check the flow rate.	_____	_____	_____
29. Reported and recorded your observations.	_____	_____	_____

Date of Satisfactory Completion _____   Instructor's Initials _____

Giving the Bedpan

Name: _____   Date: _____

Quality of Life	S	U	Comments
• Knocked before entering the person's room.	_____	_____	_____
• Addressed the person by name.	_____	_____	_____
• Introduced yourself by name and title.	_____	_____	_____
• Explained the procedure to the person before starting and during the procedure.	_____	_____	_____
• Protected the person's rights during the procedure.	_____	_____	_____
• Handled the person gently during the procedure.	_____	_____	_____

Pre-Procedure

	S	U	Comments
1. Followed *Delegation Guidelines: Bedpans.* Reviewed *Promoting Safety and Comfort:* a. *Urinary Needs* b. *Bedpans*	_____	_____	_____
2. Provided for privacy.	_____	_____	_____
3. Practiced hand hygiene.	_____	_____	_____
4. Put on gloves.	_____	_____	_____
5. Collected the following.			
• Bedpan	_____	_____	_____
• Bedpan cover	_____	_____	_____
• Toilet tissue	_____	_____	_____
• Waterproof pad if required	_____	_____	_____
• Bath blanket (optional)	_____	_____	_____
6. Arranged equipment on the chair or bed.	_____	_____	_____

Procedure

	S	U	Comments
7. Raised the bed for body mechanics (if the person's needs are not urgent). Lowered the bed rail near you if up.	_____	_____	_____
8. Lowered the head of the bed. Positioned the person supine. Raised the head of the bed slightly for the person's comfort.	_____	_____	_____
9. Covered the person with a bath blanket if time allowed. Folded the top linens and gown out of the way. Kept the lower body covered.	_____	_____	_____
10. Asked the person to flex the knees and raise the buttocks by pushing against the mattress with his or her feet.	_____	_____	_____
11. Slid your hand under the lower back. Helped raise the buttocks. If using a waterproof under-pad, placed it under the person's buttocks.	_____	_____	_____
12. Slid the bedpan under the person. Made sure the bedpan was centered under the person.	_____	_____	_____
13. If the person could not assist in getting on the bedpan:			
a. Placed the waterproof pad under the person's buttocks if using one.	_____	_____	_____
b. Turned the person onto the side away from you.	_____	_____	_____
c. Placed the bedpan firmly against the buttocks.	_____	_____	_____
d. Held the bedpan securely. Turned the person onto his or her back.	_____	_____	_____
e. Made sure the bedpan was centered under the person.	_____	_____	_____

Date of Satisfactory Completion _____   Instructor's Initials _____

Procedure—cont'd	S	U	Comments
14. Covered the person.	_____	_____	_____
15. Raised the head of the bed so that the person was in a sitting position (if the person used a standard bedpan). (If required by state competency tests, removed the gloves and washed your hands before raising the head of the bed.)	_____	_____	_____
16. Made sure the person was correctly positioned on the bedpan.	_____	_____	_____
17. Raised the bed rail if used. Lowered the bed.	_____	_____	_____
18. Placed the toilet tissue and call light within reach.	_____	_____	_____
19. Asked the person to signal when done or when help was needed. (Stayed with the person if necessary and was respectful. Provided as much privacy as possible.)	_____	_____	_____
20. Removed the gloves. Practiced hand hygiene.	_____	_____	_____
21. Left the room and closed the door.	_____	_____	_____
22. Returned when the person signaled. Or checked on the person every 5 minutes. Knocked before entering.	_____	_____	_____
23. Practiced hand hygiene. Put on gloves.	_____	_____	_____
24. Raised the bed for body mechanics. Lowered the bed rail (if used) and lowered the head of the bed.	_____	_____	_____
25. Asked the person to raise the buttocks. Removed the bedpan. Or held the bedpan and turned the person onto the side away from you.	_____	_____	_____
26. Cleaned the genital area if the person could not do so.	_____	_____	_____
a. Cleaned from front (meatus) to back (anus) with toilet tissue. Used fresh tissue for each wipe.	_____	_____	_____
b. Provided perineal care if needed.	_____	_____	_____
c. Removed and discarded the waterproof under-pad if using one.	_____	_____	_____
27. Covered the bedpan. Took it to the bathroom. Raised the bed rail (if used) before leaving the bedside.	_____	_____	_____
28. Noted the color, amount, and character of urine or feces.	_____	_____	_____
29. Emptied the bedpan contents into the toilet and flushed.	_____	_____	_____
30. Rinsed the bedpan. Poured the rinse into the toilet and flushed.	_____	_____	_____
31. Cleaned the bedpan with a disinfectant. Poured disinfectant into the toilet and flushed.	_____	_____	_____
32. Returned the bedpan and clean cover to the bedside stand.	_____	_____	_____
33. Removed soiled gloves. Practiced hand hygiene and put on clean gloves. Dried the bedpan with clean, dry paper towels.	_____	_____	_____
34. Helped the person with hand washing.	_____	_____	_____
35. Removed and discarded the gloves. Practiced hand hygiene.	_____	_____	_____
36. Covered the person with the top linens. Removed the bath blanket if used.	_____	_____	_____
Post-Procedure			
37. Provided for comfort as noted on the inside of the front textbook cover.	_____	_____	_____
38. Placed the call light within reach.	_____	_____	_____

Date of Satisfactory Completion _____   Instructor's Initials _____

Post-Procedure—cont'd	**S**	**U**	**Comments**
39. Lowered the bed to a safe and comfortable level appropriate for the person. Followed the care plan.			
40. Raised or lowered bed rails. Followed the care plan.			
41. Unscreened the person.			
42. Completed a safety check of the room as noted on the inside of the front textbook cover.			
43. Followed agency policy for soiled linen.			
44. Practiced hand hygiene.			
45. Reported and recorded your observations.			

Date of Satisfactory Completion _____   Instructor's Initials _____

Giving the Urinal

Name: _____   Date: _____

Quality of Life	S	U	Comments
• Knocked before entering the person's room.	___	___	___
• Addressed the person by name.	___	___	___
• Introduced yourself by name and title.	___	___	___
• Explained the procedure to the person before starting and during the procedure.	___	___	___
• Protected the person's rights during the procedure.	___	___	___
• Handled the person gently during the procedure.	___	___	___

Pre-Procedure

	S	U	Comments
1. Followed *Delegation Guidelines: Urinals.* Reviewed *Promoting Safety and Comfort:* a. *Urinary Needs* b. *Urinals*	___	___	___
2. Provided for privacy.	___	___	___
3. Determined if the man would stand, sit, or lie in bed.	___	___	___
4. Practiced hand hygiene.	___	___	___
5. Put on gloves.	___	___	___
6. Collected the following. • Urinal	___	___	___
• Non-skid footwear if the man would stand to void	___	___	___

Procedure

	S	U	Comments
7. *Using the urinal in bed:* a. Gave him the urinal.	___	___	___
b. Reminded him to tilt the bottom down to prevent spills.	___	___	___
8. *Standing to use the urinal:* a. Helped him sit on the side of the bed.	___	___	___
b. Put non-skid footwear on him.	___	___	___
c. Helped him stand. Provided support if he was unsteady.	___	___	___
d. Gave him the urinal.	___	___	___
9. *Positioning the urinal (in bed or standing):* a. Helped the person stand (step 8) if he will stand.	___	___	___
b. Positioned the urinal.	___	___	___
c. Placed the penis in the urinal if he could not do so.	___	___	___
d. Covered him for privacy.	___	___	___
10. Placed the call light within reach. Asked him to signal when done or if he needed help.	___	___	___
11. Provided for privacy.	___	___	___
12. Removed the gloves. Practiced hand hygiene.	___	___	___
13. Left the room and closed the door.	___	___	___
14. Returned when he signaled. Or checked on him every 5 minutes. Knocked before entering.	___	___	___
15. Practiced hand hygiene. Put on gloves.	___	___	___
16. Closed the cap on the urinal. Took it to the bathroom.	___	___	___
17. Noted the color, amount, and character of the urine.	___	___	___
18. Emptied the urinal into the toilet and flushed.	___	___	___
19. Rinsed the urinal with cold water. Poured the rinse into the toilet and flushed.	___	___	___

Date of Satisfactory Completion _____   Instructor's Initials _____

Procedure—cont'd	S	U	Comments
20. Cleaned the urinal with a disinfectant. Poured disinfectant into the toilet and flushed. Dried the urinal with clean, dry paper towels.			
21. Returned the urinal to its proper place.			
22. Removed soiled gloves. Practiced hand hygiene and put on clean gloves.			
23. Assisted with hand washing.			
24. Removed the gloves. Practiced hand hygiene.			
Post-Procedure			
25. Provided for comfort as noted on the inside of the front textbook cover.			
26. Placed the call light within reach.			
27. Raised or lowered bed rails. Followed the care plan.			
28. Unscreened him.			
29. Completed a safety check of the room as noted on the inside of the front textbook cover.			
30. Followed agency policy for soiled linen.			
31. Practiced hand hygiene.			
32. Reported and recorded your observations.			

Date of Satisfactory Completion _____   Instructor's Initials _____

Helping the Person to the Commode

Name: _____   Date: _____

Quality of Life	S	U	Comments
• Knocked before entering the person's room.			
• Addressed the person by name.			
• Introduced yourself by name and title.			
• Explained the procedure to the person before starting and during the procedure.			
• Protected the person's rights during the procedure.			
• Handled the person gently during the procedure.			

Pre-Procedure

	S	U	Comments
1. Followed *Delegation Guidelines: Commodes.* Reviewed *Promoting Safety and Comfort:* a. *Urinary Needs* b. *Commodes*			
2. Provided for privacy.			
3. Practiced hand hygiene.			
4. Put on gloves.			
5. Collected the following.			
• Commode			
• Toilet tissue			
• Bath blanket			
• Transfer belt			
• Robe and non-skid footwear			

Procedure

	S	U	Comments
6. Brought the commode next to the bed.			
7. Helped the person sit on the side of the bed. Lowered the bed rail if used.			
8. Helped the person put on a robe and non-skid footwear.			
9. Applied the transfer belt.			
10. Assisted the person to the commode. Used the transfer belt.			
11. Removed the transfer belt. Covered the person with a bath blanket for warmth.			
12. Placed the toilet tissue and call light within reach.			
13. Asked the person to signal when done or when help was needed. (Stayed with the person if necessary. Was respectful and provided as much privacy as possible.)			
14. Removed the gloves. Practiced hand hygiene.			
15. Left the room. Closed the door.			
16. Returned when the person signaled. Or checked on the person every 5 minutes. Knocked before entering.			
17. Practiced hand hygiene. Put on the gloves.			
18. Helped the person clean the genital area as needed. Removed and discarded the gloves and practiced hand hygiene.			
19. Applied the transfer belt. Helped the person back to bed using the transfer belt. Removed the transfer belt, robe, and footwear. Raised the bed rail if used.			
20. Put on clean gloves. Removed and covered the commode container.			

Date of Satisfactory Completion _____   Instructor's Initials _____

Procedure—cont'd

	S	U	Comments
21. Took the container to the bathroom.	_____	_____	_____
22. Observed urine and feces for color, amount, and character.	_____	_____	_____
23. Emptied the container contents into the toilet and flushed.	_____	_____	_____
24. Rinsed the container. Poured the rinse into the toilet and flushed.	_____	_____	_____
25. Cleaned and disinfected the container. Poured disinfectant into the toilet and flushed. Dried the container with clean, dry paper towels.	_____	_____	_____
26. Returned the container to the commode. Closed the lid on the commode. Cleaned other parts of the commode if necessary.	_____	_____	_____
27. Returned other supplies to their proper place.	_____	_____	_____
28. Removed and discarded soiled gloves. Practiced hand hygiene and put on clean gloves.	_____	_____	_____
29. Assisted with hand washing.	_____	_____	_____
30. Removed the gloves. Practiced hand hygiene.	_____	_____	_____

Post-Procedure

	S	U	Comments
31. Provided for comfort as noted on the inside of the front textbook cover.	_____	_____	_____
32. Placed the call light within reach.	_____	_____	_____
33. Raised or lowered bed rails. Followed the care plan.	_____	_____	_____
34. Unscreened the person.	_____	_____	_____
35. Completed a safety check of the room as noted on the inside of the front textbook cover.	_____	_____	_____
36. Followed agency policy for dirty linen.	_____	_____	_____
37. Practiced hand hygiene.	_____	_____	_____
38. Reported and recorded your observations.	_____	_____	_____

Date of Satisfactory Completion _____   Instructor's Initials _____

Applying an Incontinence Brief

Name: _____   Date: _____

Quality of Life	S	U	Comments

Quality of Life
- Knocked before entering the person's room.
- Addressed the person by name.
- Introduced yourself by name and title.
- Explained the procedure before starting and during the procedure.
- Protected the person's rights during the procedure.
- Handled the person gently during the procedure.

Pre-Procedure
1. Followed *Delegation Guidelines: Applying Incontinence Products.*
   Reviewed *Promoting Safety and Comfort:*
   a. *Urinary Needs*
   b. *Applying Incontinence Products*
2. Practiced hand hygiene.
3. Collected the following.
   - Incontinence brief
   - Barrier cream as directed by the nurse
   - Cleanser
   - Items for perineal care (Chapter 18)
   - Paper towels
   - Trash bag
   - Gloves
4. Covered the over-bed table with paper towels. Arranged items on top of them.
5. Identified the person. Checked the ID bracelet against the assignment sheet. Used 2 identifiers. Also called the person by name.
6. Marked the date, time, and your initials on the new product. Followed agency policy.
7. Provided for privacy.
8. Filled the wash basin. Water temperature is usually 105° F to 109° F (40.5° C to 42.7° C). Measured water temperature according to agency policy. Asked the person to check the water temperature. Adjusted water temperature as needed.
9. Raised the bed for body mechanics. Bed rails were up if used.

Procedure
10. Lowered the head of the bed. The bed is as flat as possible.
11. Lowered the bed rail near you if up.
12. Practiced hand hygiene. Put on the gloves.
13. Covered the person with a bath blanket. Lowered top linens to the foot of the bed.
14. Placed a waterproof under-pad under the buttocks. Asked the person to raise the buttocks off the bed. Or turned the person from side to side.
15. Loosened the tabs on each side of the product.
16. Turned the person onto the side away from you.
17. Removed the product from front to back. Observed the urine as you rolled the product up.

Date of Satisfactory Completion _____   Instructor's Initials _____

Procedure—cont'd

	S	U	Comments
18. Placed the product in the trash bag. Set the bag aside.	___	___	___
19. Performed perineal care. Put on clean gloves. Applied the barrier cream or moisturizer.	___	___	___
20. Removed and discarded the gloves. Practiced hand hygiene. Put on clean gloves.	___	___	___
21. Opened the new brief. Folded it in half length-wise along the center.	___	___	___
22. Inserted the product between the legs from front to back. (top to bottom)	___	___	___
23. Unfolded and spread the back panel.	___	___	___
24. Centered the product in the perineal area.	___	___	___
25. Turned the person onto his or her back.	___	___	___
26. Unfolded and spread the front panel. Provided a "cup" shape in the perineal area. For a man, positioned the penis downward.	___	___	___
27. Made sure the product was positioned high in the groin folds. The brief fit the shape of the body.	___	___	___
28. Secured the product.			
a. Pulled the lower tape tab forward on the side near you. Attached it at a slightly upward angle. Did the same for the other side.	___	___	___
b. Pulled the upper tape tab forward on the side near you. Attached it in a horizontal manner. Did the same for the other side.	___	___	___
29. Smoothed out all wrinkles and folds.	___	___	___
30. Asked about comfort. Asked if the product felt too loose or too tight. Checked for wrinkles or creases. Made sure the product didn't rub or irritate the groin. Adjusted the product as needed.	___	___	___
31. Removed and discarded the gloves. Practiced hand hygiene.	___	___	___
32. Raised or put on pants or slacks.	___	___	___
Post-Procedure			
33. Provided for comfort as noted on the inside of the front textbook cover.	___	___	___
34. Placed the call light within reach.	___	___	___
35. Lowered the bed to a safe and comfortable level appropriate for the person. Followed the care plan.	___	___	___
36. Raised or lowered bed rails. Followed the care plan.	___	___	___
37. Unscreened the person.	___	___	___
38. Practiced hand hygiene. Put on clean gloves.	___	___	___
39. Estimated the amount of urine in the old product: small, moderate, large. Opened the product to observe for urine color and blood.	___	___	___
40. Cleaned, rinsed, dried, and returned the wash basin and other equipment. Used a clean, dry paper towel for drying. Returned items to their proper place.	___	___	___
41. Removed and discarded the gloves. Practiced hand hygiene.	___	___	___
42. Completed a safety check of the room as noted on the inside of the front textbook cover.	___	___	___
43. Followed agency policy for used linens.	___	___	___
44. Practiced hand hygiene.	___	___	___
45. Reported and recorded your observations.	___	___	___

Date of Satisfactory Completion _____   Instructor's Initials _____

Giving Catheter Care

Name: _____   Date: _____

	S	U	Comments
Quality of Life			
• Knocked before entering the person's room.	_____	_____	_____
• Addressed the person by name.	_____	_____	_____
• Introduced yourself by name and title.	_____	_____	_____
• Explained the procedure to the person before starting and during the procedure.	_____	_____	_____
• Protected the person's rights during the procedure.	_____	_____	_____
• Handled the person gently during the procedure.	_____	_____	_____

Pre-Procedure

1. Followed *Delegation Guidelines:*   _____ _____ _____
   a. *Perineal Care*
   b. *Catheter Care*
   Reviewed *Promoting Safety and Comfort:*   _____ _____ _____
   a. *Perineal Care*
   b. *Urinary Catheters*
   c. *Catheter Care*
2. Practiced hand hygiene.   _____ _____ _____
3. Collected the following.
   • Items for perineal care (Chapter 18)   _____ _____ _____
   • Gloves   _____ _____ _____
   • Bath blanket   _____ _____ _____
4. Covered the over-bed table with paper towels. Arranged items on top of them.   _____ _____ _____
5. Identified the person. Checked the ID bracelet against the assignment sheet. Called the person by name.   _____ _____ _____
6. Provided for privacy.   _____ _____ _____
7. Filled the wash basin. Water temperature is usually 105° F to 109° F (40.5° C to 42.7° C). Measured water temperature according to agency policy. Asked the person to check the water temperature. Adjusted water temperature as needed.   _____ _____ _____
8. Raised the bed for body mechanics. Bed rails were up if used.   _____ _____ _____
9. Lowered the bed rail near you if up.   _____ _____ _____

Procedure

10. Practiced hand hygiene. Put on gloves.   _____ _____ _____
11. Covered the person with a bath blanket. Fanfolded top linens to the foot of the bed.   _____ _____ _____
12. Draped the person for perineal care (Chapter 18).   _____ _____ _____
13. Folded back the bath blanket to expose the genital area.   _____ _____ _____
14. Asked the person to flex the knees and raise the buttocks off the bed. Placed the waterproof pad under the buttocks.   _____ _____ _____
15. Checked the drainage tubing. Made sure it was not kinked and that urine could flow freely.   _____ _____ _____
16. Separated the labia (female). In an uncircumcised male, retracted the foreskin. Checked for crusts, abnormal drainage, or secretions.   _____ _____ _____
17. Gave perineal care. (See procedure: *Giving Female Perineal Care* or *Giving Male Perineal Care* in Chapter 18.) Kept the foreskin of the uncircumcised male retracted until step 25.   _____ _____ _____

Date of Satisfactory Completion _____   Instructor's Initials _____

Procedure—cont'd	S	U	Comments
18. Applied soap to a clean, wet washcloth.	___	___	___
19. Held the catheter near the meatus. Did so for steps 20 through 24.	___	___	___
20. Washed around the catheter at the meatus. Used a circular motion.	___	___	___
21. Cleaned the catheter from the meatus down the catheter about 4 inches. Cleaned downward, away from the meatus with 1 stroke. Did not tug or pull on the catheter. Repeated as needed with a clean area of the washcloth. Used a clean washcloth if needed.	___	___	___
22. Rinsed the catheter at the meatus with a clean washcloth.	___	___	___
23. Rinsed from the meatus down the catheter about 4 inches. Rinsed downward, away from the meatus with 1 stroke. Did not tug or pull on the catheter. Repeated as needed with a clean area of the washcloth. Used a clean washcloth if needed.	___	___	___
24. Patted dry the areas washed. Dried from the meatus down the catheter about 4 inches. Did not tug or pull on the catheter.	___	___	___
25. Returned the foreskin (uncircumcised male) to its natural position.	___	___	___
26. Patted dry the perineal area. Dried from front to back.	___	___	___
27. Secured the catheter. Positioned the tubing in a straight line or coiled on the bed. Followed the nurse's directions. Secured the tubing to the bottom linens.	___	___	___
28. Removed the waterproof under-pad.	___	___	___
29. Covered the person. Removed the bath blanket.	___	___	___
30. Removed and discarded the gloves. Practiced hand hygiene.	___	___	___
Post-Procedure			
31. Provided for comfort as noted on the inside of the front textbook cover.	___	___	___
32. Placed the call light within reach.	___	___	___
33. Lowered the bed to a safe and comfortable level appropriate for the person. Followed the care plan.	___	___	___
34. Raised or lowered bed rails. Followed the care plan.	___	___	___
35. Cleaned, rinsed, dried, and returned equipment to its proper place. Used clean, dry paper towels for drying. Discarded disposable items. Wore gloves for this step.	___	___	___
36. Unscreened the person.	___	___	___
37. Completed a safety check of the room as noted on the inside of the front textbook cover.	___	___	___
38. Followed agency policy for soiled linen.	___	___	___
39. Removed and discarded the gloves. Practiced hand hygiene.	___	___	___
40. Reported and recorded your observations.	___	___	___

Date of Satisfactory Completion _____   Instructor's Initials _____

Emptying a Urinary Drainage Bag

Name: _____   Date: _____

Quality of Life	S	U	Comments
• Knocked before entering the person's room.	___	___	___
• Addressed the person by name.	___	___	___
• Introduced yourself by name and title.	___	___	___
• Explained the procedure to the person before starting and during the procedure.	___	___	___
• Protected the person's rights during the procedure.	___	___	___
• Handled the person gently during the procedure.	___	___	___

Pre-Procedure

	S	U	Comments
1. Followed *Delegation Guidelines: Drainage Systems.* Reviewed *Promoting Safety and Comfort:*	___	___	___
a. *Urinary Catheters.*			
b. *Urine Drainage Systems*			
2. Collected the following.			
• Graduate (measuring container)	___	___	___
• Gloves	___	___	___
• Paper towels	___	___	___
• Antiseptic wipes	___	___	___
3. Practiced hand hygiene.	___		
4. Identified the person. Checked the ID bracelet against the assignment sheet. Used 2 identifiers. Called the person by name.	___		
5. Provided for privacy.	___		___

Procedure

	S	U	Comments
6. Put on the gloves.	___	___	___
7. Placed a paper towel on the floor. Placed the graduate on top of it.	___	___	___
8. Positioned the graduate under the collection bag.	___	___	___
9. Opened the clamp on the drain.	___	___	___
10. Let all urine drain into the graduate. Did not let the drain touch the graduate.	___	___	___
11. Cleaned the end of the drain with an antiseptic wipe.	___	___	___
12. Clamped and positioned the drain in the holder.	___	___	___
13. Measured urine. Reviewed procedure: *Measuring Intake and Output* in Chapter 24.	___	___	___
14. Removed and discarded the paper towel.	___	___	___
15. Emptied the contents of the graduate into the toilet and flushed.	___	___	___
16. Rinsed the graduate. Emptied the rinse into the toilet and flushed.	___	___	___
17. Cleaned, disinfected the graduate. Used clean, dry paper towels for drying.	___	___	___
18. Returned the graduate to its proper place.	___	___	___
19. Removed and discarded the gloves. Practiced hand hygiene.	___	___	___
20. Recorded the time and amount on the intake and output (I&O) record (Chapter 24).	___	___	___

Post-Procedure

	S	U	Comments
21. Provided for comfort as noted on the inside of the front textbook cover.	___	___	___

Date of Satisfactory Completion _____   Instructor's Initials _____

Post-Procedure—cont'd   S   U   Comments

22. Placed the call light within reach.

23. Unscreened the person.

24. Completed a safety check of the room as noted on
    the inside of the front textbook cover.

25. Reported and recorded the amount and other
    observations.

Date of Satisfactory Completion _____   Instructor's Initials _____

Applying a Condom Catheter

Name: _____   Date: _____

	S	U	Comments
Quality of Life			
• Knocked before entering the person's room.			
• Addressed the person by name.			
• Introduced yourself by name and title.			
• Explained the procedure to the person before starting and during the procedure.			
• Protected the person's rights during the procedure.			
• Handled the person gently during the procedure.			

Pre-Procedure

1. Followed *Delegation Guidelines:*
   a. *Perineal Care* (Chapter 18)
   b. *Condom Catheters*
   Reviewed *Promoting Safety and Comfort:*
   a. *Perineal Care* (Chapter 18)
   b. *Urinary Catheters*
   c. *Condom Catheters*
2. Practiced hand hygiene.
3. Collected the following.
   • Condom catheter
   • Elastic tape
   • Drainage bag or leg bag
   • Cap for the drainage bag
   • Basin of warm water
   • Soap
   • Towel and washcloths
   • Bath blanket
   • Gloves
   • Waterproof under-pad
   • Paper towels
4. Arranged paper towels and equipment on the over-bed table.
5. Identified the person. Checked the ID bracelet against the assignment sheet. Used 2 identifiers. Called the person by name.
6. Provided for privacy.
7. Raised the bed for body mechanics. Bed rails were up if used.

Procedure

8. Lowered the bed rail near you if up.
9. Practiced hand hygiene. Put on the gloves.
10. Covered the person with a bath blanket. Lowered top linens to the knees.
11. Asked the person to raise his buttocks off the bed or turned him onto his side away from you.
12. Slid the waterproof pad under his buttocks.
13. Had the person lower his buttocks or turned him onto his back.
14. Secured the drainage bag to the bed frame or had a leg bag ready. Closed the drain.

Date of Satisfactory Completion _____   Instructor's Initials _____

Procedure—cont'd

	S	U	Comments
15. Exposed the genital area.	___	___	___
16. Removed the condom catheter. Put on clean gloves.	___	___	___
a. Removed the tape. Rolled the sheath off the penis.	___	___	___
b. Disconnected the drainage tubing from the condom. Capped the drainage tube.	___	___	___
c. Discarded the tape and condom.	___	___	___
17. Provided perineal care (Chapter 18). Observed the penis for reddened areas, skin breakdown, and irritation.	___	___	___
18. Removed the gloves and practiced hand hygiene. Put on clean gloves.	___	___	___
19. Removed the protective backing from the condom to expose the adhesive strip.	___	___	___
20. Held the penis firmly. Rolled the condom onto the penis. Left a 1-inch space between the penis and the end of the catheter.	___	___	___
21. Secured the condom.			
a. For a self-adhering condom, pressed the condom to the penis.	___	___	___
b. For a condom secured with elastic tape, applied elastic tape in a spiral. Did not apply the tape completely around the penis.	___	___	___
22. Made sure the penis tip did not touch the condom. Made sure the condom was not twisted.	___	___	___
23. Connected the condom to the drainage tubing. Coiled and secured excess tubing on the bed or attached a leg bag.	___	___	___
24. Removed the waterproof under-pad and gloves. Discarded them. Practiced hand hygiene.	___	___	___
25. Covered the person. Removed the bath blanket.	___	___	___

Post-Procedure

	S	U	Comments
26. Provided for comfort as noted on the inside of the front textbook cover.	___	___	___
27. Placed the call light within reach.	___	___	___
28. Lowered the bed to a safe and comfortable level appropriate for the person. Followed the care plan.	___	___	___
29. Raised or lowered bed rails. Followed the care plan.	___	___	___
30. Unscreened the person.	___	___	___
31. Practiced hand hygiene. Put on clean gloves.	___	___	___
32. Measured and recorded the amount of urine in the bag. Cleaned or discarded the collection bag.	___	___	___
33. Cleaned, rinsed, dried, and returned the wash basin and other equipment. Used clean, dry paper towels for drying. Returned items to their proper place.	___	___	___
34. Removed and discarded the gloves. Practiced hand hygiene.	___	___	___
35. Completed a safety check of the room as noted on the inside of the front textbook cover.	___	___	___
36. Reported and recorded your observations.	___	___	___

Date of Satisfactory Completion _____   Instructor's Initials _____

Giving a Small-Volume Enema

Name: _____   Date: _____

Quality of Life	S	U	Comments
• Knocked before entering the person's room.	_____	_____	_____
• Addressed the person by name.	_____	_____	_____
• Introduced yourself by name and title.	_____	_____	_____
• Explained the procedure to the person before starting and during the procedure.	_____	_____	_____
• Protected the person's rights during the procedure.	_____	_____	_____
• Handled the person gently during the procedure.	_____	_____	_____

Pre-Procedure

	S	U	Comments
1. Follow *Delegation Guidelines:*	_____	_____	_____
a. *Bowel Needs*			
b. *The Small-Volume Enema*			
See *Promoting Safety and Comfort:*	_____	_____	_____
a. *Bowel Needs*			
b. *Enemas*			
2. Practiced hand hygiene.			
3. Collected the following before going to the person's room.			
• Small-volume enema	_____	_____	_____
• Waterproof under-pad	_____	_____	_____
• Gloves	_____	_____	_____
4. Arranged items in the person's room.	_____	_____	_____
5. Practiced hand hygiene.	_____	_____	_____
6. Identified the person. Checked the ID bracelet against the assignment sheet. Called the person by name.	_____	_____	_____
7. Put on gloves.	_____	_____	_____
8. Collected the following.			
• Commode or bedpan	_____	_____	_____
• Toilet tissue	_____	_____	_____
• Robe and non-skid footwear	_____	_____	_____
• Bath blanket	_____	_____	_____
9. Removed and discarded the gloves. Practiced hand hygiene. Put on clean gloves.	_____	_____	_____
10. Provided for privacy.	_____	_____	_____
11. Raised the bed for body mechanics. Bed rails were up if used.	_____	_____	_____

Procedure

	S	U	Comments
12. Lowered the bed rail near you if up.	_____	_____	_____
13. Covered the person with a bath blanket. Fanfolded top linens to the foot of the bed.	_____	_____	_____
14. Positioned the person in the Sims' or a left side-lying position.	_____	_____	_____
15. Placed the waterproof pad under the buttocks.	_____	_____	_____
16. Exposed the anal area.	_____	_____	_____
17. Positioned the bedpan near the person.	_____	_____	_____
18. Removed the cap from the enema tip.	_____	_____	_____
19. Separated the buttocks to see the anus.	_____	_____	_____
20. Asked the person to take a deep breath through the mouth.	_____	_____	_____

Date of Satisfactory Completion _____   Instructor's Initials _____

	S	U	Comments

Procedure—cont'd

21. Inserted the enema tip 2 inches into the adult's rectum. Did this when the person was exhaling. Inserted the tip gently. Stopped if the person complained of pain, you felt resistance, or bleeding occurred.

22. Squeezed and rolled the container gently. Released pressure on the bottle after you removed the tip from the rectum.

23. Put the bottle into the box, tip first. Discarded the container and box.

24. Assisted the person to the bathroom or commode when he or she had the urge to have a BM. The person wore a robe and non-skid footwear when up. The bed was at a low level that was comfortable and safe for the person. Or helped the person onto the bedpan and raised the head of the bed. Raised or lowered bed rails according to the care plan.

25. Placed the call light and toilet tissue within reach. Reminded the person not to flush the toilet.

26. Discarded disposable items.

27. Removed the gloves. Practiced hand hygiene.

28. Left the room if the person could be left alone.

29. Returned when the person signaled. Or checked on the person every 5 minutes. Knocked before entering the room or bathroom.

30. Practiced hand hygiene. Put on gloves.

31. Lowered the bed rail if up.

32. Observed enema results for amount, color, consistency, shape, and odor. Called for the nurse to observe the results.

33. Provided perineal care as needed.

34. Removed the waterproof pad.

35. Emptied, rinsed, cleaned, disinfected and dried the equipment. Used clean, dry paper towels for drying. Flushed the toilet after the nurse observed the results.

36. Returned equipment to its proper place.

37. Removed the gloves and practiced hand hygiene.

38. Assisted the person with hand washing. Wore gloves. Practiced hand hygiene after removing and discarding the gloves.

39. Covered the person. Removed the bath blanket.

Post-Procedure

40. Provided for comfort as noted on the inside of the front textbook cover.

41. Placed the call light within reach.

42. Lowered the bed to a safe and comfortable level appropriate for the person. Followed the care plan.

43. Raised or lowered bed rails. Followed the care plan.

44. Unscreened the person.

45. Completed a safety check of the room as noted on the inside of the front textbook cover.

46. Followed agency policy for dirty linen and used supplies.

47. Practiced hand hygiene.

48. Reported and recorded your observations.

Date of Satisfactory Completion _____   Instructor's Initials _____

Preparing the Person for a Meal

Name: _____ Date: _____

	S	U	Comments
Quality of Life			
• Knocked before entering the person's room.	____	____	____
• Addressed the person by name.	____	____	____
• Introduced yourself by name and title.	____	____	____
• Explained the procedure to the person before starting and during the procedure.	____	____	____
• Protected the person's rights during the procedure.	____	____	____
• Handled the person gently during the procedure.	____	____	____
Pre-Procedure			
1. Followed *Delegation Guidelines: Preparing for Meals.* Reviewed *Promoting Safety and Comfort: Preparing for Meals.*	____	____	____
2. Practiced hand hygiene.	____	____	____
3. Collected the following.			
• Equipment for oral hygiene	____	____	____
• Bedpan and cover, urinal, commode, or specimen pan	____	____	____
• Toilet tissue	____	____	____
• Wash basin	____	____	____
• Soap	____	____	____
• Washcloth and towel	____	____	____
• Gloves	____	____	____
4. Provided for privacy.	____	____	____
Procedure			
5. Made sure eyeglasses and hearing aids were in place.	____	____	____
6. Assisted with oral hygiene. Made sure dentures were in place. Wore gloves and practiced hand hygiene after removing them.	____	____	____
7. Assisted with elimination. Made sure the incontinent person was clean and dry. Wore gloves and practiced hand hygiene after removing them.	____	____	____
8. Assisted the person with hand washing. Wore gloves and practiced hand hygiene after removing them.	____	____	____
9. Did the following if the person would sit in a chair.			
a. Positioned the person in a chair or wheelchair.	____	____	____
b. Removed items from the over-bed table. Cleaned the table.	____	____	____
c. Adjusted the over-bed table in front of the person.	____	____	____
10. Assisted the person to the dining area (if the person would eat in the dining area).	____	____	____
11. Did the following if the person would eat in bed.			
a. Raised the head of the bed to a comfortable position.	____	____	____
b. Removed items from the over-bed table. Cleaned the over-bed table.	____	____	____
c. Adjusted the over-bed table in front of the person.	____	____	____
Post-Procedure			
12. Provided for comfort as noted on the inside of the front textbook cover.	____	____	____
13. Placed the call light within reach.	____	____	____

Date of Satisfactory Completion _____   Instructor's Initials _____

Post-Procedure—cont'd

	S	U	Comments
14. Emptied, cleaned, disinfected equipment. Used clean, dry paper towels for drying. Returned equipment to its proper place. Wore gloves, and practiced hand hygiene after removing and discarding them.	_____	_____	_____
15. Straightened the room. Eliminated unpleasant noise, odors, or equipment.	_____	_____	_____
16. Unscreened the person.	_____	_____	_____
17. Completed a safety check of the room as noted on the inside of the front textbook cover.	_____	_____	_____
18. Practiced hand hygiene.	_____	_____	_____

Date of Satisfactory Completion _____   Instructor's Initials _____

Serving Meal Trays

Name: _____   Date: _____

Quality of Life	S	U	Comments
• Knocked before entering the person's room.	____	____	____
• Addressed the person by name.	____	____	____
• Introduced yourself by name and title.	____	____	____
• Explained the procedure to the person before starting and during the procedure.	____	____	____
• Protected the person's rights during the procedure.	____	____	____
• Handled the person gently during the procedure.	____	____	____

Pre-Procedure

	S	U	Comments
1. Followed *Delegation Guidelines: Serving Meals.*	____	____	____
Reviewed *Promoting Safety and Comfort: Serving Meals.*	____	____	____
2. Practiced hand hygiene.	____	____	____
3. Prepared the person for the meal if was not already done according to the procedure *Preparing the Person for a Meal.*	____	____	____

Procedure

	S	U	Comments
4. Made sure the tray was complete. Checked items on the tray with the dietary card. Made sure assistive devices were included.	____	____	____
5. Identified the person. Checked the ID bracelet against the dietary card. Used 2 identifiers. Called the person by name.	____	____	____
6. Placed the tray within the person's reach. Adjusted the over-bed table as needed.	____	____	____
7. Removed food covers. Opened cartons, cut food into bite-sized pieces, buttered bread, and so on as needed. Seasoned food as the person preferred and as allowed on the care plan.	____	____	____
8. Placed the napkin, clothes protector, assistive devices, and eating utensils within reach. Helped the person apply the clothes protector if needed.	____	____	____
9. Placed the call light within reach.	____	____	____
10. Did the following when the person was done eating.			
a. Measured and recorded intake if ordered (Chapter 24).	____	____	____
b. Noted the amount and type of foods eaten.	____	____	____
c. Checked for and removed any food in the mouth (pocketing). Wore gloves. Practiced hand hygiene after removing them.	____	____	____
d. Removed the tray.	____	____	____
e. Cleaned spills. Changed soiled linen and clothing.	____	____	____
f. Helped the person return to bed if needed.	____	____	____
g. Assisted the person with oral hygiene and hand washing. Wore gloves. Practiced hand hygiene after removing and discarding the gloves.	____	____	____

Post-Procedure

	S	U	Comments
11. Provided for comfort as noted on the inside of the front textbook cover.	____	____	____
12. Placed the call light within reach.	____	____	____
13. Raised or lowered bed rails. Followed the care plan.	____	____	____
14. Completed a safety check of the room as noted on the inside of the front textbook cover.	____	____	____
15. Followed agency policy for soiled linen.	____	____	____
16. Practiced hand hygiene.	____	____	____
17. Reported and recorded your observations.	____	____	____

Date of Satisfactory Completion _____   Instructor's Initials _____

Feeding the Person

Name: _____   Date: _____

	S	U	Comments

Quality of Life

- Knocked before entering the person's room.
- Addressed the person by name.
- Introduced yourself by name and title.
- Explained the procedure to the person before starting and during the procedure.
- Protected the person's rights during the procedure.
- Handled the person gently during the procedure.

Pre-Procedure

1. Followed *Delegation Guidelines: Feeding the Person.* Reviewed *Promoting Safety and Comfort: Feeding the Person.*
2. Practiced hand hygiene.
3. Positioned the person in a comfortable position for eating—usually sitting in a chair or Fowler's or high-Fowler's.
4. Got the tray. Placed it on the over-bed table or dining table where the person could reach it.

Procedure

5. Checked items on the tray with the dietary card. Made sure the tray was complete.
6. Identified the person. Checked the ID bracelet against the dietary card. Called the person by name.
7. Draped a napkin across the person's chest and underneath the chin. Or applied a clothes protector. Cleaned the person's hands with a hand wipe.
8. Told the person what foods and fluids were on the tray.
9. Prepared food for eating. Cut food into bite-sized pieces. Seasoned food as the person preferred and as allowed on the care plan.
10. Placed the chair where you could sit comfortably. Sat facing the person at eye level.
11. Served foods in the order the person preferred. Identified foods as you served them. Alternated between solid and liquid foods. Used a spoon for safety. Allowed enough time for chewing and swallowing. Did not rush the person. Offered water, coffee, tea, or other beverage on the tray.
12. Checked the person's mouth before offering more food or fluids. Made sure the person's mouth was empty between bites and swallows. Asked if the person was ready for the next bite or drink.
13. Used straws (if allowed) for liquids if the person could not drink out of a glass or cup. Had one straw for each liquid. Provided short straws for weak persons. Followed the care plan for using straws.
14. Wiped the person's hands, face, and mouth as needed during the meal. Used the napkin or hand wipe.
15. Followed the care plan if the person had dysphagia. Gave thickened liquid with a spoon.

Date of Satisfactory Completion _____   Instructor's Initials _____

Procedure—cont'd	S	U	Comments
16. Conversed with the person in a pleasant manner.	___	___	___
17. Encouraged the person to eat as much as possible.	___	___	___
18. Wiped the person's mouth with a napkin. Discarded the napkin or hand wipe.	___	___	___
19. Noted how much and which foods were eaten.	___	___	___
20. Measured and recorded intake if ordered (Chapter 24).	___	___	___
21. Removed the tray.	___	___	___
22. Took the person back to his or her room (if in a dining area).	___	___	___
23. Assisted with oral hygiene and hand washing. Provided for privacy and put on gloves. Practiced hand hygiene after removing and discarding the gloves.	___	___	___

Post-Procedure

	S	U	Comments
24. Provided for comfort as noted on the inside of the front textbook cover.	___	___	___
25. Placed the call light within reach.	___	___	___
26. Raised or lowered bed rails. Followed the care plan.	___	___	___
27. Completed a safety check of the room as noted on the inside of the front textbook cover.	___	___	___
28. Returned the food tray to the food cart.	___	___	___
29. Practiced hand hygiene.	___	___	___
30. Reported and recorded your observations.	___	___	___

Date of Satisfactory Completion _____ Instructor's Initials _____

Measuring Intake and Output

Name: _____   Date: _____

	S	U	Comments

Quality of Life
- Knocked before entering the person's room.
- Addressed the person by name.
- Introduced yourself by name and title.
- Explained the procedure to the person before starting and during the procedure.
- Protected the person's rights during the procedure.
- Handled the person gently during the procedure.

Pre-Procedure
1. Followed *Delegation Guidelines: Measuring Intake and Output.*
   Reviewed *Promoting Safety and Comfort: Measuring Intake and Output.*
2. Practiced hand hygiene.
3. Collected the following.
   - I&O record
   - 2 Graduates
     - For intake
     - For output
   - Gloves
   - Paper towels

Procedure
4. Put on gloves.
5. Measured intake as follows.
   a. Poured liquid remaining in a container into the graduate. Avoided spills and splashes on the outside of the graduate.
   b. Measured the amount at eye level or on a flat surface. Kept the graduate level.
   c. Checked the serving amount on the I&O record. Or checked the serving size of each container.
   d. Subtracted the remaining amount from the full serving amount. Noted the amount.
   e. Poured the fluid in the graduate back into the container.
   f. Repeated steps 5, a–e for each liquid.
   g. Added the amounts from each liquid together.
   h. Recorded the time and amount on the I&O record.
6. Measured output as follows.
   a. Poured the fluid into the graduate used to measure output. Avoided spills and splashes on the outside of the graduate.
   b. Measured the amount at eye level or on a flat surface. Kept the graduate level.
   c. Disposed of fluid in the toilet. Avoided splashes.
7. Cleaned, rinsed, disinfected, and dried the graduates. Disposed of rinse into the toilet and flushed. Used clean, dry paper towels for drying. Returned the graduates to their proper place.

Date of Satisfactory Completion _____   Instructor's Initials _____

Procedure—cont'd	S	U	Comments
8. Cleaned, rinsed, disinfected, and dried the voiding receptacle or drainage container. Disposed of the rinse into the toilet and flushed. Used clean, dry paper towels for drying. Returned the item to its proper place.	_____	_____	_____
9. Removed and discarded the gloves. Practiced hand hygiene.	_____	_____	_____
10. Recorded the amount on the I&O record.	_____	_____	_____
Post-Procedure			
11. Provided for comfort as noted on the inside of the front textbook cover.	_____	_____	_____
12. Made sure the call light was within reach.	_____	_____	_____
13. Completed a safety check of the room as noted on the inside of the front textbook cover.	_____	_____	_____
14. Reported and recorded your observations.	_____	_____	_____

Date of Satisfactory Completion _____   Instructor's Initials _____

Providing Drinking Water

NATCEP

Name: _____   Date: _____

Quality of Life	S	U	Comments
• Knocked before entering the person's room.	___	___	___
• Addressed the person by name.	___	___	___
• Introduced yourself by name and title.	___	___	___
• Explained the procedure to the person before starting and during the procedure.	___	___	___
• Protected the person's rights during the procedure.	___	___	___
• Handled the person gently during the procedure.	___	___	___

Pre-Procedure

1. Followed *Delegation Guidelines: Providing Drinking Water.*   ___ ___ ___

   Reviewed *Promoting Safety and Comfort: Providing Drinking Water.*   ___ ___ ___
2. Obtained a list of persons with special fluid orders from the nurse or used your assignment sheet.   ___ ___ ___
3. Practiced hand hygiene.
4. Collected the following.
   - Cart   ___ ___ ___
   - Ice chest filled with ice   ___ ___ ___
   - Cover for the ice chest   ___ ___ ___
   - Scoop   ___ ___ ___
   - Paper towels   ___ ___ ___
   - Water mugs   ___ ___ ___
   - Large water pitcher filled with cold water (optional depending on agency procedure)   ___ ___ ___
   - Towel for the scoop   ___ ___ ___
5. Covered the cart with paper towels. Arranged equipment on top of the paper towels.   ___ ___ ___

Procedure

6. Took the cart to the person's room door. Did not take the cart into the room.   ___ ___ ___
7. Checked the person's fluid orders. Used the list from the nurse.   ___ ___ ___
8. Identified the person. Checked the ID bracelet against the fluid orders sheet or your assignment sheet. Used 2 identifiers. Called the person by name.   ___ ___ ___
9. Took the pitcher from the person's over-bed table. Emptied it into the bathroom sink.   ___ ___ ___
10. Determined if a new mug was needed.   ___ ___ ___
11. Used the scoop to fill the mug with ice. Did not let the scoop touch the rim or inside of the mug, lid, or straw.   ___ ___ ___
12. Placed the ice scoop on the towel.
13. Filled the mug with water. Got water from the bathroom or used the larger water pitcher on the cart.   ___ ___ ___
14. Placed the mug on the over-bed table.   ___ ___ ___
15. Made sure the mug was within the person's reach.   ___ ___ ___

Date of Satisfactory Completion _____   Instructor's Initials _____

Post-Procedure	**S**	**U**	**Comments**
16. Provided for comfort as noted on the inside of the front textbook cover.	_____	_____	_____
17. Placed the call light within reach.	_____	_____	_____
18. Completed a safety check of the room as noted on the inside of the front textbook cover.	_____	_____	_____
19. Practiced hand hygiene.	_____	_____	_____
20. Repeated steps 6 through 19 for each person.	_____	_____	_____

Date of Satisfactory Completion _____ Instructor's Initials _____

Taking a Temperature with an Electronic Thermometer

Name: _____   Date: _____

	S	U	Comments

Quality of Life
- Knocked before entering the person's room.
- Addressed the person by name.
- Introduced yourself by name and title.
- Explained the procedure to the person before starting and during the procedure.
- Protected the person's rights during the procedure.
- Handled the person gently during the procedure.

Pre-Procedure
1. Followed *Delegation Guidelines: Taking Temperatures.* Reviewed *Promoting Safety and Comfort: Taking Temperatures.*
2. For an oral temperature, asked the person not to eat, drink, smoke, or chew gum for at least 15 to 20 minutes before the measurement or as required by agency policy.
3. Practiced hand hygiene.
4. Collected the following.
   - Thermometer—electronic or tympanic membrane
   - Probe (blue for an oral or axillary temperature; red for a rectal temperature.)
   - Probe covers
   - Toilet tissue (rectal temperature)
   - Water-soluble lubricant (rectal temperature)
   - Gloves
   - Towel (axillary temperature)
5. Plugged the probe into the thermometer if using a standard electronic thermometer.
6. Practiced hand hygiene.
7. Identified the person. Checked the ID bracelet against the assignment sheet. Used 2 identifiers. Called the person by name.

Procedure
8. Provided for privacy. Positioned the person for an oral, rectal, axillary, or tympanic membrane temperature. The Sims' position was used for a rectal temperature.
9. Put on gloves if contact with blood, body fluids, secretions, or excretions was likely.
10. Inserted the probe into a probe cover.
11. *For an oral temperature:*
    a. Asked the person to open the mouth and raise the tongue.
    b. Placed the covered probe at the base of the tongue and to one side.
    c. Asked the person to lower the tongue and close the mouth.
12. *For a rectal temperature:*
    a. Placed some lubricant on toilet tissue.
    b. Lubricated the end of the covered probe.

Date of Satisfactory Completion _____   Instructor's Initials _____

Procedure—cont'd	S	U	Comments
c. Exposed the anal area.	_____	_____	_____
d. Raised the upper buttock.	_____	_____	_____
e. Inserted the probe ½ inch into the rectum.	_____	_____	_____
f. Held the probe in place.	_____	_____	_____
13. *For an axillary temperature:*			
a. Helped the person remove an arm from the gown. Did not expose the person.	_____	_____	_____
b. Dried the axilla with the towel.	_____	_____	_____
c. Placed the covered probe in the center of the axilla.	_____	_____	_____
d. Placed the person's arm over the chest.	_____	_____	_____
e. Held the probe in place.	_____	_____	_____
14. *For a tympanic membrane temperature:*			
a. Asked the person to turn his or her head so that the ear was in front of you.	_____	_____	_____
b. Pulled back on the adult's ear to straighten the ear canal.	_____	_____	_____
c. Inserted the covered probe gently.	_____	_____	_____
15. Started the thermometer.	_____	_____	_____
16. Held the probe in place until you heard a tone or you saw a flashing or steady light.	_____	_____	_____
17. Read the temperature on the display.	_____	_____	_____
18. Removed the probe. Pressed the eject button to discard the cover.	_____	_____	_____
19. Noted the person's name and temperature on your note pad or assignment sheet.	_____	_____	_____
20. Returned the probe to the holder.	_____	_____	_____
21. Helped the person put the gown back on (axillary temperature). For a rectal temperature:			
a. Wiped the anal area with toilet tissue to remove lubricant.	_____	_____	_____
b. Covered the person.	_____	_____	_____
c. Disposed of used toilet tissue.	_____	_____	_____
d. Removed the gloves. Practiced hand hygiene.	_____	_____	_____
Post-Procedure			
22. Provided for comfort as noted on the inside of the front textbook cover.	_____	_____	_____
23. Placed the call light within reach.	_____	_____	_____
24. Unscreened the person.	_____	_____	_____
25. Completed a safety check of the room as noted on the inside of the front textbook cover.	_____	_____	_____
26. Returned the thermometer to the charging unit.	_____	_____	_____
27. Practiced hand hygiene.	_____	_____	_____
28. Reported and recorded the temperature. Noted the temperature site. Reported an abnormal temperature at once.	_____	_____	_____

Date of Satisfactory Completion _____   Instructor's Initials _____

Taking a Temperature with a Glass Thermometer

Name: _____   Date: _____

	S	U	Comments

Quality of Life
- Knocked before entering the person's room.
- Addressed the person by name.
- Introduced yourself by name and title.
- Explained the procedure to the person before starting and during the procedure.
- Protected the person's rights during the procedure.
- Handled the person gently during the procedure.

Pre-Procedure
1. Followed *Delegation Guidelines: Taking Temperatures.* Reviewed *Promoting Safety and Comfort:*
   a. *Glass Thermometers*
   b. *Taking Temperatures*
2. For an oral temperature, asked the person not to eat, drink, smoke, or chew gum for at least 15 to 20 minutes before the measurement or as required by agency policy.
3. Practiced hand hygiene.
4. Collected the following.
   - Oral or rectal thermometer and holder
   - Tissues
   - Plastic covers if used
   - Gloves
   - Toilet tissue (rectal temperature)
   - Water-soluble lubricant (rectal temperature)
   - Towel (axillary temperature)
5. Practiced hand hygiene.
6. Identified the person. Checked the ID bracelet against the assignment sheet. Used 2 identifiers. Called the person by name.
7. Provided for privacy.

Procedure
8. Put on the gloves.
9. Rinsed the thermometer in cold running water if it was soaking in a disinfectant. Dried it with tissues.
10. Checked for breaks, cracks, or chips.
11. Shook down the thermometer below the lowest number. Held the device by the stem.
12. Inserted it into a plastic cover if used.
13. *For an oral temperature:*
    a. Asked the person to moisten his or her lips.
    b. Placed the bulb end of the thermometer under the tongue and to one side.
    c. Asked the person to close the lips around the thermometer to hold it in place.
    d. Asked the person not to talk. Reminded the person not to bite down on the thermometer.
    e. Left it in place for 2 to 3 minutes or as required by agency policy.

Date of Satisfactory Completion _____   Instructor's Initials _____

Procedure—cont'd	S	U	Comments
14. *For a rectal temperature:*			
a. Positioned the person in the Sims' position.	_____	_____	_____
b. Put a small amount of lubricant on a tissue.	_____	_____	_____
c. Lubricated the bulb end of the thermometer.	_____	_____	_____
d. Folded back top linens to expose the anal area.	_____	_____	_____
e. Raised the upper buttock to expose the anus.	_____	_____	_____
f. Inserted the thermometer 1 inch into the rectum. Did not force the thermometer.	_____	_____	_____
g. Held the thermometer in place for 2 minutes or as required by agency policy. Did not let go of it while it was in the rectum.	_____	_____	_____
15. *For an axillary temperature:*			
a. Helped the person remove an arm from the gown. Did not expose the person.	_____	_____	_____
b. Dried the axilla with the towel.	_____	_____	_____
c. Placed the bulb end of the thermometer in the center of the axilla.	_____	_____	_____
d. Asked the person to place the arm over the chest to hold the thermometer in place. Held it and the arm in place if he or she could not help.	_____	_____	_____
e. Left the thermometer in place for 5 to 10 minutes or as required by agency policy.	_____	_____	_____
16. Removed the thermometer.	_____	_____	_____
17. *For an oral or axillary temperature:*			
a. Used a tissue to remove the plastic cover.	_____	_____	_____
b. Wiped the thermometer with a tissue if no cover was used. Wiped from the stem to the bulb end.	_____	_____	_____
c. Discarded the tissue and cover (if used).	_____	_____	_____
d. Read the thermometer.	_____	_____	_____
e. Helped the person put the gown back on (axillary temperature).	_____	_____	_____
18. *For a rectal temperature:*			
a. Used toilet tissue to remove the plastic cover.	_____	_____	_____
b. Wiped the thermometer with toilet tissue if no cover was used. Wiped from the stem to the bulb end.	_____	_____	_____
c. Placed used toilet tissue on several thicknesses of clean toilet tissue. Discarded the cover (if used).	_____	_____	_____
d. Read the thermometer.	_____	_____	_____
e. Placed the thermometer on clean toilet tissue.	_____	_____	_____
f. Wiped the anal area with toilet tissue to remove lubricant and any feces. Set the used toilet tissue on several thicknesses of clean toilet tissue.	_____	_____	_____
g. Covered the person.	_____	_____	_____
h. Discarded tissue and disposed of toilet tissue in the toilet.	_____	_____	_____
i. Remove and discarded the gloves. Practiced hand hygiene.	_____	_____	_____
19. Noted the person's name and temperature on your note pad or assignment sheet.	_____	_____	_____
20. Shook down the thermometer.	_____	_____	_____

Date of Satisfactory Completion _____   Instructor's Initials _____

Procedure—cont'd	S	U	Comments
21. Cleaned the thermometer according to agency policy. Returned it to the holder.	_____	_____	_____
22. Removed the gloves. Practiced hand hygiene.	_____	_____	_____
Post-Procedure			
23. Provided for comfort as noted on the inside of the front textbook cover.	_____	_____	_____
24. Placed the call light within reach.	_____	_____	_____
25. Unscreened the person.	_____	_____	_____
26. Completed a safety check of the room as noted on the inside of the front textbook cover.	_____	_____	_____
27. Practiced hand hygiene.	_____	_____	_____
28. Reported and recorded the temperature. Noted the temperature site. Reported an abnormal temperature at once.	_____	_____	_____

Date of Satisfactory Completion _____   Instructor's Initials _____

Taking a Radial Pulse

Name: _____   Date: _____

Quality of Life	S	U	Comments
• Knocked before entering the person's room.	_____	_____	_____
• Addressed the person by name.	_____	_____	_____
• Introduced yourself by name and title.	_____	_____	_____
• Explained the procedure to the person before starting and during the procedure.	_____	_____	_____
• Protected the person's rights during the procedure.	_____	_____	_____
• Handled the person gently during the procedure.	_____	_____	_____

Pre-Procedure

	S	U	Comments
1. Followed *Delegation Guidelines: Taking Pulses.* Reviewed *Promoting Safety and Comfort: Taking Pulses.*	_____ _____	_____ _____	_____ _____
2. Practiced hand hygiene.	_____	_____	_____
3. Identified the person. Checked the ID bracelet against the assignment sheet. Used 2 identifiers. Called the person by name.	_____	_____	_____
4. Provided for privacy.	_____	_____	_____

Procedure

	S	U	Comments
5. Had the person sit or lie down.	_____	_____	_____
6. Located the radial pulse on the thumb side of the person's wrist. Used your first two or three middle fingertips.	_____	_____	_____
7. Noted if the pulse was strong or weak, and regular or irregular.	_____	_____	_____
8. Counted the pulse for 30 seconds. Multiplied the number of beats by 2 for the number of pulses in 60 seconds (1 minute).	_____	_____	_____
9. Counted the pulse for 1 minute if:			
a. Directed by the nurse and care plan	_____	_____	_____
b. Required by agency policy	_____	_____	_____
c. The pulse was irregular	_____	_____	_____
d. Required for your state competency test	_____	_____	_____
10. Noted the following on your note pad or assignment sheet.			
a. The person's name	_____	_____	_____
b. Pulse rate	_____	_____	_____
c. Pulse strength	_____	_____	_____
d. If the pulse was regular or irregular	_____	_____	_____

Post-Procedure

	S	U	Comments
11. Provided for comfort as noted on the inside of the front textbook cover.	_____	_____	_____
12. Placed the call light within reach.	_____	_____	_____
13. Unscreened the person.	_____	_____	_____
14. Completed a safety check of the room as noted on the inside of the front textbook cover.	_____	_____	_____
15. Practiced hand hygiene.	_____	_____	_____
16. Reported and recorded the pulse rate and your observations. Reported an abnormal pulse at once.	_____	_____	_____

Date of Satisfactory Completion _____   Instructor's Initials _____

Taking an Apical Pulse

Name: _____   Date: _____

Quality of Life	S	U	Comments
• Knocked before entering the person's room.	_____	_____	_____
• Addressed the person by name.	_____	_____	_____
• Introduced yourself by name and title.	_____	_____	_____
• Explained the procedure to the person before starting and during the procedure.	_____	_____	_____
• Protected the person's rights during the procedure.	_____	_____	_____
• Handled the person gently during the procedure.	_____	_____	_____

Pre-Procedure

1. Followed *Delegation Guidelines: Taking Pulses.* Reviewed *Promoting Safety and Comfort: Using a Stethoscope.*   _____ _____ _____
2. Practiced hand hygiene.   _____ _____ _____
3. Collected a stethoscope and antiseptic wipes.   _____ _____ _____
4. Practiced hand hygiene.   _____ _____ _____
5. Identified the person. Checked the ID bracelet against the assignment sheet. Used 2 identifiers. Called the person by name.   _____ _____ _____
6. Provided for privacy.   _____ _____ _____

Procedure

7. Cleaned the stethoscope ear-pieces and chest-piece with the wipes.   _____ _____ _____
8. Had the person sit or lie down.   _____ _____ _____
9. Exposed the upper part area of the left chest. Limited exposure of a woman's breasts to the extent necessary.   _____ _____ _____
10. Warmed the diaphragm in your palm.   _____ _____ _____
11. Placed the earpieces in your ears.   _____ _____ _____
12. Found the apical pulse. Placed the diaphragm 2 to 3 inches to the left of the breastbone.   _____ _____ _____
13. Counted the pulse for 1 minute. Counted each lub-dub as 1 beat. Noted if it was regular or irregular.   _____ _____ _____
14. Covered the person. Removed the earpieces.   _____ _____ _____
15. Noted the person's name and pulse on your note pad or assignment sheet. Noted if the pulse was regular or irregular.   _____ _____ _____

Post-Procedure

16. Provided for comfort as noted on the inside of the front textbook cover.   _____ _____ _____
17. Placed the call light within reach.   _____ _____ _____
18. Unscreened the person.   _____ _____ _____
19. Completed a safety check of the room as noted on the inside of the front textbook cover.   _____ _____ _____
20. Cleaned the stethoscope ear-pieces and chest-piece with the wipes.   _____ _____ _____
21. Returned the stethoscope to its proper place.   _____ _____ _____
22. Practiced hand hygiene.   _____ _____ _____
23. Reported and recorded your observations. Recorded the pulse rate with *Ap* for apical pulse. Reported an abnormal pulse rate at once.   _____ _____ _____

Date of Satisfactory Completion _____   Instructor's Initials _____

Counting Respirations

Name: _____   Date: _____

Procedure	S	U	Comments
1. Followed *Delegation Guidelines: Respirations.*	_____	_____	_____
2. Kept your fingers or the stethoscope over the pulse site.	_____	_____	_____
3. Did not tell the person you were counting respirations.	_____	_____	_____
4. Began counting when the chest rose. Counted each rise and fall of the chest as one respiration.	_____	_____	_____
5. Noted the following.			
a. If respirations were regular	_____	_____	_____
b. If both sides of the chest rose equally	_____	_____	_____
c. The depth of respirations	_____	_____	_____
d. If the person had any pain or difficulty breathing	_____	_____	_____
e. An abnormal respiratory pattern	_____	_____	_____
6. Counted respirations for 30 seconds. Multiplied the number by 2 for the number of respirations in 60 seconds (1 minute).	_____	_____	_____
7. Counted respirations for 1 minute if:			
a. Directed by the nurse and the care plan.	_____	_____	_____
b. Required by agency policy.	_____	_____	_____
c. They were abnormal or irregular.	_____	_____	_____
d. Required for your state competency test.	_____	_____	_____
8. Noted the person's name, respiratory rate, and other observations on your note pad or assignment sheet.	_____	_____	_____

Post-Procedure

	S	U	Comments
9. Provided for comfort as noted on the inside of the front textbook cover.	_____	_____	_____
10. Placed the call light within reach.	_____	_____	_____
11. Unscreened the person.	_____	_____	_____
12. Completed a safety check of the room as noted on the inside of the front textbook cover.	_____	_____	_____
13. Practiced hand hygiene.	_____	_____	_____
14. Reported and recorded the respiratory rate and your observations. Reported abnormal respirations at once.	_____	_____	_____

Date of Satisfactory Completion _____   Instructor's Initials _____

Measuring Blood Pressure

Name: _____   Date: _____

Quality of Life	S	U	Comments
• Knocked before entering the person's room.			
• Addressed the person by name.			
• Introduced yourself by name and title.			
• Explained the procedure to the person before starting and during the procedure.			
• Protected the person's rights during the procedure.			
• Handled the person gently during the procedure.			

Pre-Procedure

	S	U	Comments
1. Followed *Delegation Guidelines: Measuring Blood Pressure.*			
Reviewed *Promoting Safety and Comfort:*			
a. *Using a Stethoscope*			
b. *Blood Pressure Equipment*			
2. Practiced hand hygiene.			
3. Collected the following.			
• Sphygmomanometer			
• Stethoscope			
• Antiseptic wipes			
4. Practiced hand hygiene.			
5. Identified the person. Checked the ID bracelet against the assignment sheet. Used 2 identifiers. Called the person by name.			
6. Provided for privacy.			

Procedure

	S	U	Comments
7. Had the person sit or lie down.			
8. Positioned the person's arm level with the heart. The palm was up.			
9. Wiped the stethoscope stethoscope ear-pieces and chest-piece with the wipes. Warmed the diaphragm in your palm. Discarded the wipes.			
10. Stood no more than 3 feet away from the manometer. The mercury type was vertical, on a flat surface, and at eye level. The aneroid type was directly in front of you.			
11. Exposed the upper arm.			
12. Squeezed the cuff to expel any remaining air. Closed the valve on the bulb.			
13. Found the brachial artery at the inner aspect of the elbow (on the little finger side of the arm). Used your fingertips.			
14. Located the arrow on the cuff. Placed the arrow over the brachial artery. Wrapped the cuff around the upper arm at least 1 inch above the elbow. It was even and snug.			
15. Placed the stethoscope earpieces in your ears. Placed the diaphragm over the brachial artery. Did not place it under the cuff.			
16. Found the radial pulse.			

Date of Satisfactory Completion _____   Instructor's Initials _____

Procedure—cont'd	S	U	Comments

17. *Method 1:*
    a. Inflated the cuff until you could no longer feel the pulse. Noted this point. _____ _____ _____
    b. Inflated the cuff 30 mm Hg beyond the point where you last felt the pulse. _____ _____ _____
18. *Method 2:*
    a. Inflated the cuff until you could no longer feel the pulse. Noted this point. _____ _____ _____
    b. Inflated the cuff 30 mm Hg beyond the point where you last felt the pulse. _____ _____ _____
    c. Deflated the cuff slowly. Noted the point when you felt the pulse. _____ _____ _____
    d. Waited 30 seconds. _____ _____ _____
    e. Inflated the cuff again, 30 mm Hg beyond the point where you felt the pulse return. _____ _____ _____
19. *Method 3:*
    a. Inflated the cuff 160 mm Hg to 180 mm Hg. _____ _____ _____
    b. Deflated the cuff if you heard a blood pressure sound. Reinflated the cuff to 200 mm Hg. _____ _____ _____
20. Deflated the cuff at an even rate of 2 to 4 millimeters per second. Turned the valve counterclockwise to deflate the cuff. _____ _____ _____
21. Noted the point where you heard the first sound. This was the systolic reading. It is near the point where the pulse disappeared (Method 1) or returned (Method 2). _____ _____ _____
22. Continued to deflate the cuff. Noted the point where the sound disappeared. This was the diastolic reading. _____ _____ _____
23. Deflated the cuff completely. Removed it from the person's arm. Removed the stethoscope earpieces from your ears. _____ _____ _____
24. Noted the person's name and blood pressure on your note pad or assignment sheet. _____ _____ _____
25. Returned the cuff to the case or wall holder. _____ _____ _____

Post-Procedure
26. Provided for comfort as noted on the inside of the front textbook cover. _____ _____ _____
27. Placed the call light within reach. _____ _____ _____
28. Unscreened the person. _____ _____ _____
29. Completed a safety check of the room as noted on the inside of the front textbook cover. _____ _____ _____
30. Cleaned the earpieces and diaphragm with the wipes. Discarded the wipes. _____ _____ _____
31. Returned the equipment to its proper place. _____ _____ _____
32. Practiced hand hygiene. _____ _____ _____
33. Reported and recorded the blood pressure. Noted which arm was used. Reported an abnormal blood pressure at once. _____ _____ _____

Date of Satisfactory Completion _____   Instructor's Initials _____

Measuring Weight and Height

Name: _____   Date: _____

Quality of Life	S	U	Comments
• Knocked before entering the person's room.	___	___	___
• Addressed the person by name.	___	___	___
• Introduced yourself by name and title.	___	___	___
• Explained the procedure to the person before starting and during the procedure.	___	___	___
• Protected the person's rights during the procedure.	___	___	___
• Handled the person gently during the procedure.	___	___	___

Pre-Procedure

1. Followed Delegation *Guidelines: Weight and Height.* ___ ___ ___
   Reviewed *Promoting Safety and Comfort: Weight and Height.* ___ ___ ___
2. Asked the person to void. ___ ___ ___
3. Practiced hand hygiene. ___ ___ ___
4. Brought the scale and paper towels (for a standing scale) to the person's room. ___ ___ ___
5. Practiced hand hygiene. ___ ___ ___
6. Identified the person. Checked the ID bracelet against the assignment sheet. Used 2 identifiers. Called the person by name. ___ ___ ___
7. Provided for privacy. ___ ___ ___

Procedure

8. Placed the paper towels on the scale platform. ___ ___ ___
9. Raised the height rod. ___ ___ ___
10. Moved the weights to zero (0). The pointer was in the middle. ___ ___ ___
11. Had the person remove the robe and footwear. Assisted as needed. ___ ___ ___
12. Helped the person stand on the scale. The person stood in the center of the scale. Arms were at the sides. The person didn't hold on to anyone or anything. ___ ___ ___
13. Moved the weights until the balance pointer was in the middle. ___ ___ ___
14. Noted the weight on your note pad or assignment sheet. ___ ___ ___
15. Asked the person to stand very straight. ___ ___ ___
16. Lowered the height rod until it rested on the person's head. ___ ___ ___
17. Read the height at the movable part of the height rod. Recorded the height in inches or in feet and inches to the nearest ¼ inch. ___ ___ ___
18. Noted the height on your note pad or assignment sheet. ___ ___ ___
19. Raised the height rod. Helped the person step off of the scale. ___ ___ ___
20. Helped the person put on a robe and non-skid footwear if he or she would be up. Or helped the person back to bed. ___ ___ ___

Date of Satisfactory Completion _____   Instructor's Initials _____

Procedure—cont'd	S	U	Comments
21. Lowered the height rod. Adjusted the weights to zero (0) according to agency policy.	_____	_____	_____
Post-Procedure			
22. Provided for comfort as noted on the inside of the front textbook cover.	_____	_____	_____
23. Placed the call light within reach.	_____	_____	_____
24. Raised or lowered bed rails. Followed the care plan.	_____	_____	_____
25. Unscreened the person.	_____	_____	_____
26. Completed a safety check of the room as noted on the inside of the front textbook cover.	_____	_____	_____
27. Discarded the paper towels.	_____	_____	_____
28. Returned the scale to its proper place.	_____	_____	_____
29. Practiced hand hygiene.	_____	_____	_____
30. Reported and recorded the measurements.	_____	_____	_____

Date of Satisfactory Completion _____   Instructor's Initials _____

Collecting a Random Urine Specimen

Name: _____   Date: _____

Quality of Life	S	U	Comments
• Knocked before entering the person's room.	_____	_____	_____
• Addressed the person by name.	_____	_____	_____
• Introduced yourself by name and title.	_____	_____	_____
• Explained the procedure to the person before starting and during the procedure.	_____	_____	_____
• Protected the person's rights during the procedure.	_____	_____	_____
• Handled the person gently during the procedure.	_____	_____	_____

Pre-Procedure

1. Followed *Delegation Guidelines: Urine Specimens.*
   Reviewed *Promoting Safety and Comfort:*
   a. *Collecting Specimens*
   b. *Urine Specimens*
2. Practiced hand hygiene.
3. Collected the following before going to the person's room.
   - Laboratory requisition slip
   - Specimen container and lid
   - Voiding device—bedpan and cover, urinal, or specimen pan
   - Specimen label
   - Plastic bag
   - *BIOHAZARD* label (if needed)
   - Gloves
4. Arranged your work area.
5. Practiced hand hygiene.
6. Identified the person. Checked the ID bracelet against the requisition slip. Compared all information. Called the person by name. Asked the person to state his or her first and last name and birthdate.
7. Labeled the container in the person's presence.
8. Put on gloves.
9. Collected a commode (if needed) and a graduate to measure output.
10. Provided for privacy.

Procedure

11. Placed the specimen pan on the toilet or commode container.
12. Asked the person to urinate into the receptacle. Reminded him or her to put toilet tissue into the wastebasket or toilet (not in the bedpan or specimen pan).
13. Took the voiding device or commode container to the bathroom.
14. Poured about 120 mL (4 oz) of urine into the specimen container.
15. Placed the lid on the specimen container. Put the container in the plastic bag. Did not let the container touch the outside of the bag. Applied a *BIOHAZARD* label.

Date of Satisfactory Completion _____   Instructor's Initials _____

Procedure—cont'd	S	U	Comments
16. Measured urine if I&O was ordered. Included the amount in the specimen container.	___	___	___
17. Emptied, rinsed, cleaned, and disinfected equipment. Returned equipment to its proper place.	___	___	___
18. Removed and discarded the gloves and practiced hand hygiene. Put on clean gloves.	___	___	___
19. Assisted with hand washing.	___	___	___
20. Removed the gloves. Practiced hand hygiene.	___	___	___

Post-Procedure

	S	U	Comments
21. Provided for comfort as noted on the inside of the front textbook cover.	___	___	___
22. Placed the call light within reach.	___	___	___
23. Raised or lowered bed rails. Followed the care plan.	___	___	___
24. Unscreened the person.	___	___	___
25. Completed a safety check of the room as noted on the inside of the front textbook cover.	___	___	___
26. Practiced hand hygiene.	___	___	___
27. Delivered the specimen and the requisition slip to the laboratory or storage area. Followed agency policy. Wore gloves.	___	___	___
28. Removed and discarded the gloves. Practiced hand hygiene.	___	___	___
29. Reported and recorded your observations.	___	___	___

Date of Satisfactory Completion _____   Instructor's Initials _____

Collecting a Midstream Specimen

Name: _____   Date: _____

	S	U	Comments

Quality of Life
- Knocked before entering the person's room.
- Addressed the person by name.
- Introduced yourself by name and title.
- Explained the procedure to the person before starting and during the procedure.
- Protected the person's rights during the procedure.
- Handled the person gently during the procedure.

Pre-Procedure
1. Followed *Delegation Guidelines: Urine Specimens.* Reviewed *Promoting Safety and Comfort:*
   a. *Collecting Specimens*
   b. *Urine Specimens*
2. Practiced hand hygiene.
3. Collected the following before going to the person's room.
   - Laboratory requisition slip
   - Midstream specimen kit—includes specimen container, label, towelettes sterile gloves
   - Plastic bag
   - Sterile gloves (if not part of the kit)
   - Disposable gloves
   - *BIOHAZARD* label (if needed)
4. Arranged work area.
5. Practiced hand hygiene.
6. Identified the person. Checked the ID bracelet against the requisition slip. Compared all information. Called the person by name. Asked the person to state his or her first and last name and birthdate.
7. Put on disposable gloves.
8. Collected the following.
   - Voiding device—bedpan and cover, urinal, commode, or specimen pan if needed
   - Supplies for perineal care
   - Graduate to measure output
   - Paper towel
9. Provided for privacy.

Procedure
10. Provided perineal care. (Wore gloves. Practiced hand hygiene after removing them.)
11. Opened the sterile kit.
12. Put on the sterile gloves.
13. Opened the packet of towelettes.
14. Opened the sterile specimen container. Did not touch the inside of the container or lid. Set the lid down so that the inside was up.

Date of Satisfactory Completion _____   Instructor's Initials _____

	S	U	Comments
Procedure—cont'd			
15. *For a female*—cleaned the perineal area with towelettes.			
a. Spread the labia with your thumb and index finger. Used your non-dominant hand (then this hand did not touch anything sterile).	_____	_____	_____
b. Cleaned down the urethral area from front to back. Used a clean towelette for each stroke.	_____	_____	_____
c. Kept the labia separated to collect the urine specimen (steps 17 through 20).	_____	_____	_____
16. *For a male*—cleaned the penis with the towelettes.			
a. Held the penis with your non-dominant hand (then this hand did not touch anything sterile).	_____	_____	_____
b. Cleaned the penis starting at the meatus. (Retracted the foreskin if the male is uncircumcised.) Cleaned in a circular motion. Started at the center and worked outward.	_____	_____	_____
c. Kept holding the penis until the specimen was collected (steps 17 through 20).	_____	_____	_____
17. Asked the person to void into the receptacle.	_____	_____	_____
18. Passed the specimen container into the stream of urine. Kept the labia separated.	_____	_____	_____
19. Collected about 30 to 60 mL (1 to 2 oz) of urine.	_____	_____	_____
20. Removed the specimen container before the person stopped voiding. Released the foreskin of the uncircumcised male.	_____	_____	_____
21. Released the labia or penis. Let the person finish voiding into the receptacle.	_____	_____	_____
22. Put the lid on the specimen container. Touched only the outside of the container and lid. Wiped the outside of the container. Set the container on a paper towel.	_____	_____	_____
23. Provided toilet tissue after the person was done voiding.	_____	_____	_____
24. Took the voiding device to the bathroom.	_____	_____	_____
25. Measured urine if I&O was ordered. Included the amount in the specimen container.	_____	_____	_____
26. Emptied, rinsed, cleaned, and disinfected equipment. Used clean, dry paper towels for drying. Returned equipment to its proper place.	_____	_____	_____
27. Removed the gloves and practiced hand hygiene. Put on clean disposable gloves.	_____	_____	_____
28. Labeled the specimen container in the person's presence. Placed the container in a plastic bag. Did not let the container touch the outside of the bag. Applied a *BIOHAZARD* label according to agency policy.	_____	_____	_____
29. Assisted with hand washing.	_____	_____	_____
30. Removed the gloves. Practiced hand hygiene.	_____	_____	_____
Post-Procedure			
31. Provided for comfort as noted on the inside of the front textbook cover.	_____	_____	_____
32. Placed the call light within reach.	_____	_____	_____
33. Raised or lowered bed rails. Followed the care plan.	_____	_____	_____

Date of Satisfactory Completion _____   Instructor's Initials _____

Post-Procedure—cont'd

	S	U	Comments
34. Unscreened the person.	_____	_____	_____
35. Completed a safety check of the room as noted on the inside of the front textbook cover.	_____	_____	_____
36. Practiced hand hygiene.	_____	_____	_____
37. Delivered the specimen and the requisition slip to the laboratory or storage area. Followed agency policy. Wore gloves.	_____	_____	_____
38. Removed and discarded the gloves. Practiced hand hygiene.	_____	_____	_____
39. Reported and recorded your observations.	_____	_____	_____

Date of Satisfactory Completion _____   Instructor's Initials _____

Testing Urine with Reagent Strips

Name: _____   Date: _____

Quality of life	S	U	Comments
• Knocked before entering the person's room.	_____	_____	_____
• Addressed the person by name.	_____	_____	_____
• Introduced yourself by name and title.	_____	_____	_____
• Explained the procedure to the person before starting and during the procedure.	_____	_____	_____
• Protected the person's rights during the procedure.	_____	_____	_____
• Handled the person gently during the procedure.	_____	_____	_____

Pre-Procedure

	S	U	Comments
1. Followed *Delegation Guidelines: Testing Urine.* Reviewed *Promoting Safety and Comfort:* a. *Collecting Specimens* b. *Testing Urine*	_____	_____	_____
2. Practiced hand hygiene.	_____	_____	_____
3. Collected gloves and the reagent strips ordered.	_____	_____	_____
4. Practiced hand hygiene.	_____	_____	_____
5. Identified the person. Checked the ID bracelet against the assignment sheet. Used 2 identifiers. Called the person by name. Asked the person to state his or her first and last name and birthdate.	_____	_____	_____
6. Put on gloves.	_____	_____	_____
7. Collected equipment for the urine specimen.	_____	_____	_____
8. Provided for privacy.	_____	_____	_____

Procedure

	S	U	Comments
9. Collected the urine specimen.	_____	_____	_____
10. Removed the strip from the bottle. Put the cap on the bottle at once. The cap was on tight.	_____	_____	_____
11. Dipped the strip test areas into the urine.	_____	_____	_____
12. Removed the strip after the correct amount of time. Followed the manufacturer's instructions.	_____	_____	_____
13. Tapped the strip gently against the container to remove excess urine.	_____	_____	_____
14. Waited the required amount of time. Followed the manufacturer's instructions.	_____	_____	_____
15. Compared the strip with the color chart on the bottle. Read the results.	_____	_____	_____
16. Discarded disposable items and the specimen.	_____	_____	_____
17. Emptied, rinsed, cleaned, and disinfected equipment. Used clean, dry paper towels for drying. Returned equipment to its proper place.	_____	_____	_____
18. Removed the gloves. Practiced hand hygiene.	_____	_____	_____

Post-Procedure

	S	U	Comments
19. Provided for comfort as noted on the inside of the front textbook cover.	_____	_____	_____
20. Placed the call light within reach.	_____	_____	_____
21. Raised or lowered the bed rails. Followed the care plan.	_____	_____	_____

Date of Satisfactory Completion _____   Instructor's Initials _____

Post-Procedure—cont'd

		S	U	Comments
22.	Unscreened the person.			
23.	Completed a safety check of the room as noted on the inside of the front textbook cover.			
24.	Practiced hand hygiene.			
25.	Reported and recorded the results and other observations.			

Date of Satisfactory Completion _____   Instructor's Initials _____

Collecting a Stool Specimen

Name: _____		Date: _____

Quality of life	S	U	Comments
• Knocked before entering the person's room.	_____	_____	_____
• Addressed the person by name.	_____	_____	_____
• Introduced yourself by name and title.	_____	_____	_____
• Explained the procedure to the person before starting and during the procedure.	_____	_____	_____
• Protected the person's rights during the procedure.	_____	_____	_____
• Handled the person gently during the procedure.	_____	_____	_____

Pre-Procedure

	S	U	Comments
1. Followed *Delegation Guidelines: Stool Specimens.* Reviewed *Promoting Safety and Comfort:*	_____	_____	_____
a. *Collecting Specimens*			
b. *Stool Specimens*			
2. Practiced hand hygiene.	_____	_____	_____
3. Collected the following before going to the person's room.			
• Laboratory requisition slip	_____	_____	_____
• Specimen pan for the toilet	_____	_____	_____
• Stool specimen container and lid	_____	_____	_____
• Specimen label	_____	_____	_____
• Tongue blades	_____	_____	_____
• Disposable bag	_____	_____	_____
• Plastic bag	_____	_____	_____
• *BIOHAZARD* label (if needed)	_____	_____	_____
• Gloves	_____	_____	_____
4. Arranged collected items in the person's bathroom.	_____	_____	_____
5. Practiced hand hygiene.	_____	_____	_____
6. Identified the person. Checked the ID bracelet against the requisition slip. Compared all information. Called the person by name. Asked the person to state his or her first and last name and birthdate.	_____	_____	_____
7. Labeled the specimen container in the person's presence.	_____	_____	_____
8. Put on gloves.	_____	_____	_____
9. Collected the following.			
• Device for voiding—bedpan and cover, urinal, commode, or specimen pan	_____	_____	_____
• Toilet tissue	_____	_____	_____
10. Provided for privacy.	_____	_____	_____

Procedure

	S	U	Comments
11. Asked the person to void. Provided the receptacle for voiding if the person did not use the bathroom. Emptied, rinsed, cleaned, and disinfected the device. Used clean, dry paper towels for drying. Returned it to its proper place.	_____	_____	_____
12. Put the specimen pan on the toilet if the person would use the bathroom. Placed it at the back of the toilet or provided a bedpan or commode.	_____	_____	_____

Date of Satisfactory Completion _____		Instructor's Initials _____

	S	U	Comments
Procedure—cont'd			
13. Asked the person not to put toilet tissue into the bedpan, commode, or specimen pan. Provided a bag for toilet tissue.			
14. Placed the call light and toilet tissue within reach. Raised or lowered bed rails. Followed the care plan.			
15. Removed and discarded the gloves. Practiced hand hygiene. Left the room.			
16. Returned when the person signaled. Or checked on the person every 5 minutes. Knocked before entering.			
17. Practiced hand hygiene. Put on clean gloves.			
18. Lowered the bed rail near you if up. Removed the bedpan (if used). Or assisted the person off the toilet or commode if used. Provided perineal care if needed.			
19. Noted the color, amount, consistency, and odor of stools.			
20. Collected the specimen.			
a. Used a tongue blade to take about 2 tablespoons of formed or liquid stool to the specimen container. Take the sample from:			
(1) Took the sample from the middle of a formed stool.			
(2) Areas of pus, mucus, or blood and watery areas			
(3) The middle and both ends of a hard stool			
b. Put the lid on the specimen container.			
c. Placed the container in the plastic bag. Did not let the container touch the outside of the bag. Applied a *BIOHAZARD* label according to agency policy.			
d. Wrapped the tongue blade in toilet tissue. Discarded it into the disposable bag.			
21. Removed and discarded the gloves. Practiced hand hygiene. Put on clean gloves.			
22. Emptied, rinsed, cleaned, disinfected, and dried equipment. Used clean, dry paper towels for drying. Returned equipment to its proper place.			
23. Removed and discarded the gloves and practiced hand hygiene. Put on clean gloves.			
24. Assisted with hand washing.			
25. Removed the gloves. Practiced hand hygiene.			
Post-Procedure			
26. Provided for comfort as noted on the inside of the front textbook cover.			
27. Placed the call light within reach.			
28. Raised or lowered bed rails. Followed the care plan.			
29. Unscreened the person.			
30. Completed a safety check of the room as noted on the inside of the front textbook cover.			
31. Delivered the specimen and requisition slip to the laboratory or storage area. Followed agency policy. Wore gloves.			
32. Removed and discarded the gloves. Practiced hand hygiene.			
33. Reported and recorded your observations.			

Date of Satisfactory Completion _____   Instructor's Initials _____

Collecting a Sputum Specimen

Name: _____   Date: _____

Quality of Life	S	U	Comments
• Knocked before entering the person's room.	___	___	___
• Addressed the person by name.	___	___	___
• Introduced yourself by name and title.	___	___	___
• Explained the procedure to the person before starting and during the procedure.	___	___	___
• Protected the person's rights during the procedure.	___	___	___
• Handled the person gently during the procedure.	___	___	___

Pre-Procedure

1. Followed *Delegation Guidelines: Sputum Specimens.* Reviewed *Promoting Safety and Comfort:*
   a. *Collecting Specimens*
   b. *Sputum Specimens*
2. Practiced hand hygiene.
3. Collected the following before going to the person's room.
   • Laboratory requisition slip
   • Sputum specimen container and lid
   • Specimen label
   • Plastic bag
   • *BIOHAZARD* label (if needed)
4. Arranged collected items in the person's bathroom.
5. Practiced hand hygiene.
6. Identified the person. Checked the ID bracelet against the requisition slip. Compared all information. Called the person by name. Asked the person to state his or her first and last name and birthdate.
7. Labeled the specimen container in the person's presence.
8. Collected gloves and tissues.
9. Provided for privacy. If able, the person used the bathroom for the procedure.

Procedure

10. Put on gloves.
11. Asked the person to rinse the mouth out with clear water.
12. Had the person hold the container. Only the outside was touched.
13. Asked the person to cover the mouth and nose with tissues when coughing. Followed agency policy for used tissues.
14. Asked the person to take two or three deep breaths and cough up the sputum.
15. Had the person expectorate directly into the container. Sputum did not touch the outside of the container.
16. Collected 1 to 2 teaspoons of sputum unless told to collect more.
17. Put the lid on the container.

Date of Satisfactory Completion _____   Instructor's Initials _____

Procedure—cont'd   S   U   **Comments**

18. Placed the container in the plastic bag. Did not let
    the container touch the outside of the bag. Applied
    a *BIOHAZARD* label according to agency policy.   _____   _____   _____

19. Removed the gloves and practiced hand hygiene.
    Put on clean gloves.   _____   _____   _____

20. Assisted with hand washing.   _____   _____   _____

21. Removed the gloves. Practiced hand hygiene.   _____   _____   _____

Post-Procedure

22. Provided for comfort as noted on the inside of the
    front textbook cover.   _____   _____   _____

23. Placed the call light within reach.   _____   _____   _____

24. Raised or lowered bed rails. Followed the care plan. _____   _____   _____

25. Unscreened the person.   _____   _____   _____

26. Completed a safety check of the room as noted on
    the inside of the front textbook cover.   _____   _____   _____

27. Practiced hand hygiene.   _____   _____   _____

28. Delivered the specimen and the requisition slip to
    the laboratory or storage area. Followed agency
    policy. Wore gloves.   _____   _____   _____

29. Removed and discarded the gloves. Practiced hand
    hygiene.   _____   _____   _____

30. Reported and recorded your observations.   _____   _____   _____

Date of Satisfactory Completion _____   Instructor's Initials _____

Performing Range-of-Motion Exercises

Name: _____   Date: _____

Quality of Life	S	U	Comments
• Knocked before entering the person's room.	___	___	___
• Addressed the person by name.	___	___	___
• Introduced yourself by name and title.	___	___	___
• Explained the procedure to the person before starting and during the procedure.	___	___	___
• Protected the person's rights during the procedure.	___	___	___
• Handled the person gently during the procedure.	___	___	___

Pre-Procedure

	S	U	Comments
1. Followed *Delegation Guidelines: Range-of-Motion Exercises.*	___	___	___
Reviewed *Promoting Safety and Comfort: Range-of-Motion Exercises.*	___	___	___
2. Practiced hand hygiene.	___	___	___
3. Identified the person. Checked the ID bracelet against the assignment sheet. Used 2 identifiers. Called the person by name.	___	___	___
4. Obtained a bath blanket.	___	___	___
5. Provided for privacy.	___	___	___
6. Raised the bed for body mechanics. Bed rails were up if used.	___	___	___

Procedure

	S	U	Comments
7. Lowered the bed rail near you if up.	___	___	___
8. Positioned the person supine.	___	___	___
9. Covered the person with a bath blanket. Fanfolded top linens to the foot of the bed.	___	___	___
10. Exercised the neck if allowed by your agency and if the RN instructed you to do so.			
a. Placed your hands over the person's ears to support the head. Supported the jaws with your fingers.	___	___	___
b. Flexion—brought the head forward. The chin touched the chest.	___	___	___
c. Extension—straightened the head.	___	___	___
d. Hyperextension—brought the head backward until the chin pointed up.	___	___	___
e. Rotation—turned the head from side to side.	___	___	___
f. Lateral flexion—moved the head to the right and to the left.	___	___	___
g. Repeated flexion, extension, hyperextension, rotation, and lateral flexion 5 times—or the number of times stated on the care plan.	___	___	___
11. Exercised the shoulder.			
a. Grasped the wrist with one hand. Grasped the elbow with the other hand.	___	___	___
b. Flexion—raised the arm straight in front and over the head.	___	___	___
c. Extension—brought the arm down to the side.	___	___	___

Date of Satisfactory Completion _____   Instructor's Initials _____

Procedure—cont'd	S	U	Comments

   d. Hyperextension—moved the arm behind the body. (Did this if the person was sitting in a straight-backed chair or was standing.)

   e. Abduction—moved the straight arm away from the side of the body.

   f. Adduction—moved the straight arm to the side of the body.

   g. Internal rotation—bent the elbow. Placed it at the same level as the shoulder. Moved the forearm down toward the body.

   h. External rotation—moved the forearm toward the head.

   i. Repeated flexion, extension, hyperextension, abduction, adduction, and internal and external rotation five times—or the number of times stated on the care plan.

12. Exercised the elbow.

   a. Grasped the person's wrist with one hand. Grasped the elbow with your other hand.

   b. Flexion—bent the arm so the same-side shoulder was touched.

   c. Extension—straightened the arm.

   d. Repeated flexion and extension five times—or the number of times stated on the care plan.

13. Exercised the forearm.

   a. Continued to support the wrist and elbow.

   b. Pronation—turned the hand so that the palm was down.

   c. Supination—turned the hand so that the palm was up.

   d. Repeated pronation and supination five times—or the number of times stated on the care plan.

14. Exercised the wrist.

   a. Held the wrist with both of your hands.

   b. Flexion—bent the hand down.

   c. Extension—straightened the hand.

   d. Hyperextension—bent the hand back.

   e. Radial flexion—turned the hand toward the thumb.

   f. Ulnar flexion—turned the hand toward the little finger.

   g. Repeated flexion, extension, hyperextension, radial flexion, and ulnar flexion five times—or the number of times stated on the care plan.

15. Exercised the thumb.

   a. Held the person's hand with one hand. Held the thumb with your other hand.

   b. Abduction—moved the thumb out from the inner part of the index finger.

   c. Adduction—moved the thumb back next to the index finger.

   d. Opposition—touched each fingertip with the thumb.

   e. Flexion—bent the thumb into the hand.

Date of Satisfactory Completion _____ Instructor's Initials _____

Procedure—cont'd	S	U	Comments
f. Extension—moved the thumb out to the side of the fingers.	_____	_____	_____
g. Repeated abduction, adduction, opposition, flexion, and extension five times—or the number of times stated on the care plan.	_____	_____	_____
16. Exercised the fingers.			
a. Abduction—spread the fingers and the thumb apart.	_____	_____	_____
b. Adduction—brought the fingers and thumb together.	_____	_____	_____
c. Flexion—made a fist.	_____	_____	_____
d. Extension—straightened the fingers so the fingers, hand, and arm were straight.	_____	_____	_____
e. Repeated abduction, adduction, flexion, and extension five times—or the number of times stated on the care plan.	_____	_____	_____
17. Exercised the hip.			
a. Supported the leg. Placed one hand under the knee. Placed your other hand under the ankle.	_____	_____	_____
b. Flexion—raised the leg.	_____	_____	_____
c. Extension—straightened the leg.	_____	_____	_____
d. Hyperextension—moved the leg behind the body. (Do this if the person is standing.)	_____	_____	_____
e. Abduction—moved the leg away from the body.	_____	_____	_____
f. Adduction—moved the leg toward the other leg.	_____	_____	_____
g. Internal rotation—turned the leg inward.	_____	_____	_____
h. External rotation—turned the leg outward.	_____	_____	_____
i. Repeated flexion, extension, abduction, adduction, and internal and external rotation five times—or the number of times stated on the care plan.	_____	_____	_____
18. Exercised the knee.			
a. Supported the knee. Placed one hand under the knee. Placed your other hand under the ankle.	_____	_____	_____
b. Flexion—bent the knee.	_____	_____	_____
c. Extension—straightened the knee.	_____	_____	_____
d. Repeated flexion and extension of the knee five times—or the number of times stated on the care plan.	_____	_____	_____
19. Exercised the ankle.			
a. Supported the foot and ankle. Placed one hand under the foot. Placed your other hand under the ankle.	_____	_____	_____
b. Dorsiflexion—pulled the foot forward. Pushed down on the heel at the same time.	_____	_____	_____
c. Plantar flexion—turned the foot down or pointed the toes.	_____	_____	_____
d. Repeated dorsiflexion and plantar flexion five times—or the number of times stated on the care plan.	_____	_____	_____

Date of Satisfactory Completion _____   Instructor's Initials _____

Procedure—cont'd	S	U	Comments

20. Exercised the foot.
    a. Continued to support the foot and ankle.
    b. Pronation—turned the outside of the foot up and the inside down.
    c. Supination—turned the inside of the foot up and the outside down.
    d. Repeated pronation and supination five times—or the number of times stated on the care plan.
21. Exercised the toes.
    a. Flexion—curled the toes.
    b. Extension—straightened the toes.
    c. Abduction—spread the toes apart.
    d. Adduction—pulled the toes together.
    e. Repeated flexion, extension, abduction, and adduction five times—or the number of times stated on the care plan.
22. Covered the leg. Raised the bed rail if used.
23. Went to the other side. Lowered the bed rail near you if up.
24. Repeated steps 11 through 21. Covered the leg when done.

Post-Procedure
25. Provided for comfort as noted on the inside of the front textbook cover.
26. Covered the person with the top linens. Removed the bath blanket.
27. Placed the call light within reach.
28. Lowered the bed to a safe and comfortable level appropriate for the person. Followed the care plan.
29. Raised or lowered bed rails. Followed the care plan.
30. Folded and returned the bath blanket to its proper place.
31. Unscreened the person.
32. Completed a safety check of the room as noted on the inside of the front textbook cover.
33. Practiced hand hygiene.
34. Reported and recorded your observations.

Date of Satisfactory Completion _____   Instructor's Initials _____

Helping the Person Walk

Name: _____   Date: _____

Quality of Life	S	U	Comments
• Knocked before entering the person's room.	_____	_____	_____
• Addressed the person by name.	_____	_____	_____
• Introduced yourself by name and title.	_____	_____	_____
• Explained the procedure to the person before starting and during the procedure.	_____	_____	_____
• Protected the person's rights during the procedure.	_____	_____	_____
• Handled the person gently during the procedure.	_____	_____	_____

Pre-Procedure

	S	U	Comments
1. Followed *Delegation Guidelines: Ambulation.*	_____	_____	_____
Reviewed *Promoting Safety and Comfort: Ambulation.*	_____	_____	_____
2. Practiced hand hygiene.	_____	_____	_____
3. Collected the following.			
• Robe and non-skid footwear	_____	_____	_____
• Paper or sheet to protect bottom linens	_____	_____	_____
• Gait (transfer) belt	_____	_____	_____
• Walker or cane (if needed)	_____	_____	_____
4. Identified the person. Checked the ID bracelet against the assignment sheet. Used 2 identifiers. Called the person by name.	_____	_____	_____
5. Provided for privacy.	_____	_____	_____

Procedure

	S	U	Comments
6. Lowered the bed to a safe and comfortable level appropriate for the person. Followed the care plan. Locked the bed wheels. Lowered the bed rail if up.	_____	_____	_____
7. Fanfolded top linens to the foot of the bed.	_____	_____	_____
8. Placed the paper or towel under the person's feet. Put the shoes on the person. Fastened the shoes.	_____	_____	_____
9. Helped the person sit on the side of the bed. (See procedure: *Sitting on the Side of the Bed [Dangling],* Chapter 15.)	_____	_____	_____
10. Made sure the person's feet were flat on the floor.	_____	_____	_____
11. Helped the person put on the robe.	_____	_____	_____
12. Applied the gait belt at the waist over clothing. (See procedure: *Applying a Transfer/Gait Belt,* Chapter 11.)	_____	_____	_____
13. Positioned the walker (if used) in front of the person. Or had the person hold the cane (if used) on the strong side.	_____	_____	_____
14. Helped the person stand. (See procedure: *Transferring the Person to a Chair or Wheelchair,* Chapter 11.) Grasped the belt at each side. If not using a gait belt, placed your arms under the person's arms around to the shoulder blades.	_____	_____	_____
15. Stood at the person's weak side while he or she gained balance. Held the belt at the side and back. If not using a gait belt, had one arm around the back and the other at the elbow to support the person.	_____	_____	_____
16. Encouraged the person to stand erect with the head up and back straight.	_____	_____	_____

Date of Satisfactory Completion _____   Instructor's Initials _____

Procedure—cont'd	S	U	Comments

17. *Positioned a walker or cane:*
    a. Walker—the walker is 6 to 8 inches in front of the person.
    b. Cane—the cane is held on the strong side.
       (1) The cane tip is 6 to 10 inches to the side of the strong foot.
       (2) The cane tip is 6 to 10 inches in front of the strong foot.
18. Helped the person walk. Walked to the side and slightly behind the person on the person's weak side. Provided support with the gait belt. Encouraged the person to use the hand rail on his or her strong side.
19. *If using a walker or cane:*
    a. Walker—with both hands, the person pushes the walker 6 to 8 inches in front of the feet.
    b. Cane:
       (1) The cane (on the strong side) is moved forward 6 to 10 inches.
       (2) The weak leg (opposite the cane) is moved forward even with the cane.
       (3) The strong leg is moved forward and ahead of the cane and the weak leg
20. Encouraged the person to walk normally. (The heel should strike the floor first.) Discouraged shuffling, sliding, or walking on tip-toes.
21. Walked the required distance if the person tolerated the activity. Did not rush the person.
22. Helped the person return to bed. Removed the gait belt. (See procedure: *Transferring the Person from a Chair or Wheelchair to Bed,* Chapter 16.)
23. Lowered the head of the bed. Helped the person to the center of the bed.
24. Removed the shoes. Removed and discarded the paper or towel over the bottom sheet. Followed agency policy for used linens.

Post-Procedure

25. Provided for comfort as noted on the inside of the front textbook cover.
26. Placed the call light within reach.
27. Raised or lowered bed rails. Followed the care plan.
28. Returned the robe and shoes to their proper place.
29. Unscreened the person.
30. Completed a safety check of the room as noted on the inside of the front textbook cover.
31. Practiced hand hygiene.
32. Reported and recorded your observations.

Date of Satisfactory Completion _____   Instructor's Initials _____

Applying Elastic Stockings

Name: _____   Date: _____

Quality of Life	S	U	Comments
• Knocked before entering the person's room.			
• Addressed the person by name.			
• Introduced yourself by name and title.			
• Explained the procedure to the person before starting and during the procedure.			
• Protected the person's rights during the procedure.			
• Handled the person gently during the procedure.			

Pre-Procedure

	S	U	Comments
1. Followed *Delegation Guidelines: Elastic Stockings* Reviewed *Promoting Safety and Comfort: Elastic Stockings.*			
2. Practiced hand hygiene.			
3. Obtained elastic stockings in the correct size and length. Noted location of toe opening.			
4. Identified the person. Checked the ID bracelet against the assignment sheet. Used 2 identifiers. Called the person by name.			
5. Provided for privacy.			
6. Raised the bed for body mechanics. Bed rails were up if used.			

Procedure

	S	U	Comments
7. Lowered the bed rail near you if up.			
8. Positioned the person supine.			
9. Exposed 1 leg. Fan-folded top linens to the foot of the bed or toward the other leg.			
10. Turned the stocking inside out down to the heel.			
11. Slipped the foot of the stocking over the toes, foot, and heel. Made sure the heel pocket was properly positioned on the person's heel. The toe opening was over or under the toes. Followed the manufacturer's instructions.			
12. Grasped the stocking top. Pulled the stocking up the leg. The stocking turned right side out as it was pulled up.			
13. Adjusted the stocking as needed. Made sure the stocking did not cause pressure on the toes.			
14. Removed twists, creases, or wrinkles. Made sure the stocking was even, snug, smooth, and wrinkle-free.			
15. Covered the leg. Repeated steps 9 through 14 for the other leg.			
16. Covered the person.			

Post-Procedure

	S	U	Comments
17. Provided for comfort as noted on the inside of the front textbook cover.			
18. Placed the call light within reach.			
19. Lowered the bed to its lowest position.			
20. Raised or lowered bed rails. Followed the care plan.			
21. Unscreened the person.			

Date of Satisfactory Completion _____   Instructor's Initials _____

Post-Procedure—cont'd   S   U   Comments

22. Completed a safety check of the room as noted on
    the inside of the front textbook cover.
23. Practiced hand hygiene.
24. Reported and recorded your observations.

Date of Satisfactory Completion _____   Instructor's Initials _____

Applying an Elastic Bandage

Name: _____   Date: _____

	S	U	Comments
Quality of Life			
• Knocked before entering the person's room.	_____	_____	_____
• Addressed the person by name.	_____	_____	_____
• Introduced yourself by name and title.	_____	_____	_____
• Explained the procedure to the person before starting and during the procedure.	_____	_____	_____
• Protected the person's rights during the procedure.	_____	_____	_____
• Handled the person gently during the procedure.	_____	_____	_____
Pre-Procedure			
1. Followed *Delegation Guidelines: Elastic Bandages* Reviewed *Promoting Safety and Comfort: Elastic Bandages.*	_____	_____	_____
	_____	_____	_____
2. Practiced hand hygiene.	_____	_____	_____
3. Collected the following.			
• Elastic bandage as directed by the nurse	_____	_____	_____
• Tape or clips (unless the bandage had Velcro)	_____	_____	_____
4. Identified the person. Checked the ID bracelet against the assignment sheet. Used 2 identifiers. Called the person by name.	_____	_____	_____
5. Provided for privacy.	_____	_____	_____
6. Raised the bed for body mechanics. Bed rails were up if used.	_____	_____	_____
Procedure			
7. Lowered the bed rail near you if up.	_____	_____	_____
8. Helped the person to a comfortable position. Exposed the part to be bandaged.	_____	_____	_____
9. Made sure the area was clean and dry.	_____	_____	_____
10. Held the bandage so that the roll was up. The loose end was on the bottom.	_____	_____	_____
11. Applied the bandage to the smallest part of the wrist, foot, ankle, or knee.	_____	_____	_____
12. Made two circular turns around the part.	_____	_____	_____
13. Made overlapping spiral turns in an upward direction. Each turn overlapped about ½ to ¾ of the previous turn. Made sure each overlap was equal.	_____	_____	_____
14. Applied the bandage smoothly with firm, even pressure. It was not tight.	_____	_____	_____
15. Ended the bandage with two circular turns.	_____	_____	_____
16. Secured the bandage in place with Velcro, tape, or clips. The clips were not under the body part.	_____	_____	_____
17. Checked the fingers or toes for coldness or cyanosis. Asked about pain, itching, numbness, or tingling. Removed the bandage if any were noted. Reported your observations to the nurse.	_____	_____	_____
Post-Procedure			
18. Provided for comfort as noted on the inside of the front textbook cover.	_____	_____	_____
19. Placed the call light within reach.	_____	_____	_____

Date of Satisfactory Completion _____   Instructor's Initials _____

Post-Procedure—cont'd

	S	U	Comments
20. Lowered the bed to a safe and comfortable level appropriate for the person. Followed the care plan.			
21. Raised or lowered bed rails. Followed the care plan.			
22. Unscreened the person.			
23. Completed a safety check of the room as noted on the inside of the front textbook cover.			
24. Practiced hand hygiene.			
25. Reported and recorded your observations.			

Date of Satisfactory Completion _____   Instructor's Initials _____

Applying a Dry, Non-Sterile Dressing

Name: _____ Date: _____

	S	U	Comments
Quality of Life			
• Knocked before entering the person's room.	____	____	_____
• Addressed the person by name.	____	____	_____
• Introduced yourself by name and title.	____	____	_____
• Explained the procedure to the person before starting and during the procedure.	____	____	_____
• Protected the person's rights during the procedure.	____	____	_____
• Handled the person gently during the procedure.	____	____	_____

Pre-Procedure

1. Followed *Delegation Guidelines:*
   a. *Wound Care*
   b. *Applying Dressings*
   Reviewed *Promoting Safety and Comfort:*   ____ ____ _____
   a. *Wound Care*
   b. *Applying Dressings*
2. Practiced hand hygiene.   ____ ____ _____
3. Collected the following.
   - Gloves   ____ ____ _____
   - Personal protective equipment (PPE) as needed   ____ ____ _____
   - Tape or Montgomery ties   ____ ____ _____
   - Dressings as directed by the nurse   ____ ____ _____
   - 4 × 4 gauze   ____ ____ _____
   - Saline solution as directed by the nurse   ____ ____ _____
   - Cleansing solution as directed by the nurse   ____ ____ _____
   - Adhesive remover   ____ ____ _____
   - Dressing set with scissors and forceps   ____ ____ _____
   - Plastic bag   ____ ____ _____
   - Bath blanket   ____ ____ _____
4. Practiced hand hygiene.   ____ ____ _____
5. Identified the person. Checked the ID bracelet against the assignment sheet. Used 2 identifiers. Called the person by name.   ____ ____ _____
6. Provided for privacy.   ____ ____ _____
7. Arranged the work area so that you would not have to reach over or turn your back on your work area.   ____ ____ _____
8. Raised the bed for body mechanics. Bed rails were up if used.   ____ ____ _____

Procedure

9. Lowered the bed rail near you if up.   ____ ____ _____
10. Helped the person to a comfortable position.   ____ ____ _____
11. Covered the person with a bath blanket. Fanfolded top linens to the foot of the bed.   ____ ____ _____
12. Exposed the affected body part.   ____ ____ _____
13. Made a cuff on the plastic bag. Placed it within reach.   ____ ____ _____
14. Practiced hand hygiene.   ____ ____ _____
15. Put on needed PPE. Put on gloves.   ____ ____ _____
16. Removed tape or undid Montgomery ties.
    a. *Tape:* held the skin down. Gently pulled the tape toward the wound.   ____ ____ _____

Date of Satisfactory Completion _____ Instructor's Initials _____

Procedure—cont'd	S	U	Comments
b. *Montgomery ties:* undid and folded ties away from the wound.	_____	_____	_____
17. Removed any adhesive from the skin. Picked up a gauze square with the forceps. Wet a 4 × 4 gauze dressing with the adhesive remover. Cleaned away from the wound.	_____	_____	_____
18. Removed gauze dressings. Started with the top dressing and removed each layer. Kept the soiled side of each dressing away from the person's sight. Put dressings in the plastic bag. They did not touch the outside of the bag.	_____	_____	_____
19. Removed the dressing over the wound very gently. Moistened the dressing with saline if it stuck to the wound. Discarded the dressing as in step 18.	_____	_____	_____
20. Observed the wound, drain site, and wound drainage.	_____	_____	_____
21. Removed the gloves and put them in the plastic bag. Practiced hand hygiene.	_____	_____	_____
22. Opened the new dressings.	_____	_____	_____
23. Put on clean gloves.	_____	_____	_____
24. Cleaned the wound with saline as directed by the nurse.	_____	_____	_____
25. Applied dressings as directed by the nurse.	_____	_____	_____
26. Secured the dressings in place. Used tape or Montgomery ties.	_____	_____	_____
27. Removed the gloves. Put them in the bag.	_____	_____	_____
28. Removed and discarded PPE.	_____	_____	_____
29. Practiced hand hygiene.	_____	_____	_____
30. Covered the person. Removed the bath blanket.	_____	_____	_____
Post-Procedure			
31. Provided for comfort as noted on the inside of the front textbook cover.	_____	_____	_____
32. Placed the call light within reach.	_____	_____	_____
33. Lowered the bed to a safe and comfortable level appropriate for the person. Followed the care plan.	_____	_____	_____
34. Raised or lowered bed rails. Followed the care plan.	_____	_____	_____
35. Returned equipment and supplies to the proper place. Left extra dressings and tape in the room.	_____	_____	_____
36. Discarded used supplies into the bag. Tied the bag closed. Discarded the bag following agency policy. Wore gloves.	_____	_____	_____
37. Cleaned your work area. Followed the Bloodborne Pathogen Standard.	_____	_____	_____
38. Unscreened the person.	_____	_____	_____
39. Completed a safety check of the room as noted on the inside of the front textbook cover.	_____	_____	_____
40. Removed and discarded gloves. Practiced hand hygiene.	_____	_____	_____
41. Reported and recorded your observations.	_____	_____	_____

Date of Satisfactory Completion _____   Instructor's Initials _____

Applying Heat and Cold Applications

Name: _____ Date: _____

Quality of Life	S	U	Comments
• Knocked before entering the person's room.	_____	_____	_____
• Addressed the person by name.	_____	_____	_____
• Introduced yourself by name and title.	_____	_____	_____
• Explained the procedure to the person before starting and during the procedure.	_____	_____	_____
• Protected the person's rights during the procedure.	_____	_____	_____
• Handled the person gently during the procedure.	_____	_____	_____

Pre-Procedure

	S	U	Comments

1. Followed *Delegation Guidelines:*
  a. *Wound Care*
  b. *Applying Heat and Cold*
  Reviewed *Promoting Safety and Comfort: Applying Heat and Cold.*
	_____
	
	_____
		_____
		
		_____
			_____
			
			_____

2. Practiced hand hygiene.	_____	_____	_____
3. Collected needed equipment. a. *For a hot compress:*			
• Basin	_____	_____	_____
• Water thermometer	_____	_____	_____
• Small towel, washcloth, or gauze squares	_____	_____	_____
• Plastic wrap or aquathermia pad	_____	_____	_____
• Ties, tape, or rolled gauze	_____	_____	_____
• Bath towel	_____	_____	_____
• Waterproof under-pad	_____	_____	_____
b. *For a hot soak:*			
• Water basin or arm or foot bath	_____	_____	_____
• Water thermometer	_____	_____	_____
• Waterproof under-pad	_____	_____	_____
• Bath blanket	_____	_____	_____
• Towel	_____	_____	_____
c. *For a sitz bath:*			
• Disposable sitz bath	_____	_____	_____
• Water thermometer	_____	_____	_____
• Two bath blankets, bath towels, and a clean gown	_____	_____	_____
d. *For a hot or cold pack:*			
• Commercial pack	_____	_____	_____
• Pack cover	_____	_____	_____
• Ties, tape, or rolled gauze (if needed)	_____	_____	_____
• Waterproof under-pad	_____	_____	_____
e. *For an aquathermia pad:*			
• Aquathermia pad and heating unit	_____	_____	_____
• Distilled water	_____	_____	_____
• Flannel cover or other cover as directed by the nurse	_____	_____	_____
• Ties, tape, or rolled gauze	_____	_____	_____

Date of Satisfactory Completion _____   Instructor's Initials _____

Pre-Procedure—cont'd	S	U	Comments
f. *For an ice bag, ice collar, or ice glove:*			
• Ice bag, collar, or glove	_____	_____	_____
• Crushed ice	_____	_____	_____
• Flannel cover or other cover as directed by the nurse	_____	_____	_____
• Paper towels	_____	_____	_____
g. *For a cold compress:*			
• Large basin with ice	_____	_____	_____
• Small basin with cold water	_____	_____	_____
• Gauze squares, washcloths, or small towels	_____	_____	_____
• Waterproof under-pad	_____	_____	_____
4. Identified the person. Checked the ID bracelet against the assignment sheet. Used 2 identifiers. Called the person by name.	_____	_____	_____

Procedure

	S	U	Comments
5. Provided for privacy.	_____	_____	_____
6. Positioned the person for the procedure.	_____	_____	_____
7. Placed the waterproof pad (if needed) under the body part.	_____	_____	_____
8. *For a hot compress:*			
a. Filled the basin ½ to ⅔ full with hot water as directed by the nurse. Measured water temperature.	_____	_____	_____
b. Placed the compress in the water.	_____	_____	_____
(1) Wrung out the compress.	_____	_____	_____
c. Applied the compress over the area. Noted the time.	_____	_____	_____
d. Covered the compress quickly. Did one of the following as directed by the nurse:			
(1) Applied plastic wrap and then a bath towel. Secured the towel in place with ties, tape, or rolled gauze.	_____	_____	_____
(2) Applied an aquathermia pad.	_____	_____	_____
9. *For a hot soak:*			
a. Filled the container ½ full with hot water as directed by the nurse. Measured water temperature.	_____	_____	_____
b. Placed the part into the water. Padded the edge of the container with a towel. Noted the time.	_____	_____	_____
c. Covered the person with a bath blanket for warmth.	_____	_____	_____
10. *For a sitz bath:*			
a. Placed the disposable sitz bath on the toilet seat.	_____	_____	_____
b. Filled the sitz bath ⅔ full with water as directed by the nurse. Measured water temperature.	_____	_____	_____
c. Secured the gown above the waist.	_____	_____	_____
d. Helped the person sit on the sitz bath. Noted the time.	_____	_____	_____
e. Provided for warmth. Placed a bath blanket around the shoulders. Placed another over the legs.	_____	_____	_____
f. Stayed with the person if he or she was weak or unsteady.	_____	_____	_____

Date of Satisfactory Completion _____   Instructor's Initials _____

Procedure—cont'd	S	U	Comments

11. *For an aquathermia pad:*

   a. Filled the heating unit to the fill line with distilled water. _____ _____ _____

   b. Removed the bubbles. Placed the pad and tubing below the heating unit. Tilted the heating unit from side to side. _____ _____ _____

   c. Set the temperature as the nurse directed (usually 105°F [40.5°C]). Removed the key. (Gave the key to the nurse after the procedure.) _____ _____ _____

   d. Placed the pad in the cover. _____ _____ _____

   e. Plugged in the unit. Let water warm to the desired temperature. _____ _____ _____

   f. Set the heating unit on the bedside stand. Kept the pad and connecting hoses level with the unit. Hoses did not have kinks. _____ _____ _____

   g. Applied the pad to the part. Noted the time. _____ _____ _____

   h. Secured the pad in place with ties, tape, or rolled gauze. _____ _____ _____

12. *For a hot or cold pack:*

   a. Squeezed, kneaded, or struck the pack as directed by the manufacturer. _____ _____ _____

   b. Placed the pack in the cover. _____ _____ _____

   c. Applied the pack. Noted the time. _____ _____ _____

   d. Secured the pack in place with ties, tape, or rolled gauze. (Some secure with Velcro straps.) _____ _____ _____

13. *For an ice bag, collar, or glove:*

   a. Filled the device with water. Put in the stopper. Turned the device upside down to check for leaks. _____ _____ _____

   b. Emptied the device. _____ _____ _____

   c. Filled the device ½ to ⅔ full with crushed ice or ice chips. _____ _____ _____

   d. Removed excess air. Bent, twisted, or squeezed the device or pressed it against a firm surface. _____ _____ _____

   e. Placed the cap or stopper on securely. _____ _____ _____

   f. Dried the device with paper towels. _____ _____ _____

   g. Placed the device in the cover. _____ _____ _____

   h. Applied the device. Noted the time. _____ _____ _____

   i. Secured the device in place with ties, tape, or rolled gauze. _____ _____ _____

14. *For a cold compress:*

   a. Placed the small basin with cold water into the large basin with ice. _____ _____ _____

   b. Placed the compresses into the cold water. _____ _____ _____

   c. Wrung out a compress. _____ _____ _____

   d. Applied the compress to the part. Noted the time. _____ _____ _____

15. Placed the call light within reach. Unscreened the person. _____ _____ _____

16. Raised or lowered bed rails. Followed the care plan. _____ _____ _____

17. Checked the person every 5 minutes.

   a. Checked for signs and symptoms of complications. Removed the application if any occurred. Told the nurse at once. _____ _____ _____

Date of Satisfactory Completion _____   Instructor's Initials _____

Procedure—cont'd	S	U	Comments
b. Changed the application if cooling (hot applications) or warming (cold applications) occurred.	_____	_____	_____
18. Removed the application after 15 to 20 minutes.	_____	_____	_____
Post-Procedure			
19. Provided for comfort as noted on the inside of the front textbook cover.	_____	_____	_____
20. Placed the call light within reach.	_____	_____	_____
21. Raised or lowered bed rails. Followed the care plan.	_____	_____	_____
22. Unscreened the person.	_____	_____	_____
23. Cleaned, rinsed, dried, (with clean, dry paper towels) and returned reusable items to their proper place. Followed agency policy for soiled linen. Wore gloves for this step.	_____	_____	_____
24. Completed a safety check of the room as noted on the inside of the front textbook cover.	_____	_____	_____
25. Removed and discarded the gloves. Practiced hand hygiene.	_____	_____	_____
26. Reported and recorded your observations.	_____	_____	_____

Date of Satisfactory Completion _____   Instructor's Initials _____

Using a Pulse Oximeter

Name: _____   Date: _____

Quality of Life	S	U	Comments
• Knocked before entering the person's room.	___	___	___
• Addressed the person by name.	___	___	___
• Introduced yourself by name and title.	___	___	___
• Explained the procedure before starting and during the procedure.	___	___	___
• Protected the person's rights during the procedure.	___	___	___
• Handled the person gently during the procedure.	___	___	___

Pre-Procedure

	S	U	Comments
1. Followed *Delegation Guidelines: Pulse Oximetry.* Reviewed *Promoting Safety and Comfort: Pulse Oximetry.*	___	___	___
2. Practiced hand hygiene.	___	___	___
3. Collected the following before going to the person's room.			
• Oximeter	___	___	___
• Tape (if needed)	___	___	___
• Towel	___	___	___
4. Arranged your work area.	___	___	___
5. Practiced hand hygiene.	___	___	___
6. Identified the person. Checked the ID bracelet against your assignment sheet. Used 2 identifiers. Also called the person by name.	___	___	___
7. Provided for privacy.	___	___	___

Procedure

	S	U	Comments
8. Provided for comfort.	___	___	___
9. Dried the site with a towel.	___	___	___
10. Clipped or taped the sensor to the site.	___	___	___
11. Turned on the oximeter.	___	___	___
12. For continuous monitoring:			
a. Set the high and low alarm limits for SpO_2 and pulse rate.	___	___	___
b. Turned on radio and visual alarms.	___	___	___
13. Checked the person's pulse (apical or radial) with the pulse on the display. The pulse rates were about the same. Noted both pulses on your assignment sheet.			
14. Read the SpO_2 on the display. Noted the value on the flow sheet and your assignment sheet.	___	___	___
15. Left the sensor in place for continuous monitoring. Otherwise, turned off the device and removed the sensor.	___	___	___

Post-Procedure

	S	U	Comments
16. Provided for comfort as noted on the inside of the front textbook cover.	___	___	___
17. Placed the call light within reach.	___	___	___
18. Unscreened the person.	___	___	___
19. Completed a safety check of the room as noted on the inside of the front textbook cover.	___	___	___
20. Returned the device to its proper place (unless monitoring is continuous).	___	___	___
21. Practiced hand hygiene.	___	___	___
22. Reported and recorded the SpO_2, the pulse rates, and your other observations.	___	___	___

Date of Satisfactory Completion _____   Instructor's Initials _____

VIDEO

Assisting with Deep-Breathing and Coughing Exercises

Name: _____ Date: _____

	S	U	Comments
Quality of Life			
• Knocked before entering the person's room.	_____	_____	_____
• Addressed the person by name.	_____	_____	_____
• Introduced yourself by name and title.	_____	_____	_____
• Explained the procedure to the person before starting and during the procedure.	_____	_____	_____
• Protected the person's rights during the procedure.	_____	_____	_____
• Handled the person gently during the procedure.	_____	_____	_____
Pre-Procedure			
1. Followed *Delegation Guidelines: Deep Breathing and Coughing.*	_____	_____	_____
Reviewed *Promoting Safety and Comfort: Deep Breathing and Coughing*	_____	_____	_____
2. Practiced hand hygiene.	_____	_____	_____
3. Identified the person. Checked the ID bracelet against the assignment sheet. Used 2 identifiers. Called the person by name.	_____	_____	_____
4. Provided for privacy.	_____	_____	_____
Procedure			
5. Lowered the bed rail if up.	_____	_____	_____
6. Helped the person to a comfortable sitting position: sitting on the side of the bed, semi-Fowler's, or Fowler's.	_____	_____	_____
7. Had the person deep breathe.			
a. Had the person place the hands over the rib cage.	_____	_____	_____
b. Had the person take a deep breath. It was as deep as possible. Reminded the person to inhale through the nose.	_____	_____	_____
c. Asked the person to hold the breath for 2 to 3 seconds.	_____	_____	_____
d. Asked the person to exhale slowly through pursed lips. Asked the person to exhale until the ribs moved as far down as possible.	_____	_____	_____
e. Repeated this step four more times.	_____	_____	_____
8. Asked the person to cough.			
a. *If the person did not have a productive cough:* Had the person place both hands over the incision. One hand was on top of the other. The person could hold a pillow or folded towel over the chest or abdominal incision.	_____	_____	_____
b. *If the person had a productive cough:*			
1. Had the person practice cough etiquette.	_____	_____	_____
2. Splinted the chest or abdominal incision with your hands or a pillow. Wore gloves.	_____	_____	_____
c. Had the person take in a deep breath as in step 7.	_____	_____	_____
d. Asked the person to cough strongly twice with the mouth open.	_____	_____	_____
Post-Procedure			
9. Provided for comfort as noted on the inside of the front textbook cover.	_____	_____	_____

Date of Satisfactory Completion _____ Instructor's Initials _____

Post-Procedure—cont'd   S   U   Comments

10. Placed the call light within reach.   _____   _____   _____

11. Raised or lowered bed rails. Followed the care plan.   _____   _____   _____

12. Unscreened the person.   _____   _____   _____

13. Completed a safety check of the room as noted on   _____   _____   _____
    the inside of the front textbook cover.

14. Practiced hand hygiene.   _____   _____   _____

15. Reported and recorded your observations.   _____   _____   _____

Date of Satisfactory Completion _____   Instructor's Initials _____

Caring for Eyeglasses

Name: _____   Date: _____

	S	U	Comments
Quality of Life			
• Knocked before entering the person's room.			
• Addressed the person by name.			
• Introduced self by name and title.			
• Explained the procedure to the person before starting and during the procedure.			
• Protected the person's rights during the procedure.			
• Handled the person gently during the procedure.			
Pre-Procedure			
1. Followed *Delegation Guidelines: Corrective Lenses.* Reviewed *Promoting Safety and Comfort: Corrective Lenses*			
2. Practiced hand hygiene.			
3. Collected the following.			
• Eyeglass case			
• Cleaning solution or warm water			
• Disposable lens cloth or cotton cloth			
Procedure			
4. Removed the eyeglasses.			
a. Held the frames in front of the ears.			
b. Lifted the frames from the ears. Brought the eyeglasses down away from the face.			
5. Cleaned the lenses with a cleaning solution or warm water. Cleaned in a circular motion. Dried the lenses with the cloth.			
6. *If the person will not wear the eyeglasses:*			
a. Opened the eyeglass case.			
b. Folded the glasses. Put them in the case. Do not touch the clean lenses.			
c. Placed the case in the top drawer of the bedside stand.			
7. *If the person wears the eyeglasses:*			
a. Held the frames at each side. Placed them over the ears.			
b. Adjusted the eyeglasses so the nose-piece rests on the nose.			
c. Returned the case to the top drawer of the bedside stand.			
Post-Procedure			
8. Provided for comfort.			
9. Placed the call light and other needed items within reach.			
10. Returned the cleaning solution to its proper place.			
11. Discarded the disposable cloth.			
12. Completed a safety check of the room.			
13. Practiced hand hygiene.			
14. Reported and recorded your observations.			

Date of Satisfactory Completion _____   Instructor's Initials _____

Adult CPR—1 Rescuer

Name: _____   Date: _____

Procedure	S	U	Comments
1. Made sure the scene was safe.	_____	_____	_____
2. Checked if the person was responding. Tapped or gently shook the person. Called the person by name (if known). Shouted: "Are you okay?"	_____	_____	_____
3. Called for help.	_____	_____	_____
4. Activated the EMS system or the agency's RRT.			
a. *If alone with a phone*, used it while continuing to give care.	_____	_____	_____
b. *If alone without a phone*, left the person to activate the EMS system before starting CPR.	_____	_____	_____
c. *If help arrived*, sent him or her to activate the EMS system.	_____	_____	_____
5. Got an AED.			
a. *If alone*, got the AED before starting CPR.	_____	_____	_____
b. *If help arrived*, asked him or her to get the AED.	_____	_____	_____
6. Checked for breathing and a carotid pulse at the same time. Looked for no breathing or only gasping. Started CPR for no breathing (or only gasping) and no definite pulse within 10 seconds.	_____	_____	_____
7. Positioned the person for CPR if not already done. The person was supine on a hard, flat surface.	_____	_____	_____
8. Exposed the person's chest.			
9. Gave CPR.			
a. Placed 2 hands on the lower half of the sternum. Gave 30 chest compressions at a rate of 100 to 120 per minute. Established a regular rhythm. Counted out loud. Allowed the chest to recoil between compressions.	_____	_____	_____
b. Opened the airway. Used the head tilt–chin lift method.	_____	_____	_____

c. Gave two breaths. Used a barrier device if one was available. Each breath took only 1 second. The chest rose. If the first breath didn't make the chest rise:
    (1) Opened the airway. Used the head tilt-chin lift method.
    (2) Gave another breath.
	_____	_____	_____

10. Continued the cycle of 30 chest compressions followed by 2 breaths. Limited interruptions in compressions to less than 10 seconds. Used the AED when available.	_____	_____	_____
11. Continued CPR until help took over or the person began to move. If movement occurred, placed the person in the recovery position.	_____	_____	_____

Date of Satisfactory Completion _____   Instructor's Initials _____

Adult CPR with AED—Two Rescuers

Name: _____ Date: _____

Procedure	S	U	Comments
1. Made sure the scene was safe.	___	___	___
2. *Rescuer 1*	___	___	___
a. Checked if the person was responding. Tapped or gently shook the person. Called the person by name, if known. Shouted: "Are you okay?"	___	___	___
b. Shouted for help if the person did not respond.	___	___	___
3. *Rescuer 2:*			
a. Activated the EMS system or the agency's RRT using a phone if available or left to do so.	___	___	___
b. Got a defibrillator (AED) if one was available.	___	___	___
4. *Rescuer 1:* Followed steps 6 through 10 in procedure: *Adult CPR-1 Rescuer.*	___	___	___
5. *Rescuer 2:*			
a. Opened the case with the AED.	___	___	___
b. Turned on the AED.	___	___	___
c. Applied adult electrode pads to the person's chest. Followed the instructions and diagram provided with the AED.	___	___	___
d. Attached the connecting cables to the AED.	___	___	___
e. Cleared away from the person. Made sure no one was touching the person.	___	___	___
f. Let the AED check the person's heart rhythm.	___	___	___
g. Made sure everyone was clear of the person if the AED advised a "shock." Loudly instructed others not to touch the person. Said: "I am clear, you are clear, everyone is clear!" Looked to make sure no one was touching the person.	___	___	___
h. Pressed the shock button if the AED advised a "shock."	___	___	___
6. *Rescuers 1 and 2-performed 2-rescuer CPR.*			
a. Began with compressions. One rescuer gave 30 chest compressions. The rescuer paused for the other rescuer to give 2 breaths.	___	___	___
b. The other rescuer gave 2 breaths after every 30 chest compressions.	___	___	___
7. Paused for a rhythm check when prompted by the AED. Repeated steps 5, e–h after 2 minutes of CPR. Changed positions and continued CPR beginning with compressions.	___	___	___
8. Continued until help took over or the person began to move. If movement occurred, placed the person in the recovery position.	___	___	___

Date of Satisfactory Completion _____ Instructor's Initials _____

Assisting With Post-Mortem Care

Name: _____   Date: _____

	S	U	Comments

Pre-Procedure

1. Followed *Delegation Guidelines: Care of the Body After Death.* Reviewed *Promoting Safety and Comfort: Care of the Body After Death.*
2. Practiced hand hygiene.
3. Collected the following.
   - Post-mortem kit (shroud or body bag, gown, ID tags, gauze squares, safety pins)
   - Disposable bed protectors
   - Wash basin
   - Bath towels and washcloths
   - Denture cup
   - Items for shaving facial hair
   - Tape
   - Dressings
   - Gloves
   - Cotton balls
   - Valuables envelope
4. Provided for privacy.
5. Raised the bed for body mechanics.
6. Made sure the bed was flat.

Procedure

7. Put on the gloves.
8. Positioned the body supine. Arms and legs were straight. A pillow was under the head and shoulders. Or you raised the head of the bed 15 to 20 degrees per agency policy.
9. Closed the eyes. Gently pulled the eyelids over the eyes. Applied moist cotton balls gently over the eyelids if the eyes would not stay closed.
10. Inserted dentures if it was agency policy. If not, put them in a labeled denture cup.
11. Closed the mouth. If necessary, placed a rolled towel under the chin to keep the mouth closed.
12. Removed all jewelry, except for wedding rings if this was agency policy. Listed the jewelry that you removed. Placed the jewelry and the list in a valuables envelope.
13. Placed a cotton ball over the rings. Taped them in place.
14. Removed drainage containers.
15. Removed tubes and catheters. Used the gauze squares as the nurse directed.
16. Shaved facial hair if agency policy or if desired by the family.
17. Bathed soiled areas with plain water. Dried thoroughly.
18. Placed a bed protector under the buttocks.

Date of Satisfactory Completion _____   Instructor's Initials _____

Procedure—cont'd   S   U   Comments

19. Removed soiled dressings. Replaced them with clean ones.

20. Put a clean gown on the body. Positioned the body as in step 8.

21. Brushed and combed the hair if necessary.

22. Covered the body to the shoulders with a sheet if the family would view the body.

23. Gathered the person's belongings. Put them in a bag labeled with the person's name. Made sure eyeglasses, hearing aids, and other valuables were included.

24. Removed supplies, equipment, and linens. Straightened the room. Provided soft lighting.

25. Removed and discarded the gloves. Practiced hand hygiene.

26. Let the family view the body. Provided for privacy. Returned to the room after they left.

27. Practiced hand hygiene. Put on gloves.

28. Filled out the ID tags. Tied one to the ankle or to the right big toe.

29. Placed the body in the body bag or covered it with a sheet. Or applied the shroud.
    a. Positioned the shroud under the body.
    b. Brought the top down over the head.
    c. Folded the bottom up over the feet.
    d. Folded the sides over the body.
    e. Pinned or taped the shroud in place.

30. Attached the second ID tag to the body bag, sheet, or shroud.

31. Left the denture cup with the body.

32. Pulled the privacy curtain around the bed or closed the door.

Post-Procedure

33. Removed and discarded the gloves. Practiced hand hygiene.

34. Cleaned the unit after the body was removed. Wore gloves for this step.

35. Removed the gloves. Practiced hand hygiene.

36. Reported the following.
    a. The time the body was taken by the funeral director
    b. What was done with jewelry, other valuables, and personal items
    c. What was done with dentures

Date of Satisfactory Completion _____   Instructor's Initials _____

PREPARING FOR THE COMPETENCY EVALUATION

After completing your state's training program, you need to pass the competency evaluation. The purpose of the competency evaluation is to make sure you can do your job safely. This section will help you prepare for the test.

COMPETENCY EVALUATION

The competency evaluation has a written test and a skills test. The number of questions varies with each state. Each question has four answer choices. Although some questions may appear to have more than one possible answer, there is only one best answer. You will have about 1 minute to read and answer each question. Some questions take less time to read and answer. Other questions take longer. You should have enough time to take the test without feeling rushed.

The content of the written test varies depending on your state. Content may include:
- Activities of Daily Living—hygiene, dressing and grooming, nutrition and hydration, elimination, rest/sleep/comfort
- Basic Nursing Skills—infection control, safety/ emergency, therapeutic/technical procedures (e.g., vital signs, bedmaking), data collection and reporting
- Restorative Skills—prevention, self-care/independence
- Emotional and Mental Health Needs
- Spiritual and Cultural Needs
- The Person's Rights
- Legal and Ethical Behavior
- Being a Member of the Health Care Team
- Communication

The written test is given as a paper and pencil test in most states. Some test sites may use computers. You do not need computer experience to take the test on the computer. If you have difficulty reading English, you may request to take an oral test. Talk with your instructor or employer about details for computer testing or oral testing.

The skills test involves performing five nursing skills that you learned in your training program. These skills are chosen randomly. You do not select the skills. You are allowed about 30 minutes to do the skills. See the Skills Evaluation Review for more information about the skills test.

TAKING THE COMPETENCY EVALUATION

To register for the test, you need to complete an application. Your instructor or employer tells you when and where the tests are given. There is a fee for the evaluation. If you work in a nursing center, the employer may pay this fee. If you pay the fee, you may need to purchase a money order or certified check. Make sure your name is on the money order or certified check. Cash and personal checks may not be accepted.

Plan to arrive at the test site about 15 to 30 minutes before the evaluation begins. Most centers do not admit you if you are late. Know the exact location of the test site and room. Drive or take transportation to the test site a few days or a week before the test. Making a "dry run" lets you know how much time you need to travel, park, and get to the test site. It will also help decrease your anxiety level on the test day.

To be admitted to the test, you need two pieces of identification (ID). The first form of ID is a government-issued document such as a driver's license or passport. It must have a current photo and your signature. The name on the ID must be the same as the name on your application form. If your name has changed and you have not been able to have the name changed on your identification documents, ask your instructor or employer what to do. The second form of ID must include your name and signature. Examples include a library card, hunting license, or credit card.

Take several sharpened Number 2 pencils to the test. For the skills test you will need a watch with a second hand. You may need a person to play the role of the patient or resident. Ask your instructor or employer how this is done in your state.

Taking the written test and skills test may take several hours. You may want to bring snacks or lunch and a beverage to the testing site. Eating and drinking are not allowed during the test. However, you may be told where you can eat while waiting for the test.

You cannot bring textbooks, study notes, or other materials into the testing room. The only exception may be a language translation dictionary that you show to the proctor (a person who monitors the test) before the test begins. Cell phones, pagers, calculators, or other electronic devices are not permitted during testing. Children and pets are not allowed in the testing areas.

STUDYING FOR THE COMPETENCY EVALUATION

You began to prepare for the written and skills test during your training program. You learned the basic nursing content and skills needed to provide safe, quality care. The following suggestions can help you study for the competency evaluation.

- Begin to study at least 2 to 3 weeks before the test. Plan to study for 1 to 2 hours each day.
- Decide on a specific time to study. Choose a study time that is best for you. This may be early in the morning before others are awake. It may be in the evening after others go to sleep. Try to choose a time when you are mentally alert.
- Choose a specific area to study in. This area should be quiet, well lit, and comfortable. You should have enough room to write and to spread out your books, notes, and other study aids—CD and DVD. The area does not need to be noise-free. The testing site is not absolutely quiet. You want to concentrate and not be distracted by the noise around you.
- Collect everything you need before settling down to study. This includes your textbook, notes, paper, highlighters, pens or pencils, CD, and DVD.
- Take short breaks when you need them. Take a break when your mind begins to wander or if you feel sleepy.
- Develop a study plan. Write your plan down so that you can refer to it. Study one content area before going on to the next. For example, study personal hygiene before going on to vital signs. Do not jump from one subject to another.
- Use a variety of ways to study.
  - Use index cards to help you review abbreviations and terminology. Put the abbreviation or term on the front of the card and place the meaning on the back. Take the cards with you and review them whenever you have a break or are waiting.
  - Record key points. You can listen to the recording while cooking or while riding in the car.
  - Study groups are another way to prepare for a test. Group members can quiz each other.
- To remember what you are learning, try these ideas.
  - Relax when you study. When relaxed, you learn information quickly and recall it with greater ease.
  - Repeat what you are learning. Say it out loud. This helps you remember the idea.
  - Make the information you are learning meaningful. Think about how the information will help you be a good nursing assistant.
  - Write down what you are learning. Writing helps you remember information. Prepare study sheets.
  - Be positive about what you are learning. You remember what you find interesting.
- Suggestions for studying if you have children:
  - When you first come home from work or school, spend time with your children. Then plan study time.
  - Select educational programs on TV that your children can watch as you study. Or get a DVD from the library.
  - When you take your study breaks, spend time with your children.
  - Ask other adults to take care of the children while you study.
- Take the two 75-question practice tests in this section. Each question has the correct answer and the reason why an answer is correct or incorrect. If you practice taking tests, you are more likely to pass them. Take the practice tests under conditions similar to the real test. Work within time limits.
- If your state has a practice test and a candidate handbook, study the content. Some states have practice tests online.

MANAGING ANXIETY

Almost everyone dreads taking tests. It is common and normal to experience anxiety before taking a test. If used wisely, anxiety can actually help you do well. When you are anxious, that means you are concerned. You may be concerned about how prepared you are to take the test. Or you may be concerned about how you will feel about yourself if you do not pass the test. Being concerned usually results in some action. To overcome anxiety before the test:

- Study and prepare for the test. That helps increase your confidence as you recall or clarify what you have learned. Anxiety decreases as confidence increases. When you think you know the information, keep studying. This reinforces your learning.
- Develop a positive mental attitude. You can pass this test. You took tests in your training program and passed them. Praise yourself. Talk to yourself in a positive way. If a negative thought enters your mind, stop it at once. Challenge the mental thought and tell yourself you will pass the test.
- Visualize success. Think about how wonderful you will feel when you are notified that you have passed the test.
- Perform breathing exercises. Breathe slowly and deeply.
- Perform regular exercise. Exercise helps you stay physically fit. It also helps keep you calm.
- Good nourishment helps you think clearly. Eat a nourishing meal before the test. Do not skip breakfast. Vitamin C helps fight short-term stress. Protein and calcium help overcome the effects of long-term stress. Complex carbohydrates (pasta, nuts, yogurt) can help settle your nerves. Eat familiar foods the day before and the day of the test. Do not eat foods that could cause stomach or intestinal upset.
- Maintain a normal routine the day before the test.
- Get a good night's sleep before the test. Go to bed early enough so that you do not oversleep or are too tired to get up. Set your alarm clock properly. You may want to set two alarm clocks.
- Do not "cram" the evening before or the day of the test. Last-minute cramming increases your anxiety. Do something relaxing with family and friends.
- Avoid drinking large amounts of coffee, colas, water, or other beverages. You do not want to be uncomfortable with a full bladder when you take the test.
- Wear comfortable clothes. Dress in layers so that you are prepared for a cold or warm room.

- If you are a woman, remember that worry and anxiety can affect your menstrual cycle. Wear a panty liner, sanitary napkin, or tampon if you think your period may start. This eliminates worry about soiling your clothing during the test.
- Allow plenty of time for travel, traffic, and parking.
- Arrive early enough to use the restroom before the test begins.
- Do not talk about the test with others. Their panic or anxiety may affect your self-confidence.

TAKING THE TEST

Follow these guidelines for taking the test.
- Listen carefully and follow the instructions given by the proctor (person administering the test).
- When you receive the test, make certain you have all the test pages.
- Read and follow all directions carefully.
- You are not allowed to ask questions about the content of the test questions.
- Do deep-breathing and muscle-relaxation exercises as needed.
- Cheating of any kind is not allowed. If the proctor sees you giving or receiving any type of assistance, your test booklet is taken and you must leave the testing site.
- If using a computer answer sheet, completely fill in the bubble.
- If you make a mistake, erase the wrong answer completely. Do not make any stray marks on the paper. Not erasing completely or leaving stray marks could cause the computer to misread your answer.
- Do not worry or get anxious if people finish the test before you do. Persons who finish a test early do not necessarily have a better score than those who finish later.
- You cannot take any evaluation materials or notes out of the testing room.

ANSWERING MULTIPLE-CHOICE QUESTIONS

Pace yourself during the test. First, answer all the questions that you know. Then go back and answer skipped questions. Sometimes you will remember the answer later. Or another test question may give you a clue to the one you skipped. Spending too much time on a question can cost you valuable time later. To help you answer the questions or statements:
- Always read the questions or statements carefully. Do not scan or glance at questions. Scanning or glancing can cause you to miss important key words. Read each word of the question.

- Before reading the answers, decide what the answer is in your own words. Then read all four answers to the question. Select the one best answer.
- Do not read into a question. Take the question as it is asked. Do not add your own thoughts and ideas to the question. Do not assume or suppose "what if." Just respond to the information provided.
- Trust your common sense. If unsure of an answer, select your first choice. Do not change your answer unless you are absolutely sure of the correct answer. Your first reaction is usually correct.
- Look for key words in every question. Sometimes key words are in italics, highlighted, or underlined. Common key words are: *always, never, first, except, best, not, correct, incorrect, true,* or *false.*
- Know which words can make a statement correct (e.g., *may, can, usually, most, at least, sometimes*). The word "except" can make a question a false statement.
- Be careful of answers with these key words or phrases: *always, never, every, only, all, none, at all times,* or *at no time.* These words and phrases do not allow for exceptions. In nursing, exceptions are generally present. However, sometimes answers containing these words are correct. For example, which of the following is correct and which are incorrect?
  a. Always use a turning sheet.
  b. Never shake linens.
  c. Soap is used for all baths.
  d. The signal light must always be attached to the bed.

The correct answer is b. Incorrect answers are a, c, and d.
- Omit answers that are obviously wrong. Then choose the best of the remaining answers.
- Go back to the questions you skipped. Answer all questions by eliminating or narrowing your choices. Always mark an answer even if you are not sure.
- Review the test a second time for completeness and accuracy before turning it in.
- Make sure you have answered each question. Also check that you have given only one answer for each question.
- Remember, the test is not designed to trick or confuse you. The written competency evaluation tests what you know, not what you do not know. You know more than you are asked.

ONLINE TESTING

The test may be given by computer at the test site. Ask your instructor what computer skills you will need. You usually do not need keyboard or typing skills. You will use a computer mouse to select answers. Also, you will usually receive instruction before the test begins. This will let you practice using the computer before starting the test.

TEXTBOOK CHAPTERS REVIEW

NOTE: This review covers selected chapters based on Competency Evaluation requirements.

CHAPTER 1 INTRODUCTION TO HEALTH CARE

HOSPITALS

- Hospitals provide emergency care, surgery, nursing care, x-ray procedures and treatments, and laboratory testing. They also provide respiratory, physical, occupational, speech, and other therapies. Persons cared for in hospitals are called *patients*. Hospital *patients* have acute, chronic, or terminal illnesses.

LONG-TERM CARE CENTERS

- Provide care for people who do not need hospital care but cannot care for themselves at home.
- Provide medical and nursing, dietary, recreational, rehabilitative, and social services. Housekeeping and laundry services are also provided.
- Residents are older or disabled.
- Some have chronic diseases, poor nutrition, memory problems, or poor health.
- Some residents are recovering from illness, injury, or surgery.
- Some residents return home when well enough. Some residents need nursing care until death.
- Long-term care centers include board and care homes, assisted living residences, nursing centers, skilled nursing facilities, hospices, Alzheimer's or dementia care units, and rehabilitation and subacute care units.
- Long-term care centers meet the needs of:
  - Alert, oriented persons
  - Confused and disoriented persons
  - Persons needing complete care
  - Short-term residents
  - Persons needing respite care
  - Life-long residents
  - Residents who are mentally ill
  - Terminally ill persons

THE HEALTH TEAM

- In nursing centers, it is called the interdisciplinary health care team.
- Made up of many health care workers whose skills and knowledge focus on total care.
- Works together to provide coordinated quality care to meet each person's needs.
- Follows the direction of the RN leading the team.

The Nursing Team

- All focus on the physical, social, emotional, and spiritual needs of the person and family.
- Care is coordinated by an RN.

Nursing Assistants

- Report to the nurse supervising their work.
- Perform delegated tasks under the supervision of a licensed nurse.
- Have passed a nursing assistant training and competency evaluation program.

MEETING STANDARDS

Survey Process

- Surveys are done to see if agencies meet set standards for licensure, certification, and accreditation.
  - A license is issued by the state. A center must have a license to operate and provide care.
  - Certification is required to receive Medicare and Medicaid funds.
  - Accreditation is voluntary. It signals quality and excellence.

Your Role

- Provide quality care.
- Protect the person's rights.
- Provide for the person's and your own safety.
- Help keep the center clean and safe.
- Conduct yourself in a professional manner.
- Have good work ethics.
- Follow agency policies and procedures.
- Answer questions honestly and completely.

CHAPTER 1 REVIEW QUESTIONS

Circle the BEST answer.

1. Nursing assistants do all the following *except*
   a. Provide quality care
   b. Follow agency policies and procedures
   c. Conduct themselves in an unprofessional manner
   d. Help keep the agency clean and safe

2. Nursing assistants report to
   a. Other nursing assistants
   b. Licensed nurses
   c. The administrator
   d. The medical director
3. The health team does all the following *except*
   a. Involves many health care workers
   b. Follows the direction of the nursing assistant
   c. Works together to provide coordinated care
   d. The RN leads the team

Answers to Chapter 1 questions are on p. 450.

CHAPTER 2 THE PERSON'S RIGHTS

- Centers must protect and promote residents' rights. Centers must inform residents of their rights. Residents must be free to exercise their rights without interference. If residents are not able to exercise their rights, legal representatives do so for them.
- *The Patient Care Partnership: Understanding Expectations, Rights, and Responsibilities* document explains the person's rights and expectations during hospital stays. The relationships among the doctor, health team, and patient are stressed.

THE OMNIBUS BUDGET RECONCILIATION ACT OF 1987 (OBRA)

- OBRA is a federal law. It applies to all 50 states.
- OBRA requires that nursing centers provide care in a manner and in a setting that maintains or improves each person's quality of life, health, and safety.
- OBRA requires nursing assistant training and competency evaluation.
- Residents' rights are a major part of OBRA.

INFORMATION

- The right to information includes:
  - Access to all records about the person, including medical records, incident reports, contracts, and financial records
  - Information about his or her health condition
  - Information about his or her doctor, including name, specialty, and contact information
- Report any request for information to the nurse. Do not give information described earlier to the person or family.

REFUSING TREATMENT

- The person has the right to refuse treatment.
- A person who does not give consent or refuses treatment cannot be treated against his or her wishes.

- The center must find out what the person is refusing and why.
- Advance directives are part of the right to refuse treatment. They include living wills and instructions about life support.
- Report any treatment refusal to the nurse.

PRIVACY AND CONFIDENTIALITY

- Residents have the right to:
  - Personal privacy. The person's body is not exposed unnecessarily. Only staff directly involved in care and treatments are present. The person must give consent for others to be present. A person has the right to use the bathroom in private. Privacy is maintained for all personal care measures.
  - Visit with others in private—in areas where others cannot see or hear them. This includes phone calls.
  - Send and receive mail without others interfering. No one can open mail the person sends or receives without his or her consent.
- Information about the person's care, treatment, and condition is kept confidential. So are medical and financial records.

PERSONAL CHOICE

- Residents have the right to make their own choices. They can:
  - Choose their own doctors.
  - Take part in planning and deciding their care and treatment.
  - Choose activities, schedules, and care based on their preferences.
  - Choose when to get up and go to bed, what to wear, how to spend their time, and what to eat.
  - Choose friends and visitors inside and outside the center.

GRIEVANCES

- Residents have the right to voice concerns, questions, and complaints about treatment or care.
- The center must promptly try to correct the matter.
- No one can punish the person in any way for voicing the grievance.

WORK

- The person is not required to work or perform services for the center.
- The person has the right to work or perform services if he or she wants to.

TAKING PART IN RESIDENT GROUPS

- The person has the right to:
  - Form and take part in resident groups.
  - Take part in social, cultural, religious, and community events. The resident has the right to help in getting to and from events of their choice.

PERSONAL ITEMS

- The resident has the right to:
  - Keep and use personal items, such as clothing and some furnishings.
  - Have his or her property protected and treated with care and respect. Items are labeled with the person's name.
- Protect yourself and the center from being accused of stealing a person's property. Do not go through a person's closet, drawers, purse, or other space without the person's knowledge and consent. If a nurse asks you to inspect closets and drawers, follow center policy for reporting and recording the inspection.

FREEDOM FROM ABUSE, MISTREATMENT, AND NEGLECT

- Residents have the right to be free from:
  - Verbal, sexual, physical, or mental abuse
  - Involuntary seclusion—separating a person from others against his or her will, keeping the person to a certain area, and keeping the person away from his or her room without consent
- No one can abuse, neglect, or mistreat a resident. This includes center staff, volunteers, other residents, family members, visitors, and legal representatives.
- Nursing centers must investigate suspected or reported cases of abuse. They cannot employ persons who:
  - Were found guilty of abusing, neglecting, or mistreating others by a court of law.
  - Have a finding entered into the state's nursing assistant registry about abuse, neglect, mistreatment, or wrongful acts involving the person's money or property.

FREEDOM FROM RESTRAINT

- Residents have the right not to have body movements restricted by restraints or drugs.
- Restraints are used only to protect the person or others from harm. A doctor's order is needed for restraint use.

QUALITY OF LIFE

- Residents must be cared for in a manner that promotes dignity and respect for self. Physical, social, and mental well-being must be promoted. Review

Box 2-2, OBRA Required Actions to Promote Dignity and Privacy, in the textbook.
- Centers must provide activity programs that enhance each person's physical, mental, and psycho-social well-being. Centers must provide religious services for spiritual health. You assist residents to and from activity programs. You may need to help them with activities.
- Residents have a right to a safe, clean, comfortable, and home-like setting. The center must provide a setting and services that meet the person's needs and preferences. The setting and staff must promote the person's independence, self-worth, and quality of life.

ACTIVITIES

- Residents have the *right to activities that enhance each person's physical, mental, and psycho-social well-being*. The center provides religious services for spiritual health.

ENVIRONMENT

- Residents have the *right to a safe, clean, comfortable, and home-like setting*. The person is allowed to have and use personal items to the extent possible.

CHAPTER 2 REVIEW QUESTIONS

Circle the BEST answer.
1. Residents have all the following rights *except*
   a. Refusing a treatment
   b. Making a telephone call in private
   c. Choosing activities to attend
   d. Being punished for voicing a grievance
2. The person has a right to take part in planning and deciding his or her care and treatment.
   a. True
   b. False
3. The person is required to work for the center.
   a. True
   b. False
Answers to Chapter 2 questions are on p. 450.

CHAPTER 3 THE NURSING ASSISTANT
FEDERAL AND STATE LAWS

Nurse Practice Acts
- Each state has a nurse practice act. It regulates nursing practice in that state.

NURSING ASSISTANTS

- A state's nurse practice act is used to decide what nursing assistants can do. Some nurse practice acts

also regulate nursing assistant roles, functions, education, and certification requirements. Other states have separate laws for nursing assistants.
- Nursing assistants must be able to function with skill and safety. They can have their certification, license, or registration denied, revoked, or suspended.

The Omnibus Budget Reconciliation Act of 1987 (OBRA)
- The purpose of OBRA, a federal law, is to improve the quality of life of nursing center residents.
- OBRA sets minimum training and competency evaluation requirements for nursing assistants. Each state must have a nursing assistant training and competency evaluation program (NATCEP). A nursing assistant must successfully complete a NATCEP to work in a nursing center, hospital, long-term care unit, or home care agency receiving Medicare funds. The competency evaluation has a written test and a skills test. The written test has multiple-choice questions. The skills test involves performing certain skills learned in your training program. OBRA allows at least three attempts to successfully complete the evaluation.
- OBRA requires at least 75 hours of instruction. Some states have more hours. At least 16 hours of supervised training in a laboratory or clinical setting are required.
- OBRA requires a nursing assistant registry in each state. It is an official record that lists persons who have successfully completed the NATCEP. The registry has information about each nursing assistant.
  - Full name, including maiden name and any married names
  - Last known home address
  - Registry number and the date it expires
  - Date of birth
  - Last known employer, date hired, and date employment ended
  - Date the competency evaluation was passed
  - Information about findings of abuse, neglect, or dishonest use of property
- Retraining and a new competency evaluation program are required for nursing assistants who have not worked for 24 months.
- Each state's NATCEP must meet OBRA requirements.

ROLES AND RESPONSIBILITIES
- Nurse practice acts, OBRA, state laws, and legal and advisory opinions direct what you can do.
- Rules for you to follow (see Box 3-2 in the textbook):
  - You are an assistant to the nurse.
  - A nurse assigns and supervises your work.
  - You report observations about the person's physical and mental status to the nurse. Report changes in the person's condition or behavior at once.

- The nurse decides what should be done for a person. You do not make these decisions.
- Review directions and the care plan with the nurse before going to the person.
- Perform only those nursing tasks that you are trained to do.
- Ask a nurse to supervise you if you are not comfortable performing a nursing task.
- Perform only the nursing tasks that your state and job description allow.
- Role limits for nursing assistants (see Box 3-3 in the textbook):
  - Never give drugs.
  - Never insert tubes or objects into body openings. Do not remove tubes from the body.
  - Never take oral or telephone orders from doctors.
  - Never perform procedures that require sterile technique.
  - Never tell the person or family the person's diagnosis or treatment plans.
  - Never diagnose or prescribe treatments or drugs for anyone.
  - Never supervise others, including other nursing assistants.
  - Never ignore an order or request to do something. This includes nursing tasks that you can do, those you cannot do, and those that are beyond your legal limits.
- OBRA defines the basic range of functions for nursing assistants. All NATCEPs include those functions. Some states allow other functions. NATCEPs also prepare nursing assistants to meet the standards listed in Box 3-4, Nursing Assistant Standards, in the textbook.
- The job description is a document that describes what the agency expects you to do (see Figure 3-2 in the textbook). It also states educational requirements. Always obtain a written job description when you apply for a job. Do not take a job that requires you to:
  - Act beyond the legal limits of your role.
  - Function beyond your training limits.
  - Perform acts that are against your morals or religion.
- No one can force you to do something beyond the legal limits of your role. Sometimes jobs are threatened for refusing to follow a nurse's orders. Often staff obey out of fear. That is why you must understand your job description.

DELEGATION
- Delegate means to authorize another person to perform a nursing task in a certain situation.
- RNs can delegate tasks to you. In some states, LPNs/LVNs can delegate tasks to you.
- Nursing assistants cannot delegate. You cannot delegate any task to other nursing assistants or to any other worker.

- Delegation decisions must protect the person's health and safety. The delegating nurse is legally responsible for his or her actions and the actions of others who performed the delegated tasks.
- If you perform a task that places the person at risk, you may face serious legal problems.

The Five Rights of Delegation

- *The right task.* Can the task be delegated? Is the nurse allowed to delegate the task? Is the task in your job description?
- *The right circumstances.* What are the person's physical, mental, emotional, and spiritual needs at this time?
- *The right person.* Do you have the training and experience to safely perform the task for this person?
- *The right directions and communication.* The nurse must give clear directions. The nurse tells you what to do and when to do it. The nurse tells you what observations to make and when to report back. The nurse allows questions and helps you set priorities.
- *The right supervision.* In this step, the nurse:
  - Guides, directs, and evaluates the care you give.
  - Demonstrates tasks as needed and is available to answer questions.
  - Assesses how the task affected the person and how well you performed the task.
  - Tells you what you did well and how to improve your work.

Your Role in Delegation

- When you agree to perform a task, you are responsible for your own actions. You must complete the task safely. Report to the nurse what you did and the observations you made.
- You should refuse to perform a task when:
  - The task is beyond the legal limits of your role.
  - The task is not in your job description.
  - You were not prepared to perform the task.
  - The task could harm the person.
  - The person's condition has changed.
  - You do not know how to use the supplies or equipment.
  - Directions are not ethical or legal.
  - Directions are against agency policies.
  - Directions are unclear or incomplete.
  - A nurse is not available for supervision.
- Never ignore an order or request to do something. Tell the nurse about your concerns.
- Do not refuse a task because you do not like it or do not want to do it.

CHAPTER 3 REVIEW QUESTIONS

Circle the BEST answer.

1. OBRA does not require nursing assistant training and competency evaluation.
   a. True
   b. False

2. Nursing assistants perform nursing tasks delegated to them by an RN or LPN/LVN.
   a. True
   b. False

3. A resident asks you about his or her medical condition. You
   a. Tell the nurse about the resident's request
   b. Tell the resident what is in his or her medical record
   c. Ignore the question
   d. Tell another nursing assistant about the resident's request

4. You answer the telephone. The doctor starts to give you an order. You
   a. Take the order from the doctor
   b. Politely give your name and title, ask the doctor to wait for the nurse, and promptly find the nurse
   c. Politely ask the doctor to call back later
   d. Ask the doctor if the nurse may call him or her back

5. You can have your certification revoked for all the following *except*
   a. Substance abuse or dependency
   b. Abandoning a patient or resident
   c. Performing acts beyond the nursing assistant role
   d. Giving safe care

6. When should you refuse a task?
   a. The task is not in your job description.
   b. The task is within the legal limits of your role.
   c. The directions for the task are clear.
   d. A nurse is available for questions and supervision.

7. A nurse delegates a task that you did not learn in your training. The task is in your job description. What is your appropriate response to the nurse?
   a. "I cannot do that task."
   b. "I did not learn that task in my training. Can you show me how to do it?"
   c. "I will ask the other nursing assistant to watch me do the task."
   d. "I will ask the other nursing assistant to do the task for me."

8. You are busy with a new resident. It is time for another resident's bath. You may delegate the bath to another nursing assistant.
   a. True
   b. False

Answers to Chapter 3 questions are on p. 450.

CHAPTER 4 ETHICS AND LAWS
ETHICAL ASPECTS

- Ethics is the knowledge of what is right conduct and wrong conduct. Morals are involved. It also deals with choices or judgments about what should or should not be done. An ethical person behaves and acts in the right way. An ethical person does not cause a person harm.

- Ethical behavior involves not being prejudiced or biased. To be prejudiced or biased means to make judgments and have views before knowing the facts. Judgments and views usually are based on one's values and standards. They are based on the person's culture, religion, education, and experiences. The person's situation may be very different from your own. You should not judge a person by your values and standards. Also, do not avoid persons whose standards and values differ from your own.
- Ethical problems involve making choices. You must decide what is the right thing to do.

Boundaries

- **Professional boundaries** separate helpful behaviors from behaviors that are not helpful.
- *Boundary crossing is a brief act or behavior of being over-involved with the person. The intent of the act or behavior is to meet the person's needs.* The act or behavior may be thoughtless or something you did not mean to do. Or it could have purpose if it meets the person's needs.
- A **boundary violation** is an act or behavior that meets your needs, not the person's. The act or behavior is not ethical. Boundary violations include abuse, keeping secrets with a person, or giving a lot of personal information about yourself to another. Review Box 4-1, Code of Conduct for Nursing Assistants, in the textbook.
- **Professional sexual misconduct** is an act, behavior, or comment that is sexual in nature. It is sexual misconduct even if the person consents or makes the first move.
- To maintain professional boundaries, review Box 4-2, Maintaining Professional Boundaries, in the textbook. Be alert to **boundary signs** (acts, behaviors, or thoughts that warn of a boundary crossing or violation).

LEGAL ASPECTS

- A law is a rule of conduct made by a government body.
- Criminal laws are concerned with offenses against the public and society in general. An act that violates a criminal law is called a crime.
- Civil laws are concerned with relationships between people. Examples are those that involve contracts and nursing practice. A person found guilty of breaking a civil law usually has to pay a sum of money to the injured person.
- Torts are part of civil law. A tort is a wrong committed against a person or the person's property. Some torts are unintentional. Harm was not intended. Some torts are intentional. Harm was intended.

Unintentional Torts

- **Negligence** is an unintentional wrong. The negligent person did not act in a reasonable and careful manner. As a result, the person or person's property was harmed. The person causing harm did not mean to cause harm.
- **Malpractice** is negligence by a professional person.
- You are legally responsible (liable) for your own actions. The nurse is liable as your supervisor.

Intentional Torts

- **Defamation** is injuring a person's name and reputation by making false statements to a third person. **Libel** is making false statements in print, writing, or through pictures or drawings. **Slander** is making false statements orally. Never make false statements about a patient, resident, family member, co-worker, or any other person.
- **False imprisonment** is the unlawful restraint or restriction of a person's freedom of movement. It involves threatening to restrain a person, restraining a person, and preventing a person from leaving the agency.
- **Invasion of privacy** is violating a person's right not to have his or her name, photo, or private affairs exposed or made public without giving consent. Review Box 4-4, Protecting the Right to Privacy, in the textbook.
- The Health Insurance Portability and Accountability Act (HIPAA) of 1996 protects the privacy and security of a person's health information. **Protected health information** refers to identifying information and information about the person's health care that is maintained or sent in any form (paper, electronic, oral). Direct any questions about the person or the person's care to the nurse.
- **Fraud** is saying or doing something to trick, fool, or deceive a person. The act is fraud if it does or could cause harm to a person or the person's property.
- **Assault** is intentionally attempting or threatening to touch a person's body without the person's consent. The person fears bodily harm. **Battery** is touching a person's body without his or her consent. Protect yourself from being accused of assault and battery. Explain to the person what you are going to do and get the person's consent.

Informed Consent

- A person has the right to decide what will be done to his or her body and who can touch his or her body. Consent is informed when the person clearly understands all aspects of treatment.
- Persons who cannot give consent are persons who are under the legal age (usually 18 years) or are mentally incompetent. Unconscious, sedated, or confused persons cannot give consent. Informed consent is given by a responsible party—wife, husband, parent, daughter, son, legal representative.
- There are different ways to give consent.
  - Written consent
  - Verbal consent
  - Implied consent

- Before any procedure, explain the steps to the person. This is how you obtain verbal or implied consent. Also explain each step during a procedure.
- You are never responsible for obtaining written consent.

REPORTING ABUSE

- **Abuse** is
  - The willful infliction of injury, unreasonable confinement, intimidation, or punishment that results in physical harm, pain, or mental anguish. Intimidation means to make afraid with threats of force or violence.
  - Depriving the person (or the person's caregiver) of the goods or services needed to attain or maintain well-being.
- Abuse also includes involuntary seclusion.
- **Vulnerable adults** are persons 18 years old or older who have disabilities or conditions that make them at risk to be wounded, attacked, or damaged. They have problems caring for or protecting themselves due to:
  - A mental, emotional, physical, or developmental disability
  - Brain damage
  - Changes from aging
- All residents are vulnerable. Older persons and children are at risk for abuse.
- Some persons have behaviors and ways of living that threaten their health, safety, and well-being (self-neglect). Causes include declining health and chronic disease. Report warning signs of self-neglect to the nurse.
  - Hoarding
  - Weight loss
  - Absence of food, water, or heat
  - Failing to take needed drugs
  - Refusing to seek medical treatment for serious illnesses
  - Dehydration
  - Poor hygiene
  - Skin rashes
  - Pressure ulcers
  - Not wearing the correct clothing for the weather or wearing dirty or torn clothing
  - Not having dentures, eyeglasses, hearing aids, walkers, wheelchairs, commodes, or other needed devices
  - Confusion, disorientation, hallucinations, or delusions
  - Not attending to or not being able to attend to housekeeping
  - Safety hazards in the home
  - Mis-using drugs or alcohol
- Elder abuse is any knowing, intentional, or negligent act by a caregiver or another person to an older adult. It may include physical abuse, neglect, verbal abuse, involuntary seclusion, financial exploitation or misappropriation, emotional or mental abuse, sexual abuse, or abandonment. Review Box 4-7, Signs of Elder Abuse, in the textbook.
- If you suspect a person is being abused, report your observations to the nurse.
- Federal and state laws require the reporting of elder abuse.

Child abuse and neglect is the intentional harm or mistreatment of a child under 18 years old. It involves the following.

- Any recent act or failure to act on the part of a parent or caregiver.
- The act or failure to act results in death, serious physical or emotional harm, sexual abuse, or exploitation.
- The act or failure to act presents a likely or immediate risk for harm.

Intimate Partner Violence also called domestic abuse, domestic violence, intimate partner abuse, partner abuse, and spousal abuse—IPV occurs in relationships.

CHAPTER 4 REVIEW QUESTIONS

Circle the BEST answer.

1. A resident offers you a gift certificate for being kind to her. You should
   a. Say "thank you" and accept the gift
   b. Accept the gift and give it to charity
   c. Thank the resident for thinking of you, then explain it is against policy for you to accept the gift
   d. Accept the gift and give it to your daughter
2. To protect a person's privacy, you should do the following *except*
   a. Keep all information about the person confidential
   b. Discuss the person's treatment or diagnosis with the nurse supervising your work
   c. Open the person's mail
   d. Allow the person to visit with others in private
3. What should you do if you suspect an older person is being abused?
   a. Report the situation to the health department.
   b. Notify the nurse and discuss the observations with him or her.
   c. Notify the doctor about the suspected abuse.
   d. Ask the family why they are abusing the person.
4. A resident needs help going to the bathroom. You do not answer her call light promptly. She gets up without help, falls, and breaks a leg. This is an example of
   a. Negligence
   b. Defamation
   c. False imprisonment
   d. Slander
5. Examples of defamation include all the following *except*
   a. Implying or suggesting that a person uses drugs
   b. Saying that a person is insane or mentally ill
   c. Implying that a person steals money from staff
   d. Burning a resident with water that is too hot

6. Which statement about ethics is *false*?
   a. An ethical person does not judge others by his or her values and standards.
   b. An ethical person avoids persons whose standards and values differ from his or her own.
   c. An ethical person is not prejudiced or biased.
   d. An ethical person does not cause harm to another person.
7. Examples of false imprisonment include all of the following *except*
   a. Threatening to restrain a resident
   b. Restraining a resident without a doctor's order
   c. Treating the resident with respect
   d. Preventing a resident from leaving the agency

Answers to Chapter 4 questions are on p. 450.

CHAPTER 5 STUDENT AND WORK ETHICS
HEALTH, HYGIENE, AND APPEARANCE

- To give safe and effective care, you must be physically and mentally healthy. You need a balanced diet, sleep and rest, good body mechanics, and exercise on a regular basis. Have your eyes checked. If you smoke, good hygiene is needed. Take only those drugs ordered by your doctor. Do not drink alcohol while working.
- Personal hygiene needs careful attention. Bathe daily, use deodorant or antiperspirant, and brush your teeth often. Shampoo often. Keep fingernails clean, short, and neatly shaped.
- Review Box 5-2, Professional Appearance, in the textbook.

PREPARING FOR WORK

- Someone needs to take care of your children when you leave for work, while you are at work, and before you get home. Also plan for emergencies.
- Plan for getting to and from work. Keep your car in good working order, and keep enough gas in the car. Carpooling is an option.

TEAMWORK

- Practice good work ethics—work when scheduled, be cheerful and friendly, perform delegated tasks, be kind to others, be available to help others.
- Be ready to work when your shift starts. Arrive on your nursing unit a few minutes early. Stay the entire shift. When it is time to leave, report off-duty to the nurse. Follow the attendance policy in your employee handbook.
- A good attitude is needed. Review Box 5-1, Qualities and Traits for Good Work Ethics, in the textbook.
- Gossiping is unprofessional and hurtful. To avoid being a part of **gossip:**
  - Remove yourself from a group or setting where people are gossiping.

- Do not make or repeat any comment that can hurt a person, family member, visitor, co-worker, or the agency.
- Do not make or repeat any comment that you do not know is true.
- Do not talk about residents, family members, patients, visitors, co-workers, or the agency at home or in social settings, by e-mail, instant messaging, text messages, or social networking sites (Twitter, Facebook, MySpace, and others).
- **Confidentiality** means trusting others with personal and private information. The person's information is shared only among staff involved in his or her care. Agency, family, and co-worker information also is confidential. Share information only with the nurse. Do not eavesdrop. Be careful what you say over the intercom system.

SPEECH AND LANGUAGE

- Your speech and language must be professional.
  - Do not swear or use foul, vulgar, or abusive language.
  - Do not use slang.
  - Speak softly, gently, and clearly.
  - Do not shout or yell.
  - Do not fight or argue with a person, family member, visitor, or co-worker.
- A courtesy is a polite, considerate, or helpful comment or act.
  - Address others by Miss, Mrs., Ms., Mr., or Doctor. Use a first name only if the person asks you to do so.
  - Say "please" and "thank you." Say "I'm sorry" when you make a mistake or hurt someone.
  - Let residents, families, and visitors enter elevators first.
  - Be thoughtful—compliment others, give praise.
  - Wish the person and family well when they leave the center.
  - Hold doors open for others.
  - Help others willingly when asked.
  - Do not take credit for another person's deeds. Give the person credit for the action.

PERSONAL MATTERS

- Keep personal matters out of the workplace.
  - Make personal phone calls during meals and breaks.
  - Do not let family and friends visit you on the unit.
  - Make appointments for your days off.
  - Do not use the agency's computers and other equipment for personal use.
  - Do not take agency supplies for personal use.
  - Do not discuss personal problems at work.
  - Control your emotions.

- Do not borrow money from or lend money to co-workers.
- Do not sell things or engage in fund-raising at work.
- Do not have wireless phones and other electronic devices on while at work.
- Do not send or check text messages.
- Leave for and return from breaks and meals on time. Tell the nurse when you leave and return to the unit.

MANAGING STRESS

- Stress is the response or change in the body caused by an emotional, physical, social, or economic factor. Stress affects the whole person, physically, mentally, socially, and spiritually.
- These guidelines can help you reduce or cope with stress.
  - Exercise regularly.
  - Get enough sleep or rest.
  - Eat healthy.
  - Plan personal and quiet time for yourself.
  - Use common sense about what you can and cannot do.
  - Do one thing at a time. Set priorities.
  - Do not judge yourself harshly. Do not try to be perfect.
  - Give yourself praise.
  - Have a sense of humor.
  - Talk to the nurse if your work or a person is causing too much stress.

DEALING WITH CONFLICT

- Conflict is a clash between opposing interests or ideas. Conflicts arise over issues or events. Care is affected. To solve conflict, identify the real problem. This is part of problem solving. The problem-solving process involves these steps.
  - Step 1: Define the problem.
  - Step 2: Collect information about the problem.
  - Step 3: Identify possible solutions.
  - Step 4: Select the best solution.
  - Step 5: Carry out the solution.
  - Step 6: Evaluate the results.
- These guidelines can help you deal with conflict.
  - Ask your supervisor for some time to talk privately about the problem. Explain the problem. Give facts and specific examples. Ask for advice in solving the problem.
  - Approach the person with whom you have the conflict. Ask to talk privately. Be polite and professional.
  - Agree on a time and place to talk.
  - Talk in a private setting. No one should hear you or the other person.

- Explain the problem and what is bothering you. Give facts and specific behaviors. Focus on the problem. Do not focus on the person.
- Listen to the person. Do not interrupt.
- Identify ways to solve the problem. Offer your thoughts. Ask for the co-worker's ideas.
- Set a date and time to review the matter.
- Thank the person for meeting with you.
- Carry out the solution.
- Review the matter as scheduled.

HARASSMENT

- **Harassment** means to trouble, torment, offend, or worry a person by one's behavior or comments. Harassment can be sexual. Or it can involve age, race, ethnic background, religion, or disability. You must respect others. Do not offend others by your gestures, remarks, or use of touch. Do not offend others with jokes, photos, or other pictures. Harassment is not legal in the workplace.

RESIGNING FROM A JOB

- Whatever the reason for resigning, tell your employer. Do one of the following.
  - Give a written notice.
  - Write a resignation letter.
  - Complete a form in the human resources office.
- A 2-week notice is a good practice.

LOSING A JOB

- Poor performance may cause you to lose your job.
- Failing to follow agency policy is often grounds for termination. So is failure to get along with others.
- Box 5-4, Common Reasons for Losing a Job, in your textbook lists the many reasons why you can lose your job.

DRUG TESTING

- Drug testing policies are common because drug and alcohol use affect patient, resident, and staff safety; work ethics; and quality of care.

CHAPTER 5 REVIEW QUESTIONS

Circle the BEST answer.
1. You believe you have good work ethics. This means you do the following *except*
   a. Work when scheduled
   b. Act cheerful and friendly
   c. Refuse to help others
   d. Perform tasks assigned by the nurse

2. A nursing assistant is gossiping about a co-worker. You should
   a. Stay with the group and listen to what is being said
   b. Repeat the comment to your family
   c. Remove yourself from the group where gossip is occurring
   d. Repeat the comment to another co-worker
3. You want to maintain confidentiality about others. You do the following *except*
   a. Share information about a resident with a nurse who is on another unit
   b. Avoid talking about a resident in the elevator, hallway, or dining area
   c. Avoid talking about co-workers and residents when others are present
   d. Avoid eavesdropping
4. When you are at work, you should do which of the following?
   a. Swear and use foul language.
   b. Use slang.
   c. Argue with a visitor.
   d. Speak clearly and softly.
5. To give safe and effective care, you do all the following *except*
   a. Eat a balanced diet
   b. Get enough sleep and rest
   c. Exercise on a regular basis
   d. Drink too much alcohol
6. While at work, you should do all the following *except*
   a. Be courteous to others
   b. Make personal phone calls
   c. Admit when you are wrong or make mistakes
   d. Respect others

Answers to Chapter 5 questions are on p. 450.

CHAPTER 6 HEALTH TEAM COMMUNICATIONS
COMMUNICATION

- Communication is the exchange of information.
- For good communication:
  - Use words that mean the same thing to you and the message receiver. Avoid words with more than one meaning.
  - Use familiar words.
  - Be brief and concise.
  - Give information in a logical and orderly manner.
  - Give facts and be specific.

THE MEDICAL RECORD

- The medical record or chart is a written or electronic account of a person's condition and response to treatment and care. It is a permanent legal document.
- The medical record is a way for the health team to share information about the person. If you

know a person in the agency but you do not give care to that person, you have no right to review the person's chart. To do so is an invasion of privacy.
- Only professional staff involved in a person's care can review charts.
- A person or legal representative may ask you for the chart. Report the request to the nurse.
- Follow your agency's policies about recording in the medical record.
- Common parts of the record include:
  - Admission
  - Health history
  - Flow sheets and graphic sheets
  - Progress notes and nurses' notes

THE NURSING PROCESS

- The **nursing process** is the method nurses use to plan and deliver nursing care. It has five steps: assessment, nursing diagnosis, planning, implementation, and evaluation.
- You play a key role by making observations as you care for and talk with the person.

REPORTING AND RECORDING

- The health team communicates by reporting and recording.
- Reporting is the oral account of care and observations.
- Recording (charting) is the written account of care and observations.

Reporting
- You report care and observations to the nurse. Follow these rules.
  - Be prompt, thorough, and accurate.
  - Give the person's name and room and bed numbers.
  - Give the time your observations were made or the care was given.
  - Report only what you observed or did yourself.
  - Report care measures that you expect the person to need.
  - Report expected changes in the person's condition.
  - Give reports as often as the person's condition requires or when the nurse asks you to.
  - Report any changes from normal or changes in the person's condition at once.
  - Use your written notes to give a specific, concise, and clear report.
- You also report to the nurse:
  - When the nurse asks you to do so.
  - When you leave the unit for meals, breaks, or other reasons.
  - Before the end-of-shift report.

Recording

- Rules for recording are:
  - Always use ink. Use the color required by the center.
  - Include the date and time for every recording.
  - Make sure writing is readable and neat.
  - Use only agency-approved abbreviations.
  - Use correct spelling, grammar, and punctuation.
  - Do not use ditto marks.
  - Never erase or use correction fluid. Follow agency procedure for correcting errors.
  - Sign all entries with your name and title as required by agency policy.
  - Do not skip lines.
  - Make sure each form has the person's name and other identifying information.
  - Record only what you observed and did yourself.
  - Never chart a procedure, treatment, or care measure until after it is completed.
  - Be accurate, concise, and factual. Do not record judgments or interpretations.
  - Record in a logical and sequential manner.
  - Be descriptive. Avoid terms with more than one meaning.
  - Use the person's exact words whenever possible. Use quotation marks to show that the statement is a direct quote.
  - Chart any changes from normal or changes in the person's condition. Also chart that you informed the nurse (include the nurse's name), what you told the nurse, and the time you made the report.
  - Do not omit information.
  - Record safety measures. Example: Reminding a person not to get out of bed.
- Review the 24-hour clock, Figure 6-4 and Box 6-4 in the textbook.

MEDICAL TERMS AND ABBREVIATIONS

- Medical terminology and abbreviations are used in health care. Someone may use a word or phrase that you do not understand. If so, ask the nurse to explain its meaning.
- Review Box 6-9, Medical Terminology, in the textbook.
- Use only the abbreviations accepted by the agency. If you are not sure whether using an abbreviation is acceptable, write the term out in full. See the inside back cover of the textbook for common abbreviations.

COMPUTERS AND OTHER ELECTRONIC DEVICES

- Computers contain vast amounts of information (data) about a person. Therefore the right to privacy must be protected. If allowed access, you must follow the agency's policies. You must keep information confidential. Review Box 6-7, Electronic Devices, in the textbook.

PHONE COMMUNICATIONS

- You will answer phones at the nurses' station or in the person's room. Follow the agency's policy and guidelines.
- Guidelines for answering phones:
  - Answer the call after the first ring if possible.
  - Do not answer the phone in a rushed or hasty manner.
  - Give a courteous greeting. Identify the nursing unit and your name and title.
  - When taking a message, write down the caller's name, phone number, date and time, and message.
  - Repeat the message and phone number back to the caller.
  - Ask the caller to "please hold" if necessary.
  - Do not lay the phone down or cover the receiver with your hand when not speaking to the caller. The caller may hear confidential information.
  - Return to a caller on hold within 30 seconds.
  - Do not give confidential information to any caller.
  - Transfer a call if appropriate. Tell the caller you are going to transfer the call. Give the name and phone number in case the call gets disconnected or the line is busy.
  - End the conversation politely.
  - Give the message to the appropriate person.

CHAPTER 6 REVIEW QUESTIONS

Circle the BEST answer.

1. For good communication, you should do the following *except*
   a. Use words with more than one meaning
   b. Use words familiar to the person or family
   c. Give facts in a brief and concise manner
   d. Give information in a logical and orderly manner

2. When you record in a person's chart, you do the following *except*
   a. Record what you observed and did
   b. Record the person's response to the treatment or procedure
   c. Use abbreviations that are not on the accepted list for the center
   d. Record the time the observation was made or the treatment was performed

3. When reporting care and observations to the nurse, you do the following *except*
   a. Give the person's name and room and bed numbers
   b. Report only what you observed or did yourself
   c. Report any changes from normal or changes in the person's condition at once
   d. Report any changes from normal or changes in the person's condition at the end of the shift

Answers to Chapter 6 questions are on p. 450.

CHAPTER 7 UNDERSTANDING THE PERSON

CARING FOR THE PERSON

- The whole person needs to be considered (holism) when you provide care—physical, social, psychological, and spiritual parts. These parts are woven together and cannot be separated.
- Follow these rules to address persons with dignity and respect.
  - Use their titles—Mrs. Jones, Mr. Smith, Miss Turner, Ms. Beal, or Dr. Gonzalez.
  - Do not call them by their first names unless they ask you to.
  - Do not call them by any other name unless they ask you to.
  - Do not call them Grandma, Papa, Sweetheart, Honey, or other names.

BASIC NEEDS

- A **need** is something necessary or desired for maintaining life and mental well-being.
- According to psychologist Abraham Maslow, basic needs must be met for a person to survive and function. Needs are arranged in order of importance, from lower level to higher level.
  - *Physical needs*—are required for life. They are oxygen, food, water, elimination, rest, and shelter.
  - *Safety and security needs*—relate to feeling safe from harm, danger, and fear.
  - *Love and belonging needs*—relate to love, closeness, affection, and meaningful relationships with others.
  - *Self-esteem needs*—relate to thinking well of oneself and to seeing oneself as useful and having value. People often lack self-esteem when ill, injured, older, or disabled.
  - *The need for self-actualization*—involves learning, understanding, and creating to the limit of a person's capacity. Rarely, if ever, is it totally met.

CULTURE AND RELIGION

- **Culture** is the characteristics of a group of people—language, values, beliefs, habits, dislikes, and customs. People come from many cultures, races, and nationalities. Family practices, food choices, hygiene habits, clothing styles, and language are part of their culture. The person's culture also influences health beliefs and practices. Culture is also a factor in communication.
- **Religion** relates to spiritual beliefs, needs, and practices. A person's religion influences health and illness practices. Many may want to pray and observe religious practices. Assist residents to attend religious services as needed.

- A person may not follow all the beliefs and practices of his or her culture or religion. Some people do not practice a religion.
  - Do not judge a person by your standards, and do not force your ideas on the person

COMMUNICATING WITH THE PERSON

- For effective communication between you and the person, you must:
  - Follow the rules of communication in Chapter 6.
  - Understand and respect the patient or resident as a person.
  - View the person as a physical, psychological, social, and spiritual human being.
  - Appreciate the person's problems and frustrations.
  - Respect the person's rights.
  - Respect the person's religion and culture.
  - Give the person time to understand the information that you give.
  - Repeat information as often as needed. Use the exact same words and try rephrasing if not understood after repeating.
  - Ask questions to see if the person understood you.
  - Be patient. People with memory problems may ask the same question many times.
  - Include the person in conversations when others are present.

Verbal Communication

- Verbal communication uses written or spoken words.
- When talking with a person, follow these rules.
  - Face the person. Look directly at the person.
  - Position yourself at the person's eye level. Sit or squat by the person as needed.
  - Control the loudness and tone of your voice.
  - Speak clearly, slowly, and distinctly.
  - Do not use slang or vulgar words.
  - Repeat information as needed.
  - Ask one question at a time and wait for an answer.
  - Do not shout, whisper, or mumble.
  - Be kind, courteous, and friendly.
- Use written words if the person cannot speak or hear but can read. Keep written messages simple and brief. Use a black felt pen on white paper and print in large letters.
- Some persons cannot speak or read. Ask questions that have "yes" or "no" answers. Follow the care plan.

Nonverbal Communication

- Messages are sent with gestures, facial expressions, posture, body movements, touch, and smell. Nonverbal messages more accurately reflect a person's feelings than words do. A person may say one thing but act another way. Watch the person's eyes, hand movements, gestures, posture, and other actions.

- Touch shows comfort, caring, love, affection, interest, trust, concern, and reassurance. Touch should be gentle. Touch means different things to different people. Some people do not like being touched. To use touch, follow the person's care plan. Maintain professional boundaries.
- People send messages through their **body language**—facial expressions, gestures, posture, hand and body movements, gait, eye contact, and appearance. Your body language should show interest, enthusiasm, caring, and respect for the person. Often you need to control your body language. Control reactions to odors from body fluids, secretions, excretions, or the person's body.

Communication Methods

- *Listening* means to focus on verbal and nonverbal communication. You use sight, hearing, touch, and smell. To be a good listener:
  - Face the person.
  - Have good eye contact with the person.
  - Lean toward the person. Do not sit back with your arms crossed.
  - Respond to the person. Nod your head, repeat what the person says, and ask questions.
  - Avoid communication barriers.
- *Paraphrasing* is restating the person's message in your own words.
- *Direct questions* focus on certain information. You ask the person something you need to know.
- *Open-ended questions* lead or invite the person to share thoughts, feelings, or ideas. The person chooses what to talk about.
- *Clarifying* lets you make sure that you understand the message. You can ask the person to repeat the message, say you do not understand, or restate the message.
- *Focusing* deals with a certain topic. It is useful when a person wanders in thought.
- *Silence* is a very powerful way to communicate. Silence gives time to think, organize thoughts, choose words, and gain control. The person may need silence. Silence on your part shows caring and respect for the person's situation and feelings. Just being there shows you care.

Communication Barriers

- *Unfamiliar language.* You and the person must use and understand the same language.
- *Cultural differences.* The person from another country may attach different meanings to verbal and nonverbal communication from what you intended.
- *Changing the subject.* Avoid changing the subject whenever possible.

- *Giving your opinions.* Opinions involve judging values, behaviors, or feelings. Let others express feelings and concerns without adding your opinion. Do not make judgments or jump to conclusions.
- *Talking a lot when others are silent.* Talking too much is usually because of nervousness and discomfort with silence.
- *Failure to listen.* Do not pretend to listen. It shows lack of caring and interest. You miss important complaints or other symptoms that you must report to the nurse.
- *Pat answers.* "Don't worry." "Everything will be okay." "Your doctor knows best." These make the person feel that you do not care about his or her concerns, feelings, and fears.
- *Illness and disability.* Speech, hearing, vision, cognitive function, and body movements are often affected. Verbal and nonverbal communication is affected.
- *Age.* Values and communication styles vary among age groups.

PERSONS WITH SPECIAL NEEDS

- Common courtesies and manners apply to any person with a disability. Review Box 7-2, Disability Etiquette, in the textbook.

The Person Who Is Comatose

- The person who is comatose is unconscious and cannot respond to others. Often the person can hear and can feel touch and pain. Assume that the person hears and understands you. Use touch and give care gently. Practice these measures.
- Knock before entering the person's room.
- Tell the person your name, the time, and the place every time you enter the room.
- Give care on the same schedule every day.
- Explain what you are going to do. Explain care measures step-by-step as you do them.
- Tell the person when you are finishing care.
- Use touch to communicate care, concern, and comfort.
- Tell the person what time you will be back to check on him or her.
- Tell the person when you are leaving the room.

Persons with Bariatric Needs

- Bariatrics focuses on the treatment and control of obesity. Bariatric persons are at risk for many serious health problems. Special equipment and furniture are needed to meet the person's needs.

FAMILY AND FRIENDS

- The presence or absence of family or friends affect the person's quality of life.
- If you need to give care when visitors are there, protect the person's right to privacy. Politely ask

the visitors to leave the room when you give care. A partner or family member may help you if the patient or resident consents.

- Treat family and visitors with courtesy and respect.
- Do not discuss the person's condition with family and friends. Refer questions to the nurse. A visitor may upset or tire a person. Report your observations to the nurse.
- Know your agency's visiting policies and what is allowed for the person.
- Know the location, rules, and hours of the chapel, gift shop, lounge, dining room, or business office.

BEHAVIOR ISSUES

- Many people do not adjust well to illness, injury, and disability. They have some of the following behaviors.
  - *Anger*. Anger may be communicated verbally and nonverbally. Causes include fear, pain, loss of function, and loss of control over health and life. Verbal outbursts, shouting, raised voices, and rapid speech are common. Some people are silent. Others are uncooperative and may refuse to answer questions. Nonverbal signs include rapid movements, pacing, clenched fists, and a red face. Glaring and getting close to you when speaking are other signs. Violent behaviors can occur.
  - *Demanding behavior*. Nothing seems to please the person. The person is critical of others. Loss of independence, health, and control of life are causes.
  - *Self-centered behavior*. The person cares only about his or her own needs. The needs of others are ignored. The person becomes impatient if needs are not met.
  - *Aggressive behavior*. The person may swear, bite, hit, pinch, scratch, or kick. Protect the person, others, and yourself from harm.
  - *Withdrawal*. The person has little or no contact with family, friends, and staff. Some people are generally not social and prefer to be alone. This may signal physical illness or depression.
  - *Inappropriate sexual behavior*. Some people make inappropriate sexual remarks or touch others in the wrong way. These behaviors may be on purpose. Or they are caused by disease, confusion, dementia, or drug side effects.
- You cannot avoid the person or lose control. Behaviors are addressed in the care plan. Review Box 7-3, Dealing with Behavior Issues, in the textbook.

CHAPTER 7 REVIEW QUESTIONS

Circle the BEST answer.

1. While caring for a person, you need to
   a. Consider only the person's physical and social needs
   b. Consider the person's physical, social, psychological, and spiritual needs
   c. Consider only the person's cultural needs
   d. Ignore the person's spiritual needs

2. When referring to residents, you should
   a. Refer to them by their room number
   b. Call them "Honey"
   c. Call them by their first name
   d. Call them by their name and title

3. Based on Maslow's theory of basic needs, which person's needs must be met first?
   a. The person who wants to talk about her granddaughter's wedding
   b. The person who is uncomfortable in the dining room
   c. The person who wants mail opened
   d. The person who asks for more water

4. Which statement about culture is *false*?
   a. A person's culture influences health beliefs and practices.
   b. You must respect a person's culture.
   c. You should ignore the person's culture while you give his or her care.
   d. You should learn about another person's culture that is different from yours.

5. Which statement about religion and spiritual beliefs is *false*?
   a. A person's religion influences health and illness practices.
   b. You should assist a person to attend services in the nursing center.
   c. Many people find comfort and strength from religion during illness.
   d. A person must follow all beliefs of his or her religion.

6. A person is angry and is shouting at you. You should do the following *except*
   a. Stay calm and professional
   b. Yell so that the person will listen to you
   c. Listen to what the person is saying
   d. Report the person's behavior to the nurse

7. A person tries to scratch and kick you. You should
   a. Protect yourself from harm
   b. Argue with the person
   c. Become angry with the person
   d. Refuse to care for the person

8. When speaking with another person, you do the following *except*
   a. Position yourself at the person's eye level
   b. Speak slowly, clearly, and distinctly
   c. Shout, mumble, and whisper
   d. Ask one question at a time

9. Which statement about listening is *false*?
   a. You use sight, hearing, touch, and smell when you listen.
   b. You observe nonverbal cues.
   c. You have good eye contact with the person.
   d. You sit back with your arms crossed.

10. Which statement about silence is *false*?
    a. Silence is a powerful way to communicate.
    b. Silence gives people time to think.
    c. You should talk a lot when the other person is silent.
    d. Silence helps when the person is upset and needs to gain control.

11. A person speaks a foreign language. You should do the following *except*
    a. Keep messages short and simple
    b. Use gestures and pictures
    c. Shout or speak loudly
    d. Repeat the message in other words
12. When caring for a person who is comatose, you do the following *except*
    a. Tell the person your name when you enter the room
    b. Explain what you are doing
    c. Use touch to communicate care and comfort
    d. Make jokes about how sick the person is
13. A person is in a wheelchair. You should do all the following *except*
    a. Lean on a person's wheelchair
    b. Sit or squat to talk to a person in a wheelchair or chair
    c. Think about obstacles before giving directions to a person in a wheelchair
    d. Extend the same courtesies to the person as you would to anyone else
14. A person's daughter is visiting and you need to provide care to the person. You
    a. Expose the person's body in front of the visitor
    b. Politely ask the visitor to leave the room
    c. Decide to not provide the care at all
    d. Discuss the person's condition with the visitor

Answers to Chapter 7 questions are on p. 450.

CHAPTER 8 BODY STRUCTURE AND FUNCTION

CELLS, TISSUES, AND ORGANS

- The basic unit of body structure is the cell. Cells need food, water, and oxygen to live and function.
  - Cells are the body's building blocks. **Groups of cells with similar functions combine to form tissues.** *Epithelial tissue* covers internal and external body surfaces. *Connective tissue* anchors, connects, and supports other tissues. *Muscle tissue* stretches and contracts to let the body move. *Nerve tissue* receives and carries impulses to the brain and back to body parts.
- *Groups of tissue with the same function form organs.* An organ has one or more functions. Examples of organs are the heart, brain, liver, lungs, and kidneys. *Systems are formed by organs that work together to perform special functions*

INTEGUMENTARY SYSTEM

- The *integumentary system,* or *skin,* is the largest system. It has epithelial, connective, and nerve tissue. It also has oil glands and sweat glands. There are two skin layers.
- The *epidermis* is the outer layer. It has living cells and dead cells. Living cells of the epidermis contain *pigment.* Pigment gives skin its color. The epidermis has no blood vessels and few nerve endings.
- The *dermis* is the inner layer. It is made up of connective tissue. Blood vessels, nerves, sweat glands, and oil glands are found in the dermis. So are hair roots.
- The epidermis and dermis are supported by *subcutaneous tissue.* The subcutaneous tissue is a thick layer of fat and connective tissue.
- *Oil glands* and *sweat glands, hair,* and *nails* are skin appendages.
- The skin has many functions. It is the body's protective covering. It prevents microorganisms and other substances from entering the body. It prevents excess amounts of water from leaving the body. It protects organs from injury. Nerve endings in the skin sense both pleasant and unpleasant stimulation. Nerve endings are over the entire body. They sense cold, pain, touch, and pressure to protect the body from injury. The skin helps regulate body temperature. Blood vessels *dilate* (widen) when temperature outside the body is high. More blood is brought to the body surface for cooling during evaporation. When blood vessels *constrict* (narrow), the body retains heat. This is because less blood reaches the skin. It stores fat and water.

THE MUSCULO-SKELETAL SYSTEM

The musculo-skeletal system provides the framework for the body. It lets the body move. This system also protects internal organs and gives the body shape.

BONES

- The human body has 206 bones. There are 4 types of bones. Long bones bear the body's weight. Leg bones are long bones. Short bones allow skill and ease in movement. Bones in the wrists, fingers, ankles, and toes are short bones. Flat bones protect the organs. They include the ribs, skull, pelvic bones, and shoulder blades. Irregular bones are the vertebrae in the spinal column. They allow various degrees of movement and flexibility.
- Bones are hard, rigid structures. They are made up of living cells. Calcium and phosphorus are needed for bone formation and strength. Bones store these minerals for use by the body. Inside the hollow centers of the bones is a substance called bone marrow. Blood cells are formed in the bone marrow.

JOINTS

- A joint is the point at which two or more bones meet. Joints allow movement. Cartilage is connective tissue at the end of the long bones. It cushions the joint so that the bone ends do not rub together.

The synovial membrane lines the joints. It secretes synovial fluid. Synovial fluid acts as a lubricant so the joint can move smoothly. Bones are held together at the joint by strong bands of connective tissue called *ligaments*.

- There are three major types of joints. A ball-and-socket joint allows movement in all directions. It is made of the rounded end of one bone and the hollow end of another bone. The rounded end of one fits into the hollow end of the other. The joints of the hips and shoulders are ball-and-socket joints. A hinge joint allows movement in one direction. The elbow is a hinge joint. A pivot joint allows turning from side to side. A pivot joint connects the skull to the spine. Some joints cannot move. They connect the bones of the skull.

MUSCLES

The human body has more than 500 muscles. Some are voluntary. Others are involuntary.

- Voluntary muscles can be consciously controlled. Muscles attached to bones (skeletal muscles) are voluntary. Involuntary muscles work automatically. You cannot control them. They control the action of the stomach, intestines, blood vessels, and other body organs. Involuntary muscles also are called smooth muscles. They look smooth, not streaked or striped.
- Cardiac muscle is in the heart. It is an involuntary muscle. However, it appears striated like skeletal muscle.
- Muscles have three functions. Movement of body parts. Maintenance of posture or muscle tone. Production of body heat.
- Strong, tough connective tissues called tendons connect muscles to bones. When muscles contract (shorten), tendons at each end of the muscle cause the bone to move.
- Sphincters are circular bands of muscle fibers. They constrict (narrow) a passage. Or they close a natural body opening.

THE NERVOUS SYSTEM

- The nervous system controls, directs, and coordinates body functions. Its two main divisions are the central nervous system (CNS), consisting of the brain and spinal cord, and the peripheral nervous system, which involves the nerves throughout the body.
- Nerves connect to the spinal cord. Nerves carry messages or impulses to and from the brain. A stimulus causes a nerve impulse. A reflex is the body's response (functioning or movement) to a stimulus. Reflexes are involuntary, unconscious, and immediate.
- Nerves are easily damaged and take a long time to heal. Some nerve fibers have a protective covering called a myelin sheath. The myelin sheath also insulates the nerve fiber. Nerve fibers covered with myelin conduct impulses faster than those fibers without it.

THE CENTRAL NERVOUS SYSTEM

- The brain and spinal cord make up the central nervous system. The brain is covered by the skull. The three main parts of the brain are the cerebrum, the cerebellum, and the brainstem.
- The cerebrum is the largest part of the brain. It is the center of thought and intelligence. The outside of the cerebrum is called the cerebral cortex. It controls the highest functions of the brain.
- The cerebellum regulates and coordinates body movements. It controls balance and the smooth movements of voluntary muscles.
- The brainstem connects the cerebrum to the spinal cord. The brainstem contains the midbrain, pons, and medulla. The midbrain and pons relay messages between the medulla and the cerebrum. The medulla is below the pons. The medulla controls heart rate, breathing, blood vessel size, swallowing, coughing, and vomiting.
- The spinal cord lies within the spinal column. The cord is 17 to 18 inches long. It contains pathways that conduct messages to and from the brain.
- The brain and spinal cord are covered and protected by three layers of connective tissue called meninges.

THE PERIPHERAL NERVOUS SYSTEM

- The peripheral nervous system has 12 pairs of cranial nerves and 31 pairs of spinal nerves. Cranial nerves conduct impulses between the brain and the head, neck, chest, and abdomen. Spinal nerves carry impulses from the skin, extremities, and internal structures not supplied by the cranial nerves.
- Some peripheral nerves form the autonomic nervous system. This system controls involuntary muscles and certain body functions. The autonomic nervous system is divided into the sympathetic nervous system and the parasympathetic nervous system. The sympathetic nervous system speeds up functions. The parasympathetic nervous system slows functions.

THE SENSE ORGANS

- The five senses are sight, hearing, taste, smell, and touch. Receptors for taste are in the tongue. They are called *taste buds.* Receptors for smell are in the nose. Touch receptors are in the dermis, especially in the toes and fingertips.

THE EYE.

- Receptors for vision are in the eyes. The eye has three layers.

THE EAR.

- The ear is a sense organ. It functions in hearing and balance. The ear has three parts: the external ear, middle ear, and inner ear.

THE CIRCULATORY SYSTEM

- The circulatory system (cardiovascular system) is made up of the blood, heart, and blood vessels. The heart pumps blood through the blood vessels. The circulatory system has many functions.

THE BLOOD

- The blood consists of blood cells and plasma. Plasma also carries substances that cells need to function. Red blood cells (RBCs) are called erythrocytes. Hemoglobin is a substance in RBCs that carries oxygen and gives blood its red color. White blood cells (WBCs) are called *leukocytes*. They protect the body against infection. Platelets (thrombocytes) are needed for blood clotting. They are formed by the bone marrow.

THE HEART

The heart is a muscle. It pumps blood through the blood vessels to the tissues and cells. The heart lies in the middle to lower part of the chest cavity toward the left side.

- Heart action has two phases. Diastole. It is the resting phase. Heart chambers fill with blood.
- Systole. It is the working phase. The heart contracts. Blood is pumped through the blood vessels when the heart contracts.

THE BLOOD VESSELS

- Blood flows to body tissues and cells through the blood vessels. There are 3 groups of blood vessels: arteries, capillaries, and veins.
- Arteries carry blood away from the heart. Arterial blood is rich in oxygen. The smallest branch of an artery is an arteriole. Arterioles connect to capillaries. Capillaries are very tiny blood vessels. Food, oxygen, and other substances pass from capillaries into the cells. The capillaries pick up waste products (including carbon dioxide) from the cells.
- Veins return blood to the heart. They connect to the capillaries by venules. Venules are small veins. Venules branch together to form veins. The two main veins are the inferior vena cava and the superior vena cava. Venous blood is dark red. It has little oxygen and a lot of carbon dioxide.

THE LYMPHATIC SYSTEM

- The lymphatic (lymph) system is a complex network that transports lymph throughout the body. Lymph contains proteins and fats from the intestines. Lymph also contains white blood cells (WBCs). Lymph is formed in the tissues. Lymph is transported by lymphatic vessels—lymphatic capillaries to lymphatic venules to the right lymphatic duct and the thoracic duct. Lymph then enters the blood in veins near the neck.
- Lymph nodes are shaped like beans. They swell when producing more lymphocytes to fight infection.
- The spleen is the largest structure in the lymphatic system

THE RESPIRATORY SYSTEM

- Oxygen is needed to live Respiration is the process of supplying the cells with oxygen and removing carbon dioxide from them. Respiration involves inhalation (breathing in) and exhalation (breathing out). The terms inspiration (breathing in) and expiration (breathing out) also are used.
- The trachea divides at its lower end into the right bronchus and the left bronchus. Each bronchus enters a lung. Upon entering the lungs, the bronchi divide many times into smaller branches called bronchioles. Eventually the bronchioles subdivide. They end up in tiny one-celled air sacs called alveoli. Alveoli look like small clusters of grapes. They are supplied by capillaries. Oxygen and carbon dioxide are exchanged between the alveoli and capillaries.
- The lungs are spongy tissues. They are filled with alveoli, blood vessels, and nerves. Each lung is divided into lobes. The right lung has three lobes; the left lung has two. The lungs are separated from the abdominal cavity by a muscle called the diaphragm.

THE DIGESTIVE SYSTEM

- Digestion is the process that breaks down food physically and chemically so it can be absorbed for use by the cells. The digestive system is also called the gastrointestinal (GI) system. The system also removes solid wastes from the body.
- The digestive system involves the alimentary canal (GI tract) and the accessory organs of digestion. The alimentary canal is a long tube. It extends from the mouth to the anus. Its major parts are the mouth, pharynx, esophagus, stomach, small intestine, and large intestine. Accessory organs are the teeth, tongue, salivary glands, liver, gallbladder, and pancreas.

- Digestion begins in the mouth (oral cavity). The stomach is a muscular, pouch-like sac. It is in the upper left part of the abdominal cavity. Strong stomach muscles stir and churn food to break it up into even smaller particles. Food is mixed and churned with the gastric juices to form a semi-liquid substance called chyme. Through peristalsis, the chyme is pushed from the stomach into the small intestine.
- The small intestine is about 20 feet long. It has three parts. Digestive juices chemically break down food so it can be absorbed. Peristalsis moves the chyme through the small intestine: Tiny projections called villi line the small intestine and absorb the digested food into the capillaries.

THE URINARY SYSTEM

- The urinary system: Removes waste products from the blood. Maintains water balance within the body. Maintains electrolyte balance. Maintains acid-base balance.
- The kidneys are two bean-shaped organs in the upper abdomen. They lie against the back muscles on each side of the spine. They are protected by the lower edge of the rib cage.
- Each kidney has over a million tiny nephrons. Each nephron is the basic working unit of the kidney.
- A tube called the ureter is attached to the renal pelvis of the kidney. Each ureter is about 10 to 12 inches long. The ureters carry urine from the kidneys to the bladder. The bladder is a hollow, muscular sac. It lies toward the front in the lower part of the abdominal cavity.
- Urine is stored in the bladder until the need to urinate is felt. Urine passes from the bladder through the urethra. The opening at the end of the urethra is called the meatus. Urine passes from the body through the meatus. Urine is a clear, yellowish fluid.

THE REPRODUCTIVE SYSTEM

- The Male Reproductive System. The testes (testicles) are the male sex glands. Sex glands also are called gonads. The two testes are oval or almond-shaped glands. Male sex cells are produced in the testes. Male sex cells are called sperm cells.
- Testosterone, the male hormone, is produced in the testes.
- The Female Reproductive System. The female gonads are two almond-shaped glands called ovaries. An ovary is on each side of the uterus in the abdominal cavity.
The ovaries contain ova or eggs. Ova are the female sex cells.
- Menstruation. The endometrium is rich in blood to nourish the cell that grows into a fetus. If pregnancy does not occur, menstruation begins. Menstruation is the process in which the lining of the uterus

(endometrium) breaks up and is discharged from the body through the vagina. It occurs about every 28 days. Therefore it is called the menstrual cycle.
- Fertilization. To reproduce, a male sex cell (sperm) must unite with a female sex cell (ovum). The uniting of the sperm and ovum into one cell is called fertilization.

THE ENDOCRINE SYSTEM

- The endocrine system is made up of glands called the endocrine glands. The endocrine glands secrete chemical substances called hormones into the bloodstream. Hormones regulate the activities of other organs and glands in the body.
- The pituitary gland is called the master gland. The pituitary gland is divided into the anterior pituitary lobe and the posterior pituitary lobe. The anterior lobe also secretes hormones that regulate growth, development, and function of the male and female reproductive systems.
- The thyroid gland, shaped like a butterfly, is in the neck in front of the larynx.
- The four parathyroid glands secrete parathormone. Two lie on each side of the thyroid gland. The thymus secretes the hormone thymosin. This hormone is important for the development and function of the immune system.
- The pancreas secretes insulin. Insulin regulates the amount of sugar in the blood available for use by the cells. Insulin is needed for sugar to enter the cells
- There are two adrenal glands. An adrenal gland is on the top of each kidney. The adrenal gland has two parts: the adrenal medulla and the adrenal cortex. The adrenal medulla secretes epinephrine and norepinephrine. The adrenal cortex secretes three groups of hormones needed for life.
- Small amounts of male and female sex hormones are secreted.

THE IMMUNE SYSTEM

- The immune system protects the body from disease and infection. The immune system defends against threats inside and outside the body.
- Specific immunity is the body's reaction to a certain threat.
- Non-specific immunity is the body's reaction to anything it does not recognize as a normal body substance.
- Antibodies—normal body substances that recognize other substances. They are involved in destroying abnormal or unwanted substances.
- Antigens—substances that cause an immune response. Antibodies recognize and bind with unwanted antigens. This leads to the destruction of unwanted substances and the production of more antibodies.

- Phagocytes—white blood cells (WBCs) that digest and destroy microorganisms and other unwanted substances.
- Lymphocytes—WBCs that produce antibodies. Lymphocyte production increases as the body responds to an infection.
- B lymphocytes (B cells)—cause the production of antibodies that circulate in the plasma. The antibodies react to specific antigens.
- T lymphocytes (T cells)—destroy invading cells. Killer T cells produce poisons near the invading cells. Some T cells attract other cells. The other cells destroy the invaders.

CHAPTER 8 REVIEW QUESTIONS

Circle the BEST answer.

1. The basic unit of body structure is the
   a. Tissues
   b. Cell
   c. Skin
   d. Organs
2. The outer layer of the skin is
   a. Dermis
   b. Hair
   c. Nails
   d. Epidermis
3. Functions of the skin include all of the following *except*
   a. Stores fat and water
   b. Senses stimulation
   c. Prevents temperature regulation
   d. Prevents excess amounts of water from leaving the body
4. The ball-and-socket joint allows movement in 1 direction.
   a. True
   b. False
5. Muscle function includes all of the following *except*
   a. Movement of body parts
   b. Production of heat
   c. Maintenance of muscle tone
   d. Provide body shape
6. Arteries carry blood
   a. Away from the heart
   b. Toward the heart
   c. Without oxygen
   d. With carbon dioxide
7. The air you breathe contains how much oxygen?
   a. 10%
   b. 21%
   c. 36%
   d. 52%
8. Urine is stored in the
   a. Bladder
   b. Kidneys
   c. Ureter
   d. Urethra

Answers to Chapter 8 questions are on p. 450.

CHAPTER 9 THE OLDER PERSON

- Gerontology is the study of the aging process. Geriatrics is the care of aging people.
- Aging is normal. It is not a disease. Normal changes occur in body structure and function. Psychological and social changes also occur.

SOCIAL CHANGES

- People cope with aging in their own way. The following social changes occur with aging.
  - *Retirement.* Retirement is a reward for a life-time of work. The person can relax and enjoy life. Some people retire because of poor health or disability. Retired people may have part-time jobs or do volunteer work.
  - *Reduced income.* Retirement often means reduced income. The retired person still has expenses. Severe money problems can result. Some people have income from savings, investments, retirement plans, and insurance.
  - *Social relationships.* Social relationships change throughout life. Family time helps prevent loneliness. So do hobbies, religious and community events, and new friends.
  - *Children as caregivers.* Some older persons feel more secure when children care for them. Others feel unwanted and useless. Some lose dignity and self-respect. Tensions may occur among the child, parent, and other household members. Lack of privacy is a cause. So are disagreements and criticisms about housekeeping, raising children, cooking, and friends.
  - *Death of a partner.* When death occurs, the person loses a lover, friend, companion, and confidant. Grief may be very great. The person's life will likely change. Serious physical and mental health problems result.

PHYSICAL CHANGES

- With aging, body processes slow down. Energy level and body efficiency decline.
- *The integumentary system.* The skin loses its elasticity, strength, and fatty tissue layer. Wrinkles appear. Dry skin and itching occur. The skin is fragile and easily injured. The person is more sensitive to cold. Nails become thick and tough. Feet may have poor circulation. White or gray hair is common. Hair thins. Facial hair may occur in women. Hair is drier. Protect the person from drafts and cold. A shower or bath with a mild soap or soap substitute is enough for hygiene. Partial baths are taken at other times. Lotions and creams prevent drying and itching. Do not use hot water bottles and heating pads because of the risk for burns. Hair brushing promotes circulation and oil production.

Shampoo frequency usually decreases with age. It is done as needed for hygiene and comfort.

- *The musculo-skeletal system.* Muscle and bone strength decrease. Bones become brittle and break easily. Vertebrae shorten. Joints become stiff and painful. Mobility decreases. There is a gradual loss of height. Activity, exercise, and diet help prevent bone loss and loss of muscle strength. Range-of-motion exercises are helpful. A diet high in protein, calcium, and vitamins is needed. Protect the person from injury and falls.
- *The nervous system.* Nerve cells are lost. Blood flow to the brain is reduced. Confusion, dizziness, and fatigue may occur. Responses are slower. The risk for falls increases. Forgetfulness increases. Memory is shorter. Events from long ago are easier to recall than recent ones. Older persons have a harder time falling asleep. Sleep periods are shorter. Older persons wake often during the night and have less deep sleep. Less sleep is needed. They may rest or nap during the day. They may go to bed early and get up early.
- *The senses.* Hearing and vision losses occur. Taste and smell dull. Appetite decreases. Touch and sensitivity to pain, pressure, heat, and cold are reduced.
- *The circulatory system.* The heart muscle weakens. Arteries narrow and are less elastic. Poor circulation occurs in many body parts. The number of red blood cells decreases. This can cause fatigue.
- *The respiratory system.* Respiratory muscles weaken. Lung tissue becomes less elastic. Difficult, labored, or painful breathing may occur with activity. The person may lack strength to cough and clear the airway of secretions. Respiratory infections and diseases may develop. Normal breathing is promoted. Avoid heavy bed linens over the chest. Turning, repositioning, and deep breathing are important. The person should be as active as possible.
- *The digestive system.* Less saliva is produced. The person may have difficulty swallowing (dysphagia). Secretion of digestive juices decreases. Indigestion may occur. Loss of teeth and ill-fitting dentures cause chewing problems. Peristalsis decreases. Flatulence and constipation can occur. Dry, fried, and fatty foods are avoided. Persons with chewing problems or constipation often need foods that provide soft bulk.
- *The urinary system.* Kidney function decreases. The kidneys shrink (atrophy). Urine is more concentrated. Bladder muscles weaken. Bladder size decreases. Urinary frequency or urgency may occur. Urinary tract infections are risks. Many older persons have to urinate (void) at night. Urinary incontinence (the loss of bladder control) may occur. In men, the prostate gland enlarges. This may cause difficulty voiding or frequent urination. Adequate fluids are needed. Follow the care plan. Most fluids should be taken before 1700 (5:00 PM). This reduces the need to void during the night.
- *The reproductive system.* In men, the hormone testosterone decreases slightly. An erection takes longer. Orgasm is less forceful. Women experience menopause. Female hormones of estrogen and progesterone decrease. The uterus, vagina, and genitalia shrink (atrophy). Vaginal walls thin. There is vaginal dryness. Arousal takes longer. Orgasm is less intense.

NEEDING NURSING CENTER CARE

- Some older persons cannot care for themselves. Nursing centers are options for them. While there, the nursing center is the person's home.
- The person needing nursing center care may suffer some or all of these losses.
  - Loss of identity as a productive member of a family and community
  - Loss of possessions—home, household items, car, and so on
  - Loss of independence
  - Loss of real-world experiences—shopping, traveling, cooking, driving, hobbies
  - Loss of health and mobility
- The person may feel useless, powerless, and hopeless. The health team helps the person cope with loss and improve quality of life. Treat the person with dignity and respect. Also practice good communication skills. Follow the care plan.

SEXUALITY

- Sexuality involves the personality and the body. Illness, injury, and aging can affect sexuality.
- Attitudes and sex needs change with aging and life events. Frequency of sex decreases for many older persons because of weakness, fatigue, pain, reduced mobility, and chronic illness.
- Sexual partners are lost through death, divorce, and relationship break-ups. Or a partner needs hospital or nursing center care. This does not mean loss of sexual needs or desires.
- Love, affection, and intimacy are needed throughout life. Older persons love, fall in love, hold hands, and embrace. Many have intercourse.

Meeting Sexual Needs
- The nursing team promotes the meeting of sexual needs.
- The measures in Box 9-2, Promoting Sexuality, in the textbook may be part of the person's care plan.

The Sexually Aggressive Person
- Some residents flirt or make sexual advances or comments. Some expose themselves, masturbate, or touch other staff.

- Touch may have a sexual purpose. You must be professional about the matter.
  - Ask the person not to touch you. State the places where you were touched.
  - Tell the person that you will not do what he or she wants.
  - Tell the person what behaviors make you uncomfortable. Politely ask the person not to act that way.
  - Allow privacy if the person is becoming aroused.
  - Discuss the matter with the nurse. The nurse can help you understand the behavior.
  - Follow the care plan. It has measures to deal with sexually aggressive behaviors. They are based on the cause of the behavior. Some causes include nervous system disorders, confusion, dementia, disorientation, drug side effects, fever, poor vision, urinary or reproductive system disorders, poor hygiene, and urine or feces soiling.

Protecting the Person

- The person must be protected from unwanted sexual comments and advances. This is sexual abuse (Chapter 4). Tell the nurse right away.
- No one should be allowed to sexually abuse another person. This includes staff members, patients, residents, family members or other visitors, and volunteers.

CHAPTER 9 REVIEW QUESTIONS

Circle the BEST answer.
1. Which statement is *false*?
   a. Physical changes occur with aging.
   b. Energy level and body efficiency decline with age.
   c. Some people age faster than others.
   d. Normal aging means loss of health.
2. As a person ages, the integumentary system changes. Which statement is *false*?
   a. Dry skin and itching occur.
   b. Nails become thick and tough.
   c. The person is less sensitive to cold.
   d. Skin is injured more easily.
3. Which statement about the musculo-skeletal system and aging is *false*?
   a. Strength decreases.
   b. Vertebrae shorten.
   c. Mobility increases.
   d. Bone mass decreases.
4. Which statement about the nervous system and aging is *false*?
   a. Reflexes slow.
   b. Memory may be shorter.
   c. Sleep patterns change.
   d. Forgetfulness decreases.
5. Which statement about the digestive system and aging is *false*?
   a. Appetite decreases.
   b. Less saliva is produced.
   c. Flatulence and constipation may decrease.
   d. Teeth may be lost.

6. Which statement about the urinary system and aging is *false*?
   a. Urine becomes more concentrated.
   b. Urinary frequency may occur.
   c. Urinary urgency may occur.
   d. Bladder muscles become stronger.
7. A resident touches you in a sexual way. You should do the following *except*
   a. Ask the person not to touch you
   b. Discuss the matter with the nurse
   c. Tell the person what behaviors make you uncomfortable
   d. Yell at the person immediately
8. Unwanted sexual comments and advances are forms of sexual abuse.
   a. True
   b. False

Answers to Chapter 9 questions are on p. 450.

CHAPTER 10 SAFETY NEEDS
ACCIDENT RISK FACTORS

- Certain factors increase the risk of accidents and injuries.
  - *Age.* Older persons are at risk for falls and other injuries.
  - *Awareness of surroundings.* Confused and disoriented persons may not understand what is happening to and around them.
  - *Agitated and aggressive behaviors.* Pain, confusion, fear, and decreased awareness of surroundings can cause these behaviors.
  - *Vision loss.* Persons can fall or trip over items. Some cannot read labels on containers. Poisoning may result.
  - *Hearing loss.* Persons have problems hearing explanations and instructions. They may not hear warning signals or fire alarms. Some cannot hear approaching meal carts, drug carts, stretchers, or people in wheelchairs. They do not know to move to safety.
  - *Impaired smell and touch.* Illness and aging affect smell and touch. The person may not detect smoke or gas odors or may be unaware of injury. Burns are a risk from impaired touch.
  - *Impaired mobility.* Some diseases and injuries affect mobility. A person may know there is danger but cannot move to safety. Some persons are paralyzed. Some persons cannot walk or propel wheelchairs.
  - *Drugs.* Drug side effects may include loss of balance, drowsiness, and lack of coordination. Reduced awareness, confusion, and disorientation can occur.

IDENTIFYING THE PERSON

- You must give the right care to the right person. The person may receive an identification (ID) bracelet when admitted to the agency. To identify the person:

- Compare identifying information on the assignment sheet or treatment card with that on the ID bracelet.
- Call the person by name when checking the ID bracelet. Just calling the person by name is not enough to identify him or her. Confused, disoriented, drowsy, hard-of-hearing, or distracted persons may answer to any name.

Nursing Center Residents

- Alert and oriented residents may choose not to wear ID bracelets. This is noted on the person's care plan. Follow center policy and the care plan to identify the person. Some nursing centers have photo ID systems. Use this system safely.
- Use at least two identifiers. An identifier cannot be the person's room or bed number. Some agencies require the person to state and spell his or her name and give birth date. Others require using the person's ID number. Always follow agency policy.

PREVENTING BURNS

- Smoking, spilled hot liquids, very hot water, and electrical devices are common causes of burns.
- To prevent burns:
  - Assist with eating and drinking.
  - Be careful when carrying hot food and fluid near patients or residents.
  - Keep hot food and fluids away from counter and table edges.
  - Do not pour hot liquids near a person.
  - Turn on cold water first, then hot water. Turn off hot water first, then cold water.
  - Measure bath or shower water temperature.
  - Check for "hot spots" in bath water.
  - Do not let the person sleep with a heating pad or an electric blanket.
  - Follow safety guidelines when applying heat and cold.
  - Be sure people smoke only in smoking areas.
  - Do not leave smoking materials at the bedside.
  - Supervise the smoking of persons who cannot protect themselves.
  - Do not allow smoking in bed.
  - Do not allow smoking where oxygen is used or stored.
  - Be alert to ashes that may fall onto an older person.

PREVENTING POISONING

- Drugs and household products are common poisons. Poisoning in adults may be from carelessness,

confusion, or poor vision when reading labels. To prevent poisoning:

- Make sure patients and residents cannot reach hazardous materials.
- Follow agency policy for storing personal care items.
- Keep harmful products in their original containers.
- Leave the original label on harmful products.
- Read all labels carefully before using a product.

PREVENTING SUFFOCATION

- **Suffocation** is when breathing stops from the lack of oxygen. Death occurs if the person does not start breathing. Common causes include choking, drowning, inhaling gas or smoke, strangulation, and electrical shock.
- To prevent suffocation, review Box 10-2, Preventing Suffocation, in the textbook.

Choking

- Choking or foreign-body airway obstruction (FBAO) occurs when a foreign body obstructs the airway. Air cannot pass through the air passages into the lungs. The body does not get enough oxygen. Death can result.
- Choking often occurs during eating. A large, poorly chewed piece of meat is the most common cause. Other common causes include laughing and talking while eating and excessive alcohol intake.
- Unconscious persons can choke.
- With *mild airway obstruction*, some air moves in and out of the lungs. The person is conscious. Usually the person can speak. If the person is breathing and coughing, abdominal thrusts are not needed. Often forceful coughing can remove the object. If the obstruction persists, call for help.
- With *severe airway obstruction*, the conscious person clutches at the throat—the "universal sign of choking." The person has difficulty breathing. Some persons cannot breathe, speak, or cough. The person appears pale and cyanotic (bluish color). Air does not move in and out of the lungs. If the obstruction is not removed, the person will die. Severe airway obstruction is an emergency.
- Use abdominal thrusts to relieve FBAO. Chest thrusts are used for very obese persons and pregnant women. See Box 10-3, Relieving Choking—Chest Thrusts for Obese or Pregnant Persons, and Figure 10-5, Chest Thrusts to Relieve Choking in a Pregnant Woman, in the textbook.
- Call for help when a person has an obstructed airway. Report and record what happened, what you did, and the person's response.

PREVENTING EQUIPMENT ACCIDENTS

- All equipment is unsafe if broken, not used correctly, or not working properly. Inspect all equipment before use. Review Box 10-4, Preventing Equipment Accidents, in the textbook.

WHEELCHAIR AND STRETCHER SAFETY

- When using wheelchairs and stretchers, the person can fall from the wheelchair or stretcher. Or the person can fall during transfers to and from the wheelchair or stretcher.

HANDLING HAZARDOUS SUBSTANCES

- A hazardous substance is any chemical in the workplace that can cause harm. Hazardous substances include oxygen, mercury, disinfectants, and cleaning agents.
- Hazardous substance containers must have manufacturer warning labels. If a label is removed or damaged, do not use the substance. Take the container to the nurse. Do not leave the container unattended.
- Check the material safety data sheet (MSDS) before using a hazardous substance, cleaning up a leak or spill, or disposing of the substance. Tell the nurse about a leak or spill right away. Do not leave a leak or spill unattended.

DISASTERS

- A **disaster** is a sudden catastrophic event. The agency has procedures for disasters that could occur in your area. Follow them to keep patients, residents, visitors, staff, and yourself safe.
- Natural disasters include tornadoes, hurricanes, blizzards, earthquakes, volcanic eruptions, floods, and some fires.
- Human-made disasters include auto, bus, train, and airplane accidents. They also include fires, bombings, nuclear power plant accidents, gas or chemical leaks, explosions, and wars.

Fire Safety

- Faulty electrical equipment and wiring, overloaded electrical circuits, and smoking are major causes of fires.
- Safety measures are needed where oxygen is used and stored.
  - NO SMOKING signs are placed on the door and near the person's bed.
  - The person and visitors cannot smoke in the room.
  - Smoking materials are removed from the room.
  - Safety measures to prevent equipment accidents are followed. See Box 10-4, Preventing Equipment Accidents, in the textbook.
  - Wool blankets and fabrics that cause static electricity are removed from the room.
  - The person wears a cotton gown or pajamas.

- Lit candles, incense, and other open flames are not allowed.
- Materials that ignite easily are removed from the room.
- Review Box 10-5, Fire Prevention Measures, in the textbook.
- Know your center's policies and procedures for fire emergencies. Know where to find fire alarms, fire extinguishers, and emergency exits. Remember the word RACE.
  - R—*rescue*. Rescue persons in immediate danger. Move them to a safe place.
  - A—*alarm*. Sound the nearest fire alarm. Notify the operator.
  - C—*confine*. Close doors and windows. Turn off oxygen or electrical items.
  - E—*extinguish*. Use a fire extinguisher on a small fire that has not spread.
- Remember the word PASS for using a fire extinguisher.
  - P—*pull* the safety pin.
  - A—*aim* low. Aim at the base of the fire.
  - S—*squeeze* the lever. This starts the stream of water.
  - S—*sweep* back and forth. Sweep side to side at the base of the fire.
- Do not use elevators during a fire.

WORKPLACE VIOLENCE

- **Workplace violence** is violent acts (including assault or threat of assault) directed toward persons at work or while on duty. Review Box 10-6, Workplace Violence—Safety Measures, in the textbook.

RISK MANAGEMENT

- Risk management involves identifying and controlling risks and safety hazards affecting the agency. It deals with these and other safety issues.
  - Accident and fire prevention
  - Negligence and malpractice
  - Abuse
  - Workplace violence
  - Federal and state requirements
- Risk managers look for patterns and trends in incident reports, complaints (patients, residents, staff), and accident and injury investigations. Unsafe situations are corrected. Procedure changes and training recommendations are made as needed.
- Color-coded wristbands promote the person's safety and prevent harm. They quickly communicate an alert or warning. Know the wristband colors used in your agency. Check the care plan and your assignment sheet when you see a color-coded wristband.
- The person's belongings must be kept safe. A personal belongings list is completed. Items kept at the bedside are listed in the person's record. Clothing

and shoes are labeled with the person's name. So are other items brought from home.
- Report accidents and errors at once. An *incident report* is completed as soon as possible. Incident reports are reviewed by risk management and a committee of health care workers.

CHAPTER 10 REVIEW QUESTIONS

Circle the BEST answer.
1. You see a water spill in the hallway. What will you do?
   a. Ask housekeeping to wipe up the spill right away.
   b. Wipe up the spill right away.
   c. Report the spill to the nurse.
   d. Ask the resident to walk around the spill.
2. An electrical outlet in a person's room does not work. What will you do?
   a. Tell the administrator about the problem.
   b. Tell another nursing assistant about the problem.
   c. Try to repair the electrical outlet.
   d. Follow the center's policy for reporting the problem.
3. Accident risk factors include all of the following *except*
   a. Walking without difficulty
   b. Hearing problems
   c. Dulled sense of smell
   d. Poor vision
4. To prevent a person from being burned, you should do the following *except*
   a. Supervise the smoking of persons who are confused
   b. Turn cold water on first; turn hot water off first
   c. Do not let the person sleep with a heating pad
   d. Allow smoking in bed
5. To prevent suffocation, you should do the following *except*
   a. Make sure dentures fit properly
   b. Check the care plan for swallowing problems before serving food or liquids
   c. Leave a person alone in a bathtub or shower
   d. Position the person in bed properly
6. Which statement about mild airway obstruction is *false*?
   a. Some air moves in and out of the lungs.
   b. The person is conscious.
   c. Usually the person cannot speak.
   d. Forceful coughing will often remove the object.
7. The "universal sign of choking" is
   a. Clutching at the chest
   b. Clutching at the throat
   c. Not being able to talk
   d. Not being able to breathe
8. Which of the following is *not* a safety measure with oxygen?
   a. NO SMOKING signs are placed on the resident's door and near the bed.
   b. Lit candles and other open flames are permitted in the room.
   c. Electrical items are turned off before being unplugged.
   d. The person wears a cotton gown or pajamas.
9. You have discovered a fire in the nursing center. You should do the following *except*
   a. Rescue persons in immediate danger
   b. Sound the nearest fire alarm
   c. Open doors and windows and keep oxygen on
   d. Use a fire extinguisher on a small fire that has not spread to a larger area
10. When using a fire extinguisher, you do the following *except*
   a. Pull the safety pin on the fire extinguisher
   b. Aim at the top of the flames
   c. Squeeze the lever to start the stream
   d. Sweep the stream back and forth

Answers to Chapter 10 questions are on p. 450.

CHAPTER 11 PREVENTING FALLS
- The risk of falling increases with age.
- Falls are a leading cause of injuries and deaths among older persons. A history of falls increases the risk of falling again.
- Most falls occur in resident rooms and bathrooms. Falls are the most common accidents in nursing centers.

CAUSES AND RISK FACTORS FOR FALLS
- Falls occur within the first 72 hours of admission to a hospital or nursing center. Falls occur during the night and after meals.
- Causes for falls are poor lighting, cluttered floors, throw rugs, needing to use the bathroom, and out-of-place furniture. So are wet and slippery floors, bathtubs, and showers. Review Box 11-1, Fall Risk Factors, in the textbook.

FALL PREVENTION
- Agencies have fall prevention programs. Review Box 11-2, Preventing Falls, in the textbook. The person's care plan also lists measures specific for the person.

Bed Rails
- A **bed rail** *(side rail)* is a device that serves as a guard or barrier along the side of the bed. Bed rails are half, three quarters, or the full length of the bed.
- The nurse and care plan tell you when to raise bed rails. They are needed by persons who are unconscious or sedated with drugs. Some confused and disoriented people need them. If a person needs bed rails, keep them up at all times except when giving bedside nursing care.
- Bed rails present hazards. The person can fall when trying to get out of bed. Or the person can get caught, trapped, entangled, or strangled (entrapment).

- Bed rails are considered restraints if the person cannot get out of bed or lower them without help.
- Bed rails cannot be used unless they are needed to treat a person's medical symptoms. The person or legal representative must give consent for raised bed rails. The need for bed rails is carefully noted in the person's medical record and the care plan. If a person uses bed rails, check the person often. Report to the nurse that you checked the person. Record when you checked the person and your observations.
- To prevent falls:
  - Never leave the person alone when the bed is raised.
  - Always lower the bed to its lowest position when you are done giving care.
  - If a person does not use bed rails and you need to raise the bed, ask a co-worker to stand on the far side of the bed to protect the person from falling.
  - If you raise the bed to give care, always raise the far bed rail if you are working alone.
  - Be sure the person who uses raised bed rails has access to items on the bedside stand and over-bed table. The call light, water pitcher and cup, tissues, phone, and TV and light controls should be within the person's reach.

Hand Rails and Grab Bars

- Hand rails give support to persons who are weak or unsteady when walking.
- Grab bars provide support for sitting down or getting up from a toilet. They also are used for getting in and out of the shower or tub.

Wheel Locks

- Bed wheels are locked at all times except when moving the bed. Bed wheels are locked when giving bedside care and when you transfer a person to and from bed.
- Wheelchair and stretcher wheels are locked when transferring a person.

TRANSFER/GAIT BELTS

- Use a **transfer belt (gait belt)** to support a person who is unsteady or disabled. Always follow the manufacturer's instructions. Apply the belt over clothing and under the breasts. The belt buckle is never positioned over the person's spine. Tighten the belt so it is snug. Adjust the belt as needed for the person's comfort and safety. You should be able to slide your open, flat hand under the belt. Tuck the excess strap under the belt. Remove the belt after the procedure.
- When used to transfer a person, it is called a *transfer belt*. When used to help a person walk, it is called a *gait belt*.
- Do not leave the person alone while he or she is wearing a transfer/gait belt.

- Check with the nurse and care plan before using a transfer/gait belt if the person has:
  - A colostomy, ileostomy, gastrostomy, urostomy
  - A gastric tube
  - Chronic obstructive pulmonary disease
  - An abdominal or chest wound, incision, or drainage tube
  - Monitoring equipment
  - A hernia
  - Other conditions or care equipment involving the chest or abdomen

THE FALLING PERSON

- If a person starts to fall, do not try to prevent the fall. You could injure yourself and the person. Ease the person to the floor and protect the person's head. Do not let the person move or get up before the nurse checks for injuries. If you find a person on the floor, do not move the person. Stay with the person and call for the nurse. An incident report is completed after all falls.
- When helping the falling person, follow these procedures.
  - Stand behind the person with your feet apart. Keep your back straight.
  - Bring the person close to your body as fast as possible. Use the transfer/gait belt. Or wrap your arms around the person's waist. If necessary, you can also hold the person under the arms.
  - Move your leg so that the person's buttocks rest on it. Move the leg near the person.
  - Lower the person to the floor. The person slides down your leg to the floor. Bend at your hips and knees as you lower the person.
  - Call a nurse to check the person. Stay with the person.
  - Help the nurse return the person to bed. Ask other staff to help if needed.

CHAPTER 11 REVIEW QUESTIONS

Circle the BEST answer.

1. Most falls occur in
   a. Resident rooms and bathrooms
   b. Dining rooms
   c. Hallways
   d. Activity rooms
2. Which statement about falls is *false?*
   a. Poor lighting, cluttered floors, and throw rugs may cause falls.
   b. Improper shoes and needing to use the bathroom may cause falls.
   c. Poor judgment increases the risk for falls
   d. Falls are less likely to occur during shift changes.
3. You note the following after a person got dressed. Which is unsafe?
   a. Nonskid footwear is worn.
   b. Pant cuffs are dragging on the floor.
   c. Clothing fits properly.
   d. The belt is fastened.

4. Which statement about bed rails is *false?*
   a. The nurse and care plan tell you when to raise bed rails.
   b. Bed rails are considered restraints.
   c. You may leave a person alone when the bed is raised and the bed rails are down.
   d. Bed rails can present hazards because people try to climb over them.
5. Which statement about transfer/gait belts is *false?*
   a. To use the belt safely, follow the manufacturer's instructions.
   b. Always apply the belt over clothing.
   c. Tighten the belt so that it is snug and breathing is impaired.
   d. Place the belt buckle off-center so that it is not over the spine.
6. A person becomes faint in the hallway and begins to fall. You should do the following *except*
   a. Ease the person to the floor
   b. Protect the person's head
   c. Let the person get up before the nurse checks him or her
   d. Help the nurse complete the incident report

Answers to Chapter 11 questions are on p. 450.

CHAPTER 12 RESTRAINT ALTERNATIVES AND RESTRAINTS

- The Centers for Medicare & Medicaid Services (CMS) has rules for using restraints. These rules protect the person's rights and safety. This includes the right to be free from restraint.
- Restraints may be used only to treat a medical symptom or for the immediate physical safety of the person or others. Restraints may be used only when less restrictive measures fail to protect the person or others. They must be discontinued as soon as possible.
- The CMS uses these terms.
  - A **physical restraint** is any manual method or physical or mechanical device, material, or equipment attached to or near the person's body that he or she cannot remove easily and that restricts freedom of movement or normal access to one's body.
  - A **chemical restraint** is any drug used for discipline or convenience and not required to treat medical symptoms. The drug or dosage is not a standard treatment for the person's condition.
  - **Freedom of movement** is any change in place or position of the body or any part of the body that the person is able to control.
  - **Remove easily** is the manual method, device, material, or equipment used to restrain the person that can be removed intentionally by the person in the same manner it was applied by staff.
- Restraints were once used to prevent falls. Research shows that restraints cause falls.
- Federal, state, and accrediting agencies have guidelines about restraint use. They do not forbid restraint

use. They require considering or trying all other appropriate alternatives first.
- Every agency has policies and procedures about restraints. They include identifying persons at risk for harm, harmful behaviors, restraint alternatives, and proper restraint use. Staff training is required.

RESTRAINT ALTERNATIVES

- Knowing and treating the cause for harmful behaviors can prevent restraint use. There are many alternatives to restraints, such as answering the call light promptly. For other alternatives see Box 12-1, Restraint Alternatives, in the textbook. The care plan is changed as needed.
- Restraint alternatives may not protect the person. The doctor may need to order restraints.

SAFE RESTRAINT USE

- CMS, OBRA, Food and Drug Administration (FDA), and The Joint Commission (TJC) guidelines and state laws are followed.
- Restraints are used only when necessary to treat a person's medical symptoms—physical, emotional, or behavioral problems. Sometimes restraints are needed to protect the person or others.

Physical and Chemical Restraints

- *Physical restraints* are applied to the chest, waist, elbows, wrists, hands, or ankles. They confine the person to a bed or chair. Or they prevent movement of a body part.
- Some furniture or barriers also prevent freedom of movement.
  - A device used with a chair that the person cannot remove easily. Trays, tables, bars, and belts are examples.
  - Any chair or bed placed so close to the wall that the person cannot get out of the bed or chair.
  - Bed rails that prevent the person from getting out of bed.
  - Tucking in or using Velcro to hold a sheet fabric or clothing so tightly that freedom of movement is restricted.
  - Drugs or drug dosages are *chemical restraints* if they:
  - Control behavior or restrict movement
  - Are not standard treatment for the person's condition
- An enabler is a device that limits freedom of movement but is used to promote independence, comfort, or safety. Some devices are restraints and enablers.

Risks from Restraint Use

- Injuries occur as the person tries to get free of the restraint. Injuries also occur from using the wrong restraint, applying it wrong, or keeping it on too long. Cuts, bruises, and fractures are common. The most serious risk is death from strangulation. Review Box 12-2, Risks from Restraint Use, in the textbook.

- Restraints may also affect a person's dignity and self-esteem. Depression, anger, and agitation are common. So are embarrassment, humiliation, and mistrust.

Legal Aspects

- *Restraints must protect the person.* A restraint is used only when it is the best safety measure for the person.
- *A doctor's order is required.* The doctor gives the reason for the restraint, what body part to restrain, what to use, and how long to use it. This information is in the care plan.
- *The least restrictive method is used.* It allows the greatest amount of movement or body access possible.
- *Restraints are used only after other measures fail to protect the person.* Box 12-1 in the textbook lists alternatives to restraint use.
- *Unnecessary restraint is false imprisonment.* If you apply an unneeded restraint, you could face false imprisonment charges.
- *Informed consent is required.* The person must understand the reason for the restraint. If the person cannot give consent, his or her legal representative must give consent before a restraint can be used. The doctor or nurse provides the necessary information and obtains the consent.

Safety Guidelines

- Review Box 12-3, Safety Measures for Using Restraints, in the textbook.
- *Observe for increased confusion and agitation.* Restraints can increase confusion and agitation. Restrained persons need repeated explanations and reassurance. Spending time with them has a calming effect.
- *Protect the person's quality of life.* Restraints are used for as short a time as possible. You must meet the person's physical, emotional, and social needs.
- *Follow the manufacturer's instructions.* The restraint must be snug and firm but not tight. You could be negligent if you do not apply or secure a restraint properly.
- *Apply restraints with enough help to protect the person and staff from injury.*
- *Observe the person at least every 15 minutes or more often as noted in the care plan.* Injuries and deaths can result from improper restraint use and poor observation.
- *Remove or release the restraint, reposition the person, and meet basic needs at least every 2 hours or as often as noted in the care plan.* The restraint is removed for at least 10 minutes. Provide for food, fluid, comfort, safety, hygiene, and elimination needs and give skin care. Perform range-of-motion exercises or help the person walk.

Reporting and Recording

- Restraint information is recorded in the person's medical record.
- Report and record the following:
  - Type of restraint applied.
  - Body part or parts restrained.
  - Reason for the application.
  - Safety measures taken.
  - Time you applied the restraint.
  - Time you removed or released the restraint and for how long.
  - Care given when restraint was removed and for how long.
  - Person's vital signs.
  - Skin color and condition.
  - Condition of the limbs.
  - Pulse felt in the restrained part.
  - Changes in the person's behavior.
  - Complaints of discomfort; a tight restraint; difficulty breathing; or pain, numbness, or tingling in the restrained part. Report these complaints to the nurse at once.

CHAPTER 12 REVIEW QUESTIONS

Circle the BEST answer.

1. A geriatric chair or a bed rail may be considered a restraint if free movement is restricted.
   a. True
   b. False
2. Which statement about the use of restraints is *false*?
   a. A person may be embarrassed and humiliated when restraints are on.
   b. A person may experience depression and agitation when restraints are on.
   c. Restraints can be used for staff convenience.
   d. Restraints can cause serious injury and death.
3. Restraints can increase a person's confusion and agitation.
   a. True
   b. False
4. The person with a restraint should be observed at least every
   a. 15 minutes
   b. 30 minutes
   c. Hour
   d. 2 hours
5. Restraints need to be removed at least every
   a. Hour
   b. 2 hours
   c. 3 hours
   d. 4 hours
6. You should record all the following *except*
   a. The type of restraint used
   b. The consent for the restraint
   c. The time you removed the restraint
   d. The care you gave when the restraint was removed

Answers to Chapter 12 questions are on p. 450.

CHAPTER 13 PREVENTING INFECTION

- An **infection** is a disease state resulting from the invasion and growth of microbes in the body. Infection is a major safety and health hazard. Older and disabled persons are at risk.
- The health team follows certain practices and procedures to prevent the spread of infection (**infection control**).

MICROORGANISMS

- A **microorganism (microbe)** is a small (*micro*) living thing (*organism*). It is seen only with a microscope. Microbes are everywhere.
- Some microbes are harmful and can cause infections (**pathogens**). Others do not usually cause infection (**non-pathogens**).

Requirements of Microbes

- Microbes need a *reservoir (host)*. The reservoir is the place where the microbe lives and grows. People, plants, animals, the soil, food, and water are examples. Microbes need *water* and *nourishment* from the reservoir. Most need *oxygen* to live. A *warm* and *dark* environment is needed. Most grow best at body temperature. They are destroyed by heat and light.

Multidrug-Resistant Organisms

- *Multidrug-resistant organisms (MDROs)* are microbes that can resist the effects of antibiotics. Such pathogens are able to change their structures to survive in the presence of antibiotics. The infections they cause are harder to treat.
- MDROs are caused by prescribing antibiotics when they are not needed (over-prescribing). Not taking antibiotics for the prescribed length of time is also a cause.
- Two common types of MDROs are resistant to many antibiotics.
  - *Methicillin-resistant* Staphylococcus aureus *(MRSA)*. MRSA is resistant to antibiotics often used for "staph" infections. MRSA can cause pneumonia and serious wound and blood-stream infections.
  - *Vancomycin-resistant* Enterococcus *(VRE)*. *Enterococcus* is a bacterium normally found in the intestine and in feces. It can be transmitted to others by contaminated hands, toilet seats, care equipment, and other items that the hands touch. When not in their natural state (the intestines), enterococci can cause urinary tract, pelvic, and other infections.

INFECTION

- **A local infection** is in a body part.
- **A systemic infection** involves the whole body.

Infection in Older Persons

- Older persons may not show the normal signs and symptoms of infection. The person may have only a slight fever or no fever at all. Redness and swelling may be very slight. The person may not complain of pain. Confusion and delirium may occur.
- Infections can become life-threatening before the older person has obvious signs and symptoms. Be alert to minor changes in the person's behavior or condition. Review Box 13-1, Infection—Signs and Symptoms, in the textbook. Report any changes to the nurse at once.

The Chain of Infection

- The chain of infection begins with a *source*—a pathogen. It must have a reservoir where it can grow and multiply. A **carrier** is a human or animal that is a reservoir for microbes but does not develop the infection. To leave the reservoir, the pathogen needs a *portal of exit*. Exits are respiratory, gastrointestinal (GI), urinary, and reproductive tracts; breaks in the skin; and blood. After leaving the reservoir, the pathogen must be *transmitted* to another host. The pathogen enters the body through a *portal of entry*. Portals of entry and exit are the same. A *susceptible host* is needed for the microbe to grow and multiply.

Healthcare-Associated Infection

- A **healthcare-associated infection (HAI)** is an infection that develops in a person cared for in any setting where health care is given. Review Box 13-2, Rules of Hand Hygiene, in the textbook. The infection is related to receiving health care. Hospitals, nursing centers, clinics, and home care settings are examples. HAIs also are called *nosocomial infections*.
- Common sites for HAIs are:
  - The urinary system
  - The respiratory system
  - Wounds
  - The bloodstream
- The health team must prevent the spread of HAIs by:
  - Medical asepsis. This includes hand hygiene.
  - Surgical asepsis.
  - Standard Precautions and Transmission-Based Precautions.
  - The Bloodborne Pathogen Standard.

MEDICAL ASEPSIS

- **Asepsis** is being free of disease-producing microbes.
- **Medical asepsis (clean technique)** is the practice used to:
  - Remove or destroy pathogens.
  - Prevent pathogens from spreading from one person or place to another person or place.

- **Contamination** is the process of becoming unclean. The item or area is contaminated when pathogens are present.
- **Sterile** means the absence of all microbes—pathogens and non-pathogens.

Common Aseptic Practices
- Aseptic practices break the chain of infection.
- To prevent the spread of microbes, wash your hands:
  - After elimination.
  - After changing tampons or sanitary pads.
  - After contact with your own or another person's blood, body fluids, secretions, or excretions. This includes saliva, vomitus, urine, feces, vaginal discharge, mucus, semen, wound drainage, pus, and respiratory secretions.
  - After coughing, sneezing, or blowing your nose.
  - Before and after handling, preparing, or eating food.
  - After smoking.
  - Also do the following.
  - Provide all persons with their own linens and personal care items.
  - Cover your nose and mouth when coughing, sneezing, or blowing your nose. If without tissues, cough or sneeze into your upper arm. Do not cough or sneeze into your hands.
  - Bathe, wash hair, and brush your teeth regularly.
  - Wash fruits and raw vegetables before eating or serving them.
  - Wash cooking and eating utensils with soap and water after use.

Hand Hygiene
- *Hand hygiene is the easiest and most important way to prevent the spread of infection.* Practice hand hygiene before and after giving care. Review Box 13-2, Rules of Hand Hygiene, in the textbook.

Supplies and Equipment
- Most health care equipment is disposable. Bedpans, urinals, wash basins, water pitchers, and drinking cups are multi-use items. Do not "borrow" them for another person. Label such items with the person's room and bed number.
- Non-disposable items are cleaned and then disinfected. Then they are sterilized.
- Cleaning:
  - Wear personal protective equipment (PPE). PPE includes gloves, a mask, a gown, and goggles or a face shield.
  - Work from clean to dirty areas.
  - Rinse the item in cold water.
  - Wash the item with soap and hot water.
  - Scrub thoroughly.
  - Rinse the item in warm water.
  - Dry the item.
  - Disinfect or sterilize the item.

- Disinfect equipment and the sink used in the cleaning procedure.
- Discard PPE.
- Practice hand hygiene.
- Disinfection:
  - Disinfection is the process of destroying pathogens. Chemical disinfectants are used to clean surfaces. They also are used to clean reusable items such as commodes and wheelchairs. Wear waterproof utility or rubber gloves. Do not wear disposable gloves.
- Sterilization:
  - Sterilization is the process of destroying all microbes. Very high temperatures are used. Boiling water, radiation, liquid or gas chemicals, dry heat, and *steam under pressure* are sterilization methods. An *autoclave* is a pressure steam sterilizer. Glass, surgical items, and metal objects are autoclaved.

Other Aseptic Measures
- Review Box 13-3, Aseptic Measures, in the textbook.

ISOLATION PRECAUTIONS
- Isolation precautions prevent the spread of **communicable diseases (contagious diseases)**. They are diseases caused by pathogens that spread easily.
- The Centers for Disease Control and Prevention (CDC) isolation precautions guideline has two tiers of precautions.
  - Standard Precautions
  - Transmission-Based Precautions

Standard Precautions
- Standard Precautions reduce the risk of spreading pathogens and known and unknown infections. Standard Precautions are used for all persons whenever care is given. They prevent the spread of infection from:
  - Blood.
  - All body fluids, secretions, and excretions (except sweat) even if blood is not visible. Sweat is not known to spread infection.
  - Non-intact skin (skin with open breaks).
  - Mucous membranes.
- Review Box 13-4, Standard Precautions, in the textbook.

Transmission-Based Precautions
- Some infections require Transmission-Based Precautions. They are commonly called "isolation precautions." You must understand how certain infections are spread. This helps you understand the three types of Transmission-Based Precautions. Review Box 13-5, Transmission-Based Precautions, in the textbook.
- Agency policies may differ from those in the textbook. The rules in Box 13-6, Rules for Isolation Precautions, in the textbook are a guide for giving safe care.

Protective Measures

- Isolation Precautions involve wearing PPE—gloves, a gown, a mask, and goggles or a face shield.
- Removing linens, trash, and equipment from the room may require double-bagging.
- Follow agency procedures when collecting specimens and transporting persons.
- Wear gloves whenever contact with blood, body fluids, secretions, excretions, mucous membranes, and non-intact skin is likely. Wearing gloves is the most common protective measure for Standard Precautions and Transmission-Based Precautions. When using gloves:
  - The outside of gloves is contaminated.
  - Gloves are easier to put on dry hands.
  - Do not tear gloves when putting them on. This contaminates your hand.
  - Apply a new pair for every person.
  - Remove and discard torn, cut, or punctured gloves at once. Practice hand hygiene. Then put on a new pair.
  - Wear gloves once. Discard them after use.
  - Put on clean gloves just before touching mucous membranes or non-intact skin.
  - Put on new gloves when gloves become contaminated with blood, body fluids, secretions, or excretions. A task may require more than one pair of gloves.
  - Change gloves when touching portable computer keyboards or other mobile equipment that is transported from room to room.
  - Put on gloves last when worn with other PPE.
  - Change gloves when moving from a contaminated body site to a clean body site.
  - Make sure gloves cover your wrists. If you wear a gown, gloves cover the cuffs.
  - Remove gloves so that the inside part is on the outside. The inside is clean.
  - Practice hand hygiene after removing gloves.
- Some gloves are made of latex (a rubber product). Latex allergies are common and can cause skin rashes. Difficulty breathing and shock are more serious problems. Report skin rashes and breathing problems at once. If you or a resident has a latex allergy, wear latex-free gloves.
- Gowns prevent the spread of microbes.
- Gowns must completely cover you from your neck to your knees. The gown front and sleeves are considered contaminated. A wet gown is contaminated. Gowns are used once. When removing a gown, roll it away from you. Keep it inside out. Do not let the gown touch the floor.
- Masks are disposable. A wet or moist mask is contaminated. When removing a mask, touch only the ties or elastic bands. The front of the mask is contaminated.
- The front (outside) of goggles or a face shield is contaminated. Use the device's ties, headband, or earpieces to remove the device.
- Contaminated items, linens, and trash are bagged to remove them from the person's room. Leak-proof plastic bags are used. They have the BIOHAZARD symbol. Double-bagging is not needed unless the outside of the bag is wet, soiled, or may be contaminated. Follow agency policy for bagging and transporting trash equipment, supplies, and specimens. Also follow agency procedures for a safe transport when a person is on Transmission-Based Precautions.

Meeting Basic Needs

- Love, belonging, and self-esteem needs are often unmet when Transmission-Based Precautions are used. Visitors and staff often avoid the person. The person may feel lonely, unwanted, and rejected. He or she may feel dirty and undesirable. The person may feel ashamed and guilty for having a contagious disease. You can help meet love, belonging, and self-esteem needs by doing such things as:
  - Treating the person with respect, kindness, and dignity.
  - Planning your work so that you can stay to visit with the person.

BLOODBORNE PATHOGEN STANDARD

- The health team is at risk for exposure to human immunodeficiency virus (HIV) and the hepatitis B virus (HBV). HIV and HBV are bloodborne pathogens found in the blood.
- The Bloodborne Pathogen Standard is intended to protect you from exposure. It is a regulation of the Occupational Safety and Health Administration (OSHA).
- Staff at risk for exposure to blood or other potentially infectious materials (OPIM) receive free training.
- *Hepatitis B vaccination.* You can receive the hepatitis B vaccination within 10 working days of being hired. The agency pays for it. If you refuse the vaccination, you must sign a statement. You can have the vaccination at a later date.

Engineering and Work Practice Controls

- *Engineering controls* reduce employee exposure in the workplace. There are special containers for contaminated sharps (needles, broken glass) and specimens. These containers are closable, puncture-resistant, leak-proof, and color-coded in red. They have the BIOHAZARD symbol.
- *Work practice controls* reduce exposure risk. All tasks involving blood or OPIM are done in ways to limit splatters, splashes, and sprays. OSHA requires these work practice controls.
  - Do not eat, drink, smoke, apply cosmetics or lip balm, or handle contact lenses in areas of occupational exposure.
  - Do not store food or drinks where blood or OPIM are kept.

- Practice hand hygiene after removing gloves.
- Wash hands as soon as possible after skin contact with blood or OPIM.
- Never recap, bend, or remove needles by hand.
- Never shear or break needles.
- Discard needles and sharp instruments (razors) in containers that are closable, puncture-resistant, and leak-proof. Containers are color-coded in red and have the *BIOHAZARD* symbol.

Personal Protective Equipment (PPE)
- PPE includes gloves, goggles, face shields, masks, laboratory coats, gowns, shoe covers, and surgical caps. OSHA requires these measures for PPE.
  - Remove PPE before leaving the work area.
  - Remove PPE when a garment becomes contaminated.
  - Place used PPE in marked areas or containers when being stored, washed, decontaminated, or discarded.
  - Wear gloves when you expect contact with blood or OPIM.
  - Wear gloves when handling or touching contaminated items or surfaces.
  - Replace worn, punctured, or contaminated gloves.
  - Never wash or decontaminate disposable gloves for reuse.
  - Discard utility gloves with signs of cracking, peeling, tearing, or puncturing. Utility gloves are decontaminated for reuse if the process will not ruin them.

Equipment
- Contaminated equipment is cleaned and decontaminated. Decontaminate work surfaces with a proper disinfectant:
  - Upon completing tasks
  - At once when there is obvious contamination
  - After any spill of blood or OPIM
  - At the end of the work shift when surfaces become contaminated since the last cleaning.
- Use a brush and dustpan or tongs to clean up broken glass. Never pick up broken glass with your hands, not even with gloves.

Laundry
- OSHA requires these measures for contaminated laundry.
  - Handle it as little as possible.
  - Wear gloves or other needed PPE.
  - Bag contaminated laundry where it is used.
  - Mark laundry bags or containers with the *BIOHAZARD* symbol for laundry sent off-site.
  - Place wet, contaminated laundry in leak-proof containers before transport. The containers are color-coded in red or have the *BIOHAZARD* symbol.

Exposure Incidents
- An **exposure incident** is any eye, mouth, other mucous membrane, non-intact skin, or parenteral contact with blood or OPIM. Parenteral means piercing the mucus membranes or the skin.

- Report exposure incidents at once. Medical evaluation, follow-up, and required tests are free. Your blood is tested for HIV and HBV. You are told of any medical conditions that may need treatment.

CHAPTER 13 REVIEW QUESTIONS
Circle the BEST answer.
1. A health care–associated infection (nosocomial infection) is
   a. An infection free of disease-producing microbes
   b. An infection that develops in a person cared for in any setting where health care is given
   c. An infection acquired by health care workers
   d. An infection acquired only by older persons
2. Which statement about hand hygiene is *false*?
   a. Hand hygiene is the easiest way to prevent the spread of infection.
   b. Hand hygiene is the most important way to prevent the spread of infection.
   c. Hand hygiene is practiced before and after giving care to a person.
   d. If hands are visibly soiled, hand hygiene can be done with an alcohol-based hand rub.
3. When washing your hands, you should do the following *except*
   a. Stand away from the sink so that your clothes do not touch the sink
   b. Keep your hands lower than your elbows
   c. Wash your hands for at least 15 seconds
   d. Dry your arms from the forearms to the fingertips
4. Which statement about wearing gloves is *false*?
   a. The insides of gloves are contaminated.
   b. You need a new pair of gloves for each person you care for.
   c. Change gloves when moving from a contaminated body site to a clean body site.
   d. Gloves need to cover your wrists.
5. Which statement is *false*?
   a. Gowns must cover you from your neck to your waist.
   b. A moist mask is contaminated.
   c. The outside of goggles is contaminated.
   d. You should wash your hands after removing a gown, mask, or goggles.
6. Which statement about PPE is *false*?
   a. Remove PPE when a garment becomes contaminated.
   b. Wear gloves when handling or touching contaminated items or surfaces.
   c. Wash or decontaminate disposable gloves for re-use.
   d. Remove PPE before leaving the work area.

Answers to Chapter 13 questions are on p. 450.

CHAPTER 14 BODY MECHANICS
- Body mechanics means using the body in an efficient and careful way.

PRINCIPLES OF BODY MECHANICS

- Body alignment (posture) is the way the head, trunk, arms, and legs are aligned with one another.
- Base of support is the area on which an object rests. When standing, your feet are your base of support.
- Your strongest and largest muscles are in the shoulders, upper arms, hips, and thighs. Use these muscles to lift and move persons and heavy objects. For good body mechanics:
  - Bend your knees and squat to lift a heavy object. Do not bend from your waist.
  - Hold items close to your body and base of support.
- All activities require good body mechanics.
- Review Box 14-1, Rules for Body Mechanics, in the textbook.

ERGONOMICS

- **Ergonomics** is the science of designing a job to fit the worker. The task, work station, equipment, and tools are changed to help reduce stress on the worker's body. The goal is to prevent a serious, painful, and disabling work-related musculo-skeletal disorder (MSD).

Work-Related MSDs

- MSDs can develop slowly over weeks, months, and years. Or they can occur from one event.
- MSDs are injuries and disorders of the muscles, tendons, ligaments, joints, and cartilage. They can involve the nervous system. The arms and back are often affected.
- Early signs and symptoms of injury include pain, limited joint movement, or soft tissue swelling. Always report a work-related injury as soon as possible. Early attention can help prevent the problem from becoming worse.
- The Occupational Safety and Health Administration (OSHA) has identified risk factors for MSDs.
  - *Force*—the amount of physical effort needed for a task
  - *Repeating action*—doing the same motion or series of motions often or continually
  - *Awkward postures*—assuming positions that place stress on the body
  - *Heavy lifting*
- An MSD is more likely if risk factors are combined.
- Back injuries can occur from repeated activities or from one event. Signs and symptoms of a back injury include:
  - Pain when trying to assume a normal position
  - Decreased mobility
  - Pain when standing or rising from a seated position

POSITIONING THE PERSON

- The person must always be properly positioned at all times. Regular position changes and good alignment promote comfort and well-being. Breathing is easier. Circulation is promoted. Pressure ulcers and contractures are prevented.
- Whether in bed or in a chair, the person is repositioned at least every 2 hours. To safely position a person:
  - Use good body mechanics.
  - Ask a co-worker to help you if needed.
  - Explain the procedure to the person.
  - Be gentle when moving the person.
  - Provide for privacy.
  - Use pillows as directed by the nurse for support and alignment.
  - Provide for comfort after positioning.
  - Place the call light within reach after positioning.
  - Complete a safety check before leaving the room.
- Pressure ulcers are serious threats from lying or sitting too long in one place. When you reposition a person, make sure linens are clean, dry, and wrinkle-free.
  - Use pillows and positioning devices to support body parts and keep the person in good alignment.
  - Contractures can develop from staying in one position too long. Repositioning, exercise, and activity help prevent contractures.
- **Fowler's position** is a semi-sitting position. The head of the bed is raised between 45 and 60 degrees. The knees may be slightly elevated.
- The **supine position (dorsal recumbent position)** is the back-lying position.
- A person in the **prone position** lies on the abdomen with the head turned to one side.
- A person in the **lateral position (side-lying position)** lies on one side or the other.
- The **Sims' position (semi-prone side position)** is a left side-lying position.
- Persons who sit in chairs must hold their upper bodies and heads erect. For good alignment:
  - The person's back and buttocks are against the back of the chair.
  - Feet are flat on the floor or wheelchair footplates. Never leave feet unsupported.
  - Backs of the knees and calves are slightly away from the edge of the seat.
  - Some people require postural supports if they cannot keep their upper bodies erect.

CHAPTER 14 REVIEW QUESTIONS

Circle the BEST answer.
1. To lift and move residents and heavy objects you should
   a. Use the muscles in your lower arms
   b. Use the muscles in your legs
   c. Use the muscles in your shoulders, upper arms, hips, and thighs
   d. Use the muscles in your abdomen

2. For good body mechanics, you should do all of the following *except*
   a. Bend your knees and squat to lift a heavy object
   b. Bend from your waist to lift a heavy object
   c. Hold items close to your body and base of support
   d. Bend your legs; do not bend your back
3. Which statement is *false*?
   a. A person must be properly positioned at all times.
   b. Regular position changes and good alignment promote comfort and well-being.
   c. Regular position changes and good alignment promote pressure ulcers and contractures.
   d. When a person is in good alignment, breathing is easier and circulation is promoted.
4. In Fowler's position
   a. The head of the bed is flat
   b. The head of the bed is raised to 90 degrees
   c. The head of the bed is raised between 45 and 60 degrees
   d. The head of the bed is raised between 30 and 35 degrees

Answers to Chapter 14 questions are on p. 450.

CHAPTER 15 MOVING THE PERSON
PROMOTING SAFETY AND COMFORT

- Many older persons have fragile bones and joints. To prevent injuries:
  - Follow the rules of body mechanics.
  - Always have help to move a person.
  - Move the person carefully to prevent injury or pain.
  - Keep the person in good alignment.
  - Position the person in good alignment after the procedure.
  - Make sure his or her face, nose, and mouth are not obstructed by a pillow or other device.
- To promote mental comfort when moving or transferring the person:
  - Explain what you are going to do and how the person can help.
  - Screen and cover the person to protect the right to privacy.
  - Keep the person in good alignment.
  - Do not let the person's head hit the head-board when he or she is moved up in bed.
  - Use pillows to position the person as directed by the nurse and the care plan.
  - Use other positioning devices as directed by the nurse and the care plan.

PREVENTING WORK-RELATED INJURIES

- To prevent work-related injuries:
  - Wear shoes that provide good traction.
  - Use assistive equipment and devices whenever possible.
  - Get help from other staff.
  - Plan and prepare for the task. Know what equipment you will need and on what side of the bed to place the chair or wheelchair.
  - Schedule harder tasks early in your shift.
  - Tell the resident what he or she can do to help. Give clear, simple instructions.
  - Do not hold or grab the person under the underarms.
- For additional guidelines, review boxes Focus on Older Persons: Preventing Work-Related Injuries, Delegation Guidelines: Preventing Work-Related Injuries, and Promoting Safety and Comfort: Preventing Work-Related Injuries in the textbook.

PROTECTING THE SKIN

- Protect the person's skin from friction and shearing when moving the person in bed. Friction is the rubbing of one surface against another. Shearing is when the skin sticks to a surface while muscles slide in the direction the body is moving. Both cause infection and pressure ulcers. To reduce friction and shearing:
  - Roll the person.
  - Use a lift sheet (turning sheet).
  - Use a turning pad, slide board, slide sheet, or large waterproof pad.

MOVING PERSONS IN BED

- Before moving a person in bed, you need to know from the nurse and care plan:
  - What procedure to use
  - The number of staff needed to safely move the person
  - Position limits and restrictions
  - How far you can lower the head of the bed
  - Any limits in the person's ability to move or be repositioned
  - What pillows you can remove before moving the person
  - What equipment is needed—trapeze, lift sheet, slide sheet, mechanical lift
  - How to position the person
  - If the person uses bed rails
  - What observations to report and record
  - Who helped you with the procedure
  - How much help the person needed
  - How the person tolerated the procedure
  - How you positioned the person
  - Complaints of pain or discomfort
  - When to report observations
  - What patient or resident concerns to report at once

Moving the Person Up in Bed
- You can sometimes move light-weight adults up in bed alone if they can assist using a trapeze. Two or

more staff members are needed to move heavy, weak, and very old persons up in bed. Always protect the person and yourself from injury.

- Assist devices are used to reduce shearing and friction. Such assist devices include a drawsheet (lift sheet), flat sheet folded in half, turning pad, slide sheet, and large waterproof pad.

TURNING PERSONS

- Turning persons onto their sides helps prevent complications from bedrest. Certain procedures and care measures also require the side-lying position. After the person is turned, position him or her in good alignment. Use pillows as directed to support the person in the side-lying position.
- **Logrolling** is turning the person as a unit, in alignment, with one motion. The spine is kept straight. Logrolling is used to turn:
  - Older persons with arthritic spines, hips, or knees
  - Persons recovering from hip fractures
  - Persons with spinal cord injuries and surgery

SITTING ON THE SIDE OF THE BED (DANGLING)

- Many older persons become dizzy or faint when getting out of bed too fast. They may need to sit on the side of the bed for 1 to 5 minutes before walking or transferring. Some persons increase activity in stages—bedrest, to sitting on the side of the bed, to sitting in a chair, to walking.
- While dangling, the person coughs and deep breathes. He or she moves the legs back and forth in circles to stimulate circulation. Provide for warmth during dangling.
- Before the dangling procedure, you need this information from the nurse and the care plan:
  - Areas of weakness
  - The person's dependence level
  - The amount of help the person needs
  - If you need a co-worker to help you
  - If the bed is raised or in its lowest position
  - How long the person needs to sit on the side of the bed
  - What exercises are to be done while dangling
  - If the person will walk or transfer to a chair after dangling
- Observations to report and record:
  - Pulse and respiratory rates
  - Pale or bluish skin color (cyanosis)
  - Complaints of light-headedness, dizziness, or difficulty breathing
  - Who helped you with the procedure
  - How well the activity was tolerated
  - How long the person dangled
  - The amount of help needed
  - Other observations and complaints

CHAPTER 15 REVIEW QUESTIONS

Circle the BEST answer.

1. Friction and shearing are reduced by doing the following *except*
   a. Rolling the person
   b. Using a lift sheet or turning pad
   c. Using a pillow
   d. Using a slide board or slide sheet
2. After a person is turned, you must position him or her in good alignment.
   a. True
   b. False
3. Which statement about dangling is *false?*
   a. Many older persons become dizzy or faint when they first dangle.
   b. The person should cough and deep breathe while dangling.
   c. The person moves his or her legs before dangling.
   d. You should cover the person's shoulders with a robe or blanket while dangling.

Answers to Chapter 15 questions are on p. 450.

CHAPTER 16 TRANSFERRING THE PERSON
TRANSFERRING PERSONS

- The amount of help needed and the method used vary with the person's dependency level. See Box 16-1, Functional Status—Transfers, in your textbook.
- The rules of body mechanics apply during transfers.
- Arrange the room to allow enough space for a safe transfer. Correct placement of the chair, wheelchair, or other device also is needed for a safe transfer.
- Before a transfer, you need this information from the nurse and the care plan:
  - What procedure to use
  - The person's dependency level
  - The amount of help the person needs
  - What equipment to use—transfer belt, wheelchair, mechanical assist device, positioning devices, wheelchair cushion, bed or chair alarm, and so on
  - The person's height and weight
  - The number of staff needed
  - Areas of weakness
  - What observations to report and record
- Promoting safety and comfort:
  - Have the person wear non-skid footwear for transfers.
  - Lock the wheels of the bed, wheelchair, stretcher, or other assist device.
  - After the transfer, position the person in good alignment.
  - Transfer belts (gait belts) are used to support persons during transfers and reposition persons in chairs and wheelchairs.

Bed to Chair or Wheelchair Transfers

- Safety is important for chair, wheelchair, commode, and shower chair transfers. In transferring, the strong side moves first. Help the person out of bed on his or her strong side. Help the person from the wheelchair to the bed on his or her strong side.

- Some persons are able to stand and pivot. To pivot means to turn. A stand and pivot transfer is used if:
  - A person's legs are strong enough to bear some or all of his or her weight.
  - The person is cooperative and can follow directions.
  - The person can assist with the transfer.
  - The person must not put his or her arms around your neck. Neck, back, and other injuries to you and the person are possible.

Mechanical Lifts

- Persons who cannot help themselves are transferred with mechanical lifts. So are persons who are too heavy for the staff to transfer.
- Before using a mechanical lift, you must be trained in its use. The lift must work. The sling, straps, hooks, and chains must be in good repair. The person's weight must not exceed the lift's capacity. At least two staff members are needed. Always follow the manufacturer's instructions for using the lift.
- Before using a mechanical lift, you need this information from the nurse and the care plan:
  - The person's dependency level
  - What lift to use
  - What sling to use
  - If a padded, unpadded, or mesh sling is needed
  - What size sling to use
  - The number of staff needed to perform the task safely
- Falling from the lift is a common fear. To promote the person's mental comfort, always explain the procedure before you begin. Also show the person how the lift works.

CHAPTER 16 REVIEW QUESTIONS

Circle the BEST answer.

1. You are transferring a person from the bed to a wheelchair. Which statement is *false*?
   a. The person should wear nonskid footwear.
   b. The person may put his or her arm around your neck.
   c. You should use a gait/transfer belt.
   d. You should lock the wheelchair wheels.
2. A person has a weak left side and a strong right side. In transferring the person from the bed to the wheelchair, his or her strong (right) side moves first.
   a. True
   b. False
3. Before using a mechanical lift, you do all the following *except*
   a. Check the sling, straps, and chains to ensure good repair
   b. Check the person's weight to be sure it does not exceed the lift's capacity
   c. Follow the manufacturer's instructions for using the lift
   d. Operate the lift without a co-worker

Answers to Chapter 16 questions are on p. 450.

CHAPTER 17 COMFORT NEEDS

- Comfort is a state of well-being. Many factors affect comfort.

THE PERSON'S UNIT

- A person's unit is the personal space, furniture, and equipment provided for the person by the agency. OBRA requires that resident units be as personal and home-like as possible.
- You need to keep the person's unit clean, neat, safe, and comfortable.
- See Box 17-1, Maintaining the Person's Unit, in the textbook for measures to control temperature, odors, noise, and lighting for the person's comfort.

COMFORT

- Age, illness, and activity are factors that affect comfort.
- Temperature, ventilation, noise, odors, and lighting are factors that are controlled to meet the person's needs.

Temperature and Ventilation

- Older persons and those who are ill may need higher temperatures for comfort.
- To protect older and ill persons from cool areas and drafts:
  - Have them wear the correct clothing.
  - Make sure they wear enough clothing.
  - Offer lap robes to cover the legs.
  - Provide enough blankets for warmth.
  - Cover them with bath blankets when giving care.
  - Move them from drafty areas.

Odors

- To reduce odors in nursing centers:
  - Empty, clean, and disinfect bedpans, urinals, commodes, and kidney basins promptly.
  - Make sure toilets are flushed.
  - Check incontinent persons often.
  - Clean persons who are wet or soiled from urine, feces, vomitus, or wound drainage.
  - Change wet or soiled linens and clothing promptly.
  - Keep laundry containers closed.
  - Follow agency policy for wet or soiled linens and clothing.
  - Dispose of incontinence and ostomy products promptly.
  - Provide good hygiene to prevent body and breath odors.
  - Use room deodorizers as needed and as allowed by agency policy. Do not use sprays around persons with breathing problems.
- If you smoke, practice hand washing after handling smoking materials and before giving care. Give careful attention to your uniforms, hair, and breath because of smoke odors.

Noise
- To decrease noise:
  - Control your voice.
  - Handle equipment carefully.
  - Keep equipment in good working order.
  - Answer phones, call lights, and intercoms promptly.

Lighting
- Adjust lighting and window coverings to meet the person's changing needs. Glares, shadows, and dull lighting can cause falls, headaches, and eyestrain. A bright room is cheerful. Dim light is relaxing and restful. Persons with poor vision need bright light. Always keep light controls within the person's reach.

ROOM FURNITURE AND EQUIPMENT
- Rooms are furnished and equipped to meet basic needs.

The Bed
- Beds are raised horizontally to give care. This reduces bending and reaching.
- Bed wheels are locked at all times except when moving the bed.
- Use bed rails as the nurse and care plan direct.
- Basic bed positions:
  - *Flat*—the usual sleeping position.
  - *Fowler's position*—a semi-sitting position. The head of the bed is raised between 45 and 60 degrees.
  - *High-Fowler's position*—a semi-sitting position. The head of the bed is raised 60 to 90 degrees.
  - *Semi-Fowler's position*—the head of the bed is raised 30 degrees. Some agencies define semi-Fowler's position as when the head of the bed is raised 30 degrees and the knee portion is raised 15 degrees. Know the definition used by your agency.
  - *Trendelenburg's position*—the head of the bed is lowered and the foot of the bed is raised. A doctor orders the position.
  - *Reverse Trendelenburg's position*—the head of the bed is raised and the foot of the bed is lowered. A doctor orders the position.

BED SAFETY
- *Entrapment* means the person can get caught, trapped, or entangled in spaces created by bed rails, the mattress, the bed frame, the headboard, or the footboard. Serious injuries and deaths have occurred from entrapment. If a person is at risk for entrapment, report your concerns to the nurse at once. If a person is caught, trapped, or entangled, try to release the person. Call for the nurse at once.

See Figure 17-8 for the 7 entrapment zones of hospital bed systems.
- These persons are at greatest risk for entrapment.
  - Older
  - Frail
  - Confused or disoriented
  - Restless
  - Have uncontrolled body movements
  - Have poor muscle control
  - Are small in size
  - Are restrained

The Overbed Table
- The table is used for meals, writing, reading, and other activities.
- Only clean and sterile items are placed on the table. Never place bedpans, urinals, or soiled linen on the over-bed table or on top of the bedside stand. The bedside stand holds personal items, a wash basin and kidney basin, a urinal, bedpan and cover, and toilet paper.
- Clean the table and bedside stand after using them as a work surface and before serving meal trays.

Chairs
- The person's unit has at least one chair.

Privacy Curtains
- Each person has the right to full visual privacy—to be completely free from public view while in bed.
- Always pull the curtain completely around the bed before giving care. Privacy curtains do not block sounds or voices.

The Call System
- The call light must always be kept within the person's reach—in the room, bathroom, and shower or tub room. You must:
  - Place the call light on the person's strong side.
  - Remind the person to use the call light when help is needed.
  - Answer call lights promptly.
  - Answer bathroom and shower or tub room call lights at once.
- Persons with limited hand movement or people who cannot use call lights may need special communication measures.
- Be careful when using the intercom. Remember confidentiality. Persons nearby can hear what you and the person say.

The Bathroom
- Some bathrooms have higher toilets or raised toilet seats.
- Towel racks, toilet paper, soap, paper towel dispenser, and a wastebasket are within the person's reach.
- Usually the call light is a button or pull cord next to the toilet. Someone must respond at once when a person needs help in the bathroom.

Closet and Drawer Space
- Closet and drawer space are provided.
- The person must have free access to the closet and its contents. You must have the person's permission to open or search closets or drawers.
- Agency staff can inspect a person's closet or drawers if hoarding is suspected. The person is informed of the inspection and is present when it takes place. Have a co-worker present when you inspect a person's closet.

Other Equipment
- Many agencies furnish rooms with a TV, radio, clock, phones, computer, and Internet access.

GENERAL RULES
- Keep the person's room clean, neat, safe, and comfortable. Follow the rules in Box 17-1, Maintaining the Person's Unit.

BEDMAKING
- Clean, dry, and wrinkle-free linens promote comfort. Skin breakdown and pressure ulcers are prevented.
- To keep beds neat and clean:
  - Straighten linens whenever loose or wrinkled and at bedtime.
  - Check for and remove food and crumbs after meals and snacks.
  - Check linens for dentures, eyeglasses, hearing aids, sharp objects, and other items.
  - Change linens whenever they become wet, soiled, or damp.
  - Follow Standard Precautions and the Bloodborne Pathogen Standard.

Types of Beds
- Beds are made in these ways.
  - A closed bed is not in use. Or the bed is ready for a new resident. Top linens are not folded back.
  - An open bed is in use. Top linens are fanfolded back so the person can get into bed. A closed bed becomes an open bed by fanfolding back the top linens.
  - An occupied bed is made with the person in it.
  - A surgical bed is made to transfer a person from a stretcher to bed. This includes an ambulance stretcher.

Linens
- When handling linens and making beds:
  - Practice medical asepsis. Wear gloves to remove linen.
  - Always hold linen away from your body and uniform. Your uniform is considered dirty.
  - Never shake linen.
  - Place clean linens on a clean surface.
  - Never put clean or dirty linen on the floor.
  - Collect enough linens. Do not bring unneeded linens into the person's room. Once in the room, extra linen is considered contaminated. It cannot be used for another person.
  - Roll each piece of dirty linen away from you. The side that touched the person is inside the roll and away from you.

Making Beds
- When making beds, safety and medical asepsis are important. Use good body mechanics. Follow the rules for safe resident handling, moving, and transfers. Practice hand hygiene before handling clean linen and after handling dirty linen. To save time and energy, make beds with a co-worker.
- Review Box 17-2, Rules for Bedmaking, in the textbook.

THE OCCUPIED BED
- You make an occupied bed when the person stays in bed. Keep the person in good alignment. Follow restrictions or limits in the person's movement or position. Explain each procedure step to the person before it is done. This is important even if the person cannot respond or is in a coma.

ASSISTING WITH PAIN RELIEF
- **Pain** means to ache, hurt, or be sore. Pain is subjective. You cannot see, hear, touch, or smell pain or discomfort. You must rely on what the person says.
- Report the person's complaints of pain and your observations to the nurse.
- Review Box 17-3, Comfort and Pain-Relief Measures, in the textbook.

Factors Affecting Pain
- *Past experience.* The severity of pain, its cause, how long it lasted, and if relief occurred all affect the person's current response to pain.
- *Anxiety.* Pain and anxiety are related. Pain can cause anxiety. Anxiety increases how much pain the person feels. Reducing anxiety helps lessen pain.
- *Rest and sleep.* Pain seems worse when tired and unable to rest or sleep. Pain often seems worse at night.
- *Attention.* The more a person thinks about pain, the worse it seems.
- *Personal and family duties.* Often pain is ignored when there are children to care for. Some deny pain if fearing a serious illness.
- *The value or meaning of pain.* To some people, pain is a sign of weakness. For some persons, pain is used to avoid work, daily routines, and people. Some people like doting and pampering by others. The person values and wants such attention.

- *Support from others*. Dealing with pain is often easier when family and friends offer comfort and support. Just being nearby helps. Dealing with pain alone can increase anxiety.
- *Culture*. Culture affects pain responses. Non–English-speaking persons may have problems describing pain.
- *Illness*. Some diseases cause decreased pain sensations.
- *Age*. Older persons may have decreased pain sensations. They may not feel pain or it may not feel severe. The person is at risk for undetected disease or injury. Chronic pain may mask new pain.
- *Persons with dementia*. Persons with dementia may not be able to complain of pain. Changes in usual behavior may signal pain. Loss of appetite also signals pain. Report any changes in a person's usual behavior to the nurse.

The Back Massage
- The back massage relaxes muscles and stimulates circulation.
- Massages are given after the bath and with evening care. You also can give back massages at other times, such as after repositioning a person. Massages last 3 to 5 minutes.
- Observe the skin for breaks, bruises, reddened areas, and other signs of skin breakdown.
- Lotion reduces friction during the massage. It is warmed before applying.
- Use firm strokes. Keep your hands in contact with the person's skin.
- After the massage, apply some lotion to the elbows, knees, and heels.
- Back massages are dangerous for persons with certain heart diseases, back injuries, back and other surgeries, skin diseases, and some lung disorders. Check with the nurse and the care plan before giving back massages to persons with these conditions.
- Do not massage reddened bony areas. Reddened areas signal skin breakdown and pressure ulcers. Massage can lead to more tissue damage.
- Wear gloves if the person's skin is not intact. Always follow Standard Precautions and the Bloodborne Pathogen Standard.
- Report and record skin breakdown, redness, bruising, and breaks in the skin.

SLEEP
- Sleep is a basic need. Tissue healing and repair occur during sleep. Sleep lowers stress, tension, and anxiety. It refreshes and renews the person. The person regains energy and mental alertness. The person thinks and functions better after sleep.

Factors Affecting Sleep
- *Illness*. Illness increases the need for sleep.
- *Nutrition*. Foods with caffeine prevent sleep. The protein tryptophan tends to help sleep. It is found in protein sources—milk, cheese, red meat, fish, poultry, and peanuts.
- *Exercise*. Exercise is avoided 2 hours before bedtime.
- *Environment*. People adjust to their usual sleep settings. Any change in the usual setting can affect sleep.
- *Drugs and other substances*. Sleeping pills promote sleep. Drugs for anxiety, depression, and pain may cause sleep.
- *Emotional problems*. Fear, worry, depression, and anxiety affect sleep.

Sleep Disorders
- **Insomnia** is a chronic condition in which the person cannot sleep or stay asleep all night.
- **Sleep deprivation** means the amount and quality of sleep are decreased. Sleep is interrupted.
- **Sleepwalking** is when the person leaves the bed and walks about. If a person is sleepwalking, protect the person from injury. Guide sleepwalkers back to bed. They startle easily. Awaken them gently.

Promoting Sleep
- To promote sleep, allow a flexible bedtime, provide a bedtime snack, and have the person void before going to bed. Review Box 17-4, Promoting Sleep, in the textbook for other measures.

CHAPTER 17 REVIEW QUESTIONS
Circle the BEST answer.
1. Serious injuries and death have occurred from entrapment.
   a. True
   b. False
2. You should never place bedpans, urinals, or soiled linen on the over-bed table.
   a. True
   b. False
3. You should clean the bedside stand if you use it for a work surface.
   a. True
   b. False
4. The following protect a person from drafts except
   a. Wearing enough clothing
   b. Lap robes
   c. Using a sheet when giving care
   d. Providing blankets
5. To reduce odors, you do the following except
   a. Empty bedpans and commodes promptly
   b. Keep laundry containers open
   c. Check to make sure toilets are flushed
   d. Clean persons who are wet or soiled from urine or feces
6. Which statement about the call light is false?
   a. The call light must always be within the person's reach.
   b. Place the call light on the person's strong side.
   c. You have to answer the call lights only for residents assigned to you.
   d. Answer call lights promptly.

7. You suspect a person is hoarding food in her closet. Before you inspect the closet, what do you do?
   a. Tell another nursing assistant what you suspect
   b. Inspect the closet without telling the resident
   c. Tell the family
   d. Ask the resident if you can inspect the closet
8. Once in the person's room, extra linen is considered contaminated. It can be used for another person.
   a. True
   b. False
9. Roll each piece of dirty linen away from you. The side that touched the person is inside the roll.
   a. True
   b. False
10. Wear gloves when removing linen from the person's bed.
    a. True
    b. False
11. To keep beds neat and clean, do the following *except*
    a. Straighten linens whenever loose or wrinkled
    b. Check for and remove food and crumbs after meals
    c. Check linens for dentures, eyeglasses, and hearing aids
    d. Change linen monthly
12. Which statement is *false*?
    a. Practice medical asepsis when handling linen.
    b. Always hold linens away from your body and uniform.
    c. Shake linens to remove crumbs.
    d. Put dirty linens in the dirty laundry bin.
13. Persons with dementia may not complain of pain. Which of the following might be a signal of pain for a person with dementia?
    a. Illness
    b. Mental alertness
    c. Loss of appetite
    d. Forgetfulness
14. Which statement is *false*?
    a. A back massage relaxes and stimulates circulation.
    b. Massages are given after the bath and with evening care.
    c. You can observe the person's skin before beginning the massage.
    d. You should use cold lotion for the massage.
15. To promote sleep for a person, you should do the following *except*
    a. Follow the person's wishes
    b. Follow the care plan
    c. Follow the person's rituals and routines before bedtime
    d. Tell the person when to go to bed

Answers to Chapter 17 questions are on p. 450.

CHAPTER 18 HYGIENE NEEDS

- The skin is the body's first line of defense against disease.
- Besides cleansing, good hygiene prevents body and breath odors. It is relaxing and increases circulation.
- Culture and personal choice affect hygiene.

DAILY CARE

- Most people have hygiene routines and habits. You give routine care during the day and evening. You assist with hygiene whenever it is needed. Protect the person's right to privacy and to personal choice.
- See Box 18-1, Daily Care, in the textbook for early morning or AM care, morning care, afternoon care, and evening care procedures.

ORAL HYGIENE

- Oral hygiene keeps the mouth and teeth clean. It prevents mouth odors and infections, increases comfort, and makes food taste better. Mouth care also reduces the risk for cavities and periodontal disease.
- Assist with oral hygiene after sleep, after meals, and at bedtime. Follow the care plan.
- Follow Standard Precautions and the Bloodborne Pathogen Standard.
- Report and record:
  - Dry, cracked, swollen, or blistered lips
  - Mouth or breath odor
  - Redness, swelling, irritation, sores, or white patches in the mouth or on the tongue
  - Bleeding, swelling, or redness of the gums
  - Loose teeth
  - Rough, sharp, or chipped areas on dentures

Brushing and Flossing Teeth
- Flossing removes plaque and tartar from the teeth, as well as food from between the teeth. Flossing is usually done after brushing. If done once a day, bedtime is the best time to floss.
- Some persons need help gathering and setting up equipment for oral hygiene. You may have to perform oral care for persons who are weak, cannot move or use their arms, or are too confused to brush their teeth.

Mouth Care for the Unconscious Person
- Some unconscious persons breathe with their mouths open, causing dry mouths and crusting on the tongue and mucous membranes. Oral hygiene keeps the mouth clean and moist. It also helps prevent infection.
- The care plan tells you what cleaning agent to use.
- Use sponge swabs to apply the cleaning agent. Make sure the sponge pad is tight on the stick. To

prevent cracking of the lips, apply a lubricant to the lips. Check the care plan.
- Unconscious persons usually cannot swallow. Protect from choking and aspiration. Aspiration is breathing fluid, food, vomitus, or an object into the lungs. It can cause pneumonia and death.
- To prevent aspiration for the unconscious person:
  - Position the person on one side with the head turned well to the side.
  - Use only a small amount of fluid to clean the mouth.
  - Do not insert dentures. Dentures are not worn when the person is unconscious.
- When giving oral hygiene, keep the person's mouth open with a padded tongue blade. Do not use your fingers.
- Mouth care is given at least every 2 hours. Follow the nurse's direction and the care plan.

Denture Care
- Mouth care is given and dentures are cleaned as often as natural teeth. Dentures are usually removed at bedtime. Remind people not to wrap dentures in tissues or napkins. Otherwise, they are easily discarded.
- Dentures are slippery when wet. Hold them firmly. During cleaning, hold them firmly over a basin of water lined with a towel. Use only denture cleaning products and follow the manufacturer's instructions.
- Hot water causes dentures to lose their shape. If dentures are not worn after cleaning, store them in a container with cool or warm water or a denture soaking solution.
- Label the denture cup with the person's name, room number, and bed number. Report lost or damaged dentures to the nurse at once. Losing or damaging dentures is negligent conduct.
- Never carry dentures in your hands. Always use a denture cup or kidney basin.
- Many people do not like being seen without their dentures. Privacy is important. If you clean dentures, return them to the person as quickly as possible.
- Persons with dentures may have some natural teeth. They need to brush and floss the natural teeth.

BATHING
- Bathing cleans the skin. The mucous membranes of the genital and anal areas are cleaned as well. A bath is refreshing and relaxing. Circulation is stimulated and body parts exercised. You have time to talk to the person. You also can make observations. The person's choice of bath time is respected whenever possible.
- Review Box 18-2, Rules for Bathing, in the textbook.

- Bathing frequency is a personal matter. Some people bathe daily. Others bathe 1 or 2 times a week. Partial baths are taken the other days. Some bathe daily but not with soap. Illness and dry skin may limit bathing to every 2 or 3 days. Thorough rinsing is needed when using soap. Lotions and oils keep the skin soft.
- Provide for safety.
  - Use a hand-held shower nozzle.
  - Have the person use a shower chair or shower bench.
  - Do not use bath oil. It can make the tub or shower slippery or cause a urinary tract infection.
  - Do not leave the person alone in the tub or shower.
- Water temperature for complete bed baths and partial bed baths is between 110°F and 115°F. Older persons have fragile skin and need lower water temperatures. Measure water temperature according to agency policy.
- Report and record:
  - The color of the skin, lips, nail beds, and sclera (whites of the eyes)
  - If the skin appears pale, grayish, yellow (jaundice), or bluish (cyanotic)
  - The location and description of rashes
  - Skin texture—smooth, rough, scaly, flaky, dry, moist
  - Diaphoresis—profuse (excessive) sweating
  - Bruises or open skin areas
  - Pale or reddened areas, particularly over bony parts
  - Drainage or bleeding from wounds or body openings
  - Swelling of the feet and legs
  - Corns or calluses on the feet
  - Skin temperature (cold, cool, warm, hot)
  - Complaints of pain or discomfort
- Use caution when applying powders. Do not use powders near persons with respiratory disorders. Do not sprinkle or shake powder onto the person. To safely apply powder:
  - Turn away from the person.
  - Sprinkle a small amount onto your hands or a cloth.
  - Apply the powder in a thin layer.
  - Make sure powder does not get on the floor. Powder is slippery and can cause falls.

The Complete Bed Bath
- The complete bed bath involves washing the person's entire body in bed. Wash around the person's eyes with water. Do not use soap. Gently wipe from the inner to the outer aspect of the eye. Use a clean part of the washcloth for each stroke. Ask the person if you should use soap to wash the face. Let the person wash the genital area if he or she is able.
- Give a back massage after the bath. Apply deodorant or antiperspirant, lotion, and powder as requested. Comb and brush the hair. Empty and clean the wash basin.

The Partial Bath
- The partial bath involves bathing the face, hands, axillae (underarms), back, buttocks, and perineal area. You assist the person as needed. Most need help washing the back.

Tub Baths and Showers
- Falls, burns, and chilling from water are risks. Review Box 18-2, Rules for Bathing, and Box 18-3, Tub Bath and Shower Safety, in the textbook.
- At least two staff are needed to safely assist weak persons with tub baths and showers.
- If the person is heavy, three or more staff may be needed.
- A tub bath can cause a person to feel faint, weak, or tired. The person may need a transfer bench, a tub with a side entry door, a wheelchair or stretcher lift, or a mechanical lift to get in and out of the tub.
- Some people can use a regular shower. Have the person use the grab bars for support during the shower. Use a bath mat if the shower does not have non-skid surfaces. Never let weak or unsteady persons stand in the shower. They may need to use shower chairs, shower stalls or cabinets, or shower trolleys. Some shower rooms have two or more stations. Protect the person's privacy. Properly screen and cover the person.
- Water temperature for tub baths and showers is usually 105°F. Remember to measure water temperature. Report and record dizziness and light-headedness.
- Clean and disinfect the tub or shower before and after use.

PERINEAL CARE
- Perineal care involves cleaning the genital and anal areas. Cleaning prevents infection and odors and it promotes comfort. It is done daily during the bath and whenever the area is soiled with urine or feces. The person does perineal care if able.
- Perineal care is very important for persons who:
  - Have urinary catheters.
  - Have had rectal or genital surgery.
  - Are menstruating.
  - Are incontinent of urine or feces.
  - Are uncircumcised.
- *Perineal* and *perineum* are not common terms. Most people understand privates, private parts, crotch, genitals, or the area between the legs. Use terms the person understands.
- Standard Precautions, medical asepsis, and the Bloodborne Pathogen Standard are followed.
- Work from the cleanest area to the dirtiest—commonly called cleaning from "front to back." On a woman, clean from the urethra (cleanest) to the anal area (dirtiest). On a male, start at the meatus of the urethra and work outward. This prevents the spread of bacteria from the anal area to the vagina and urinary system.
- Use warm water. Use washcloths, towelettes, cotton balls, or swabs according to agency policy. Rinse thoroughly. Pat dry. Water temperature is usually 105°F to 109°F.
- Report and record:
  - Bleeding, redness, swelling, irritation, or discharge
  - Complaints of pain, burning, or other discomfort
  - Signs of urinary or fecal incontinence
  - Odors

CHAPTER 18 REVIEW QUESTIONS
Circle the BEST answer.
1. Oral hygiene does the following *except*
   a. Keeps the mouth and teeth clean
   b. Prevents mouth odors and infections
   c. Decreases comfort
   d. Makes food taste better
2. When giving oral hygiene, you should report and record the following *except*
   a. Dry, cracked, swollen, or blistered lips
   b. Redness, sores, or white patches in the mouth
   c. Bleeding, swelling, or redness of the gums
   d. The number of fillings a person has
3. A person is unconscious. When you do mouth care, you do the following *except*
   a. Use only a small amount of fluid to clean the mouth
   b. Use your fingers to keep the mouth open
   c. Explain what you are doing
   d. Give mouth care at least every 2 hours
4. Which statement about dentures is *false*?
   a. Dentures are slippery when wet.
   b. During cleaning, hold dentures over a basin of water lined with a towel.
   c. Store dentures in cool water.
   d. Remind people to wrap their dentures in tissues or napkins.
5. Bathing does the following *except*
   a. Cleanses the skin
   b. Stimulates circulation
   c. Makes a person tense
   d. Permits you to observe the person's skin
6. The water temperature for a complete bed bath is
   a. 102°F to 108°F
   b. 110°F to 115°F
   c. 115°F to 120°F
   d. 120°F to 125°F
7. Which statement is *false*?
   a. Use powder near persons with respiratory disorders.
   b. Before applying powder, check with the nurse and the care plan.
   c. Before applying powder, sprinkle a small amount of powder onto your hands.
   d. Apply powder in a thin layer.

8. When washing a person's eyes, you should do the following *except*
   a. Use only water
   b. Gently wipe from the inner to the outer aspect of the eye
   c. Gently wipe from the outer to the inner aspect of the eye
   d. Use a clean part of the washcloth for each stroke
9. When giving female perineal care, you should work from the urethra to the anal area.
   a. True
   b. False
10. When giving male perineal care, start at the meatus and work outward.
    a. True
    b. False

Answers to Chapter 18 questions are on p. 450.

CHAPTER 19 GROOMING NEEDS

- Hair care, shaving, nail and foot care, and clean garments prevent infection and promote comfort. They also affect love, belonging, and self-esteem needs.

HAIR CARE

- You assist patients and residents to brush, comb, and shampoo hair according to the care plan. The nursing process reflects the person's culture, personal choice, skin and scalp condition, health history, and self-care ability.

Brushing and Combing Hair

- Brushing and combing daily prevent tangled and matted hair.
- When brushing and combing hair, start at the scalp and brush or comb to the hair ends.
- Never cut hair for any reason. Tell the nurse if you think the person's hair needs to be cut.
- Special measures are needed for curly, coarse, and dry hair. Check the care plan.
- When giving hair care, place a towel across the person's back and shoulders to protect garments from falling hair. If the person is in bed, give hair care before changing the linens and pillowcase.
- Sharp brush bristles can injure the scalp. So can a comb with sharp or broken teeth. Report any concerns about the person's brush or comb.

SHAMPOOING

- Oil gland secretion decreases with aging. Therefore older persons have dry hair.
- Shampooing frequency depends on the person's needs and preferences. Usually shampooing is done weekly on the person's bath or shower day.

- Hair is dried and styled as quickly as possible after the shampoo.
- During shampooing, report and record:
  - Scalp sores
  - Flaking
  - Itching
  - Presence of nits or lice
  - Patches of hair loss
  - Very dry or very oily hair
  - Matted or tangled hair
  - How the person tolerated the procedure
- Keep shampoo away from and out of eyes. Have the person hold a washcloth over the eyes.
- Remove hearing aids before shampooing.
- Return medicated products to the nurse.
- Wear gloves if the person has scalp sores.
- Follow Standard Precautions and the Bloodborne Pathogen Standard.

SHAVING

- Review Box 19-1, Rules for Shaving, in the textbook.
- Safety razors or electric razors are used. If the agency's shaver is used, clean it before and after use. Follow agency policy for cleaning electric shavers. Safety razors (blade razors) have razor blades. Do not use safety razors on persons who have healing problems or for those taking anticoagulant drugs. Soften the beard before shaving. Pat dry the face and apply talcum powder if using an electric shaver. Older persons with wrinkled skin are at risk for nicks and cuts. Safety razors are not used to shave them or persons with dementia. Safety razors are very sharp. Protect the person and yourself from nicks and cuts. Rinse the safety razor often then wipe the razor.

Caring for Mustaches and Beards

- Wash and comb mustaches and beards daily and as needed. Ask the person how to groom his mustache or beard.
- Never trim a mustache or beard without the person's consent.

Shaving Legs and Underarms

- Many women shave their legs and underarms. This practice varies among cultures. Legs and underarms are shaved after bathing when the skin is soft. Use soap and water, shaving cream, or lotion for the lather.
- Use the kidney basin to rinse the safety razor. Do not use bath water.

NAIL AND FOOT CARE

- Nail and foot care prevents infection, injury, and odors.

- Nails are easier to trim and clean right after soaking or bathing.
- Use nail clippers to cut fingernails. Never use scissors. Use extreme caution to prevent damage to nearby tissues.
- Follow Standard Precautions and the Bloodborne Pathogen Standard.
- Report and record:
  - Dry, reddened, irritated, or callused areas
  - Breaks in the skin
  - Corns on top of and between the toes
  - Blisters
  - Very thick nails
  - Loose nails
- Some states and agencies do not let nursing assistants cut and trim toenails. You do not cut or trim toenails if a person has diabetes or poor circulation to the legs and feet or takes drugs that affect blood clotting. Also, do not cut or trim toenails if the person has very thick nails or ingrown toenails. The nurse or podiatrist cuts toenails and provides foot care for these persons.
- When doing foot care, check between the toes for cracks and sores. If left untreated, a serious infection could occur.
- The feet of persons with decreased sensation or circulatory problems may easily burn because they do not feel hot temperatures.
- After soaking, apply lotion to the feet. Because the lotion can cause slippery feet, help the person put on non-skid footwear before you transfer the person or let the person walk.

CHANGING CLOTHING AND HOSPITAL GOWNS

- Garments are changed after the bath, on admission and discharge, and whenever wet or soiled. Gowns are changed daily.
- When you assist with dressing and undressing, follow the rules in Box 19-2, Rules for Dressing and Undressing, in your textbook.

Safety

- When assisting with dressing and undressing, you turn the person from side to side. If the person uses bed rails, raise the far bed rail. If bed rails are not used, ask a co-worker to help turn and position the person. This protects the person from falling.

CHAPTER 19 REVIEW QUESTIONS

Circle the BEST answer.

1. Hair care, shaving, and nail and foot care prevent infection and promote comfort.
   a. True
   b. False
2. If a person's hair is matted, you may cut the hair.
   a. True
   b. False

3. When giving hair care, place a towel across the person's back and shoulders to protect garments from falling hair.
   a. True
   b. False
4. You should wear gloves when shampooing a person who has scalp sores.
   a. True
   b. False
5. A person takes an anticoagulant. Therefore he shaves with a blade razor.
   a. True
   b. False
6. You should wear gloves when shaving a person.
   a. True
   b. False
7. Never trim a mustache or beard without the person's consent.
   a. True
   b. False
8. Mustaches and beards need daily care.
   a. True
   b. False
9. A person has diabetes. You can cut his or her toenails.
   a. True
   b. False
10. Fingernails are cut with
    a. Scissors
    b. Nail clippers
    c. An emery board
    d. A nail file
11. Which statement is *false*?
    a. Provide privacy when a person is changing clothes.
    b. Most residents wear street clothes during the day.
    c. Let the person choose what to wear.
    d. You may tear a person's clothing.

Answers to Chapter 19 questions are on p. 450.

CHAPTER 20 URINARY NEEDS
NORMAL URINATION

- Urination (voiding) means the process of emptying urine from the bladder.
- The healthy adult produces about 1500 mL (milliliters) or 3 pints of urine a day.
- The frequency of urination is affected by amount of fluid intake, habits, availability of toilet facilities, activity, work, and illness. People usually void at bedtime, after sleep, and before meals. Some people void every 2 to 3 hours. The need to void at night disturbs sleep. Review Box 20-1, Rules for Normal Urination, in the textbook.

Observations

- Observe urine for color, clarity, odor, amount, particles, and blood. Normal urine is pale yellow, straw-colored, or amber. It is clear with no particles. A faint odor is normal.

- Ask the nurse to observe urine that looks or smells abnormal.
- Report the following urinary problems.
  - **Dysuria**—painful or difficult urination
  - **Hematuria**—blood in the urine
  - **Nocturia**—frequent urination at night
  - **Oliguria**—scant amount of urine; less than 500 mL in 24 hours
  - **Polyuria**—abnormally large amounts of urine
  - **Urinary frequency**—voiding at frequent intervals
  - **Urinary incontinence**—involuntary loss or leakage of urine
  - **Urinary urgency**—the need to void at once

Bedpans

- Women use bedpans for voiding and bowel movements (BMs). Men use them for BMs.
- Follow Standard Precautions and the Bloodborne Pathogen Standard when handling urinary devices and their contents.
- Thoroughly clean and disinfect bedpans, urinals, and commodes after use.

Urinals

- Men use urinals to void. He stands to use the urinal if possible. Or he sits on the side of the bed or lies in the bed to use it.
- Some men need support when standing to use the urinal.
- You may have to place and hold the urinal for some men. This may embarrass both the person and you. Act in a professional manner at all times.
- Remind men to hang urinals on bed rails and to signal after using them.

URINARY INCONTINENCE

- **Urinary incontinence** is the involuntary loss or leakage of urine.
- The basic types of incontinence are:
  - *Stress incontinence.* Urine leaks during exercise and certain movements that cause pressure on the bladder.
  - *Urge incontinence.* Urine is lost in response to a sudden, urgent need to void.
  - *Overflow incontinence.* Small amounts of urine leak from a full bladder.
  - *Functional incontinence.* The person has bladder control but cannot use the toilet in time.
  - *Reflex incontinence.* Urine is lost at predictable intervals when the bladder is full.
  - *Mixed incontinence.* The person has a combination of stress incontinence and urge incontinence.
  - *Transient incontinence.* This refers to temporary or occasional incontinence that is reversed when the cause is treated.
- If urinary incontinence is a new problem, tell the nurse at once.

- Incontinence is embarrassing. Garments are wet and odors develop. Skin irritation, infection, and pressure ulcers are risks. The person's pride, dignity, and self-esteem are affected. Social isolation, loss of independence, and depression are common. Complications include falls, pressure ulcers, and urinary tract infections (UTIs).
- Good skin care and dry garments and linens are essential. Promoting normal urinary elimination prevents incontinence in some people. Other people may need bladder training. Check incontinent persons often. Change wet incontinence products and clothing promptly. Prevent prolonged exposure of the skin to urine. Provide hygiene measures to prevent skin breakdown.
- Review Box 20-2, Urinary Incontinence—Nursing Measures, in the textbook.
- Caring for persons with incontinence is stressful. Remember, the person does not choose to be incontinent. If you find yourself becoming short-tempered and impatient, talk to the nurse at once. Kindness, empathy, understanding, and patience are needed.
- Incontinence products help keep the person dry. The guidelines in Box 20-3, Applying Incontinence Products, in your textbook will help prevent:
  - Leakage
  - Skin irritation and blisters
  - Tearing

BLADDER TRAINING

- Bladder training may help with urinary incontinence. Control of urination is the goal. Bladder control promotes comfort and quality of life. It also increases self-esteem. You assist with bladder training as directed by the nurse and the care plan.
- Bladder training involves resisting the desire to urinate, postponing or delaying voiding, and urinating following a schedule rather than the urge to void. Prompted voiding is voiding at scheduled times when prompted to void. Habit training/scheduled voiding is voiding to match the person's voiding habits without delaying or resisting voiding, usually every 3 to 4 hours while awake.

CHAPTER 20 REVIEW QUESTIONS

Circle the BEST answer.

1. Which statement is *false?*
   a. Normal urine is yellow, straw-colored, or amber.
   b. Urine with a strong odor is normal.
   c. A person normally voids 1500 mL a day.
   d. Observe urine for color, clarity, odor, amount, and particles.
2. Which observation does *not* need to be reported to the nurse promptly?
   a. Complaints of urgency
   b. Burning on urination
   c. Painful or difficult urination
   d. Clear amber urine

3. Which statement is *false*?
   a. Incontinence is embarrassing.
   b. Caring for persons with incontinence may be stressful.
   c. Incontinence is a personal choice.
   d. Be kind and patient to persons who are incontinent.
4. The goal of bladder training is to
   a. Allow the person to use the toilet
   b. Keep the catheter
   c. Gain control of urination
   d. Decrease self-esteem

Answers to Chapter 20 questions are on p. 450.

CHAPTER 21 URINARY CATHETERS
CATHETERS
- A catheter is a tube used to drain or inject fluid through a body opening.
- An *indwelling catheter (retention or Foley catheter)* drains urine constantly into a drainage bag.
- Catheters can protect wounds and pressure ulcers from contact with urine. They also allow hourly urinary output measurements.
- The catheter must not pull at the insertion site. Hold the catheter securely during catheter care. Then properly secure the catheter. Also make sure the tubing is not under the person. Besides obstructing urine flow, lying on the tubing is uncomfortable. It can also cause skin breakdown. Provide perineal care daily or twice a day, after bowel movements, and when there is vaginal drainage.
- Follow Standard Precautions and the Bloodborne Pathogen Standard. Review Box 21-1, Indwelling Catheter Care, in the textbook.
- Report and record:
  - Complaints of pain, burning, irritation, or the need to void (report at once)
  - Crusting, abnormal drainage, or secretions
  - The color, clarity, and odor of urine
  - Particles in the urine
  - Blood in the urine
  - Cloudy urine
  - Urine leaking at the insertion site
  - Drainage system leaks

Drainage Systems
- A closed drainage system is used for indwelling catheters. The drainage bag hangs from the bed frame, chair, or wheelchair. It must not touch the floor. The bag is always kept lower than the person's bladder. Do not hang the drainage bag on a bed rail.
- If the drainage system is disconnected accidentally, tell the nurse at once. Do not touch the ends of the catheter or tubing. Do the following.
  - Practice hand hygiene. Put on gloves.
  - Wipe the end of the tube with an antiseptic wipe.
  - Wipe the end of the catheter with another antiseptic wipe.
  - Do not put the ends down. Do not touch the ends after you clean them.
  - Connect the tubing to the catheter.
  - Discard the wipes into a *BIOHAZARD* bag.
  - Remove the gloves. Practice hand hygiene.
- Check with the nurse and care plan about when to empty and measure the urine in the drainage bag. Follow Standard Precautions and the Bloodborne Pathogen Standard.
- A leg bag is a drainage system that attaches to the thigh or calf. Empty and measure a leg bag when it is half full.
- Report and record:
  - The amount of urine measured
  - The color, clarity, and odor of urine
  - Particles in the urine
- Blood in the urine
- Cloudy urine
  - Complaints of pain, burning, irritation, or the need to urinate
  - Drainage system leaks

Condom Catheters
- Condom catheters are common for incontinent men. They are also called *external catheters, Texas catheters,* and *urinary sheaths.*
- These catheters are changed daily after perineal care.
- To apply a condom catheter, follow the manufacturer's instructions. Thoroughly wash and dry the penis before applying the catheter.
- Some condom catheters are self-adhering. Other catheters are secured in place with elastic tape in a spiral manner. Never use adhesive tape or other tape to secure catheters. They do not expand. Blood flow to the penis is cut off, injuring the penis.
- When removing or applying a condom catheter, report and record the following observations.
  - Reddened or open areas on the penis
  - Swelling of the penis
  - Color, clarity, and odor of urine
  - Particles in the urine
  - Blood in urine
  - Cloudy urine

CHAPTER 21 REVIEW QUESTIONS
Circle the BEST answer.
1. A person with a catheter complains of pain. You should notify the nurse at once.
   a. True
   b. False
2. Which statement is *false*?
   a. The urine drainage system should hang from the bed frame or chair.
   b. The urine drainage system should hang on a bed rail.
   c. The urine drainage system must be off the floor.
   d. The urine drainage system must be kept lower than the person's bladder.

3. Which statement is *false*?
    a. Condom catheters are changed daily.
    b. Follow the manufacturer's instructions when applying a condom catheter.
    c. Use adhesive tape to secure a condom catheter in place.
    d. Report and record open or reddened areas on the penis at once.

Answers to Chapter 21 questions are on p. 450.

CHAPTER 22 BOWEL NEEDS

- Some people have a bowel movement (BM) every day. Others have one every 2 to 3 days. To assist with bowel elimination, you need to know these terms.
    - Defecation—the process of excreting feces from the rectum through the anus.
    - Feces—the semi-solid mass of waste products in the colon that is expelled through the anus. It is also called a stool.
    - Stool—excreted feces.

NORMAL BOWEL ELIMINATION

- Wastes are excreted from the gastro-intestinal (GI) system.

Observations

- Stools are normally brown, soft, formed, moist, and shaped like the rectum. They have a normal odor caused by bacterial action in the intestines. Certain foods and drugs cause odors.
- Carefully observe stools before disposing of them. Observe and report the color, amount, consistency, odor, and shape and size of stools. Also, observe and report the presence of blood or mucus, frequency of defecation, and any complaints of pain or discomfort.

FACTORS AFFECTING BOWEL MOVEMENTS

- *Privacy.* Bowel elimination is a private act.
- *Habits.* Many people have a bowel movement after breakfast. Some read. Defecation is easier when a person is relaxed.
- *Diet—high-fiber foods.* Fiber helps prevent constipation.
- *Diet—other foods.* Some foods cause constipation. Other foods cause frequent stools or diarrhea.
- *Fluids.* Drinking 6 to 8 glasses of water daily promotes normal bowel elimination. Warm fluids—coffee, tea, hot cider, warm water—increase peristalsis.
- *Activity.* Exercise and activity maintain muscle tone and stimulate peristalsis.
- *Drugs.* Drugs can prevent constipation or control diarrhea. Some have diarrhea or constipation as side effects.

- *Disability.* Some people cannot control bowel movements. A bowel training program is needed.
- *Aging.* Older persons are at risk for constipation. Some older persons lose bowel control and have fecal incontinence.
- To provide comfort and safety during bowel elimination, review Box 22-1, Safety and Comfort for Bowel Needs, in the textbook. Follow Standard Precautions and the Bloodborne Pathogen Standard.

COMMON PROBLEMS

- Common problems include constipation, fecal impaction, diarrhea, fecal incontinence, and flatulence.

Constipation

- **Constipation** is the passage of a hard, dry stool.
- Common causes of constipation are a low-fiber diet and ignoring the urge to defecate. Other causes include decreased fluid intake, inactivity, drugs, aging, and certain diseases.
- Dietary changes, fluids, and activity prevent or relieve constipation. So do stool softeners, laxatives, suppositories, and enemas.
- A suppository is a cone-shaped solid drug that is inserted into a body opening; it melts at body temperature. An enema is the introduction of fluid into the rectum and lower colon.

Fecal Impaction

- A **fecal impaction** is the prolonged retention and buildup of feces in the rectum.
- Fecal impaction results if constipation is not relieved. The person cannot defecate. Liquid feces pass around the hardened fecal mass in the rectum. The liquid feces seep from the anus.
- Abdominal discomfort, abdominal distention, nausea, cramping, and rectal pain are common. Older persons have poor appetite or confusion. Some persons have a fever. Report these signs and symptoms to the nurse.

Diarrhea

- **Diarrhea** is the frequent passage of liquid stools.
- The need to have a bowel movement is urgent. Some people cannot get to a bathroom in time. Abdominal cramping, nausea, and vomiting may occur.
- Assist with elimination needs promptly, dispose of stools promptly, and give good skin care. Liquid stools irritate the skin. So does frequent wiping with toilet paper. Skin breakdown and pressure ulcers are risks.
- Follow Standard Precautions and the Bloodborne Pathogen Standard when in contact with stools.
- Report signs of diarrhea at once. Ask the nurse to observe the stool.

Fecal Incontinence

- **Fecal incontinence** is the inability to control the passage of feces and gas through the anus.
- Gas or air passed through the anus is called flatus.
- Fecal incontinence affects the person emotionally. Frustration, embarrassment, anger, and humiliation are common. The person may need:
  - Bowel training
  - Help with elimination after meals and every 2 to 3 hours
  - Incontinence products to keep garments and linens clean
  - Good skin care

Flatulence

- **Flatulence** is the excessive formation of gas or air in the stomach and intestines.
- Causes include swallowing air while eating and drinking and bacterial action in the intestines. Other causes may be gas-forming foods, constipation, bowel and abdominal surgeries, and drugs that decrease peristalsis.
- If flatus is not expelled, the intestines distend (swell or enlarge from the pressure of gases). Abdominal cramping or pain, shortness of breath, and a swollen abdomen occur. "Bloating" is a common complaint. Exercise, walking, moving in bed, and the left side-lying position often expel flatus. Enemas and drugs may be ordered.

BOWEL TRAINING

- Bowel training has two goals.
  - To gain control of bowel movements.
  - To develop a regular pattern of elimination. Fecal impactions, constipation, and fecal incontinence are prevented.
- Factors that promote elimination are part of the care plan and bowel training program. The person's usual time of day for BM is noted on the plan. Offer help with elimination at the times noted.

ENEMAS

- An **enema** is the introduction of fluid into the rectum and lower colon.
- Doctors order enemas:
  - To remove feces
  - To relieve constipation, fecal impaction, or flatulence
  - To clean the bowel of feces before certain surgeries and diagnostic procedures
- Review Box 22-2, Giving a Small-Volume Enema, in the textbook.
- The common enema solutions are:
  - *Tap water enema*—water obtained from a faucet.
  - *Saline enema*—a solution of salt and water. For adults, add 1 to 2 teaspoons of table salt to 500 to 1000 mL (milliliters) of tap water.

- *Soapsuds enema (SSE)*—for adults, add 3 to 5 mL of castile soap to 500 to 1000 mL of tap water.
- *Small-volume enema*—the adult size contains about 120 mL (4 ounces [oz]) of solution.
- *Oil-retention enema*—has mineral, olive, or cotton-seed oil. The adult size contains about 120 mL (4 oz) of solution.

THE PERSON WITH AN OSTOMY

- Sometimes part of the intestines is removed surgically. An ostomy is sometimes necessary. An **ostomy** is a surgically created opening. The opening is called a **stoma.** The person wears a pouch over the stoma to collect stools and flatus.
- Stools irritate the skin. Skin care prevents skin breakdown around the stoma. The skin is washed and dried. Then a skin barrier is applied around the stoma. It prevents stools from having contact with the skin. The skin barrier is part of the pouch or a separate device.
- The pouch has an adhesive backing that is applied to the skin. Some pouches are secured to ostomy belts.
- The pouch is changed every 3 to 7 days and when it leaks. Frequent pouch changes can damage the skin.
- Pouches have a drain at the bottom that closes with a clip, clamp, or wire closure. The drain is opened to empty the pouch. The drain is wiped with toilet tissue before it is closed.

CHAPTER 22 REVIEW QUESTIONS

Circle the BEST answer

1. Which statement is *false?*
   a. Lack of privacy can prevent defecation.
   b. Low-fiber foods promote defecation.
   c. Drinking 6 to 8 glasses of water daily promotes normal bowel elimination.
   d. Exercise stimulates peristalsis.
2. Which of the following does *not* prevent constipation?
   a. A high-fiber diet
   b. Increased fluid intake
   c. Exercise
   d. Ignoring the urge to defecate
3. A person has fecal incontinence. You should do the following *except*
   a. Be patient
   b. Help with elimination after meals
   c. Provide good skin care
   d. Scold the person for being incontinent
4. The preferred position for an enema is the
   a. Sims' position or the left side-lying position
   b. Prone position
   c. Supine position
   d. Trendelenburg's position

Answers to Chapter 22 questions are on p. 450.

CHAPTER 23 NUTRITION NEEDS

- Food and water are necessary for life. A poor diet and poor eating habits:
  - Increase the risk for infection
  - Cause healing problems
  - Increase the risk for accidents and injuries

BASIC NUTRITION

- **Nutrition** is the process involved in the ingestion, digestion, absorption, and use of foods and fluids by the body. Good nutrition is needed for growth, healing, and body functions.
- A *nutrient* is a substance that is ingested, digested, absorbed, and used by the body.
- A *calorie* is the fuel or energy value of food.

MyPlate

- The MyPlate symbol encourages healthy eating from five food groups:
  - Grains
  - Vegetables
  - Fruits
  - Dairy
  - Protein foods
- See Figure 23-1, The MyPlate Symbol, in your textbook.

Nutrients

- A well-balanced diet ensures an adequate intake of essential nutrients.
- *Protein*—is needed for tissue growth and repair. Sources include meat, fish, poultry, eggs, milk and milk products, cereals, beans, peas, and nuts.
- *Carbohydrates*—provide energy and fiber for bowel elimination. They are found in fruits, vegetables, breads, cereals, and sugar.
- *Fats*—provide energy, add flavor to food, and help the body use certain vitamins. Sources include meats, lard, butter, shortening, oils, milk, cheese, egg yolks, and nuts.
- *Vitamins*—are needed for certain body functions. The body stores vitamins A, D, E, and K. The vitamin C and the B complex vitamins are not stored and must be ingested daily.
- *Minerals*—are needed for bone and tooth formation, nerve and muscle function, fluid balance, and other body processes.
- *Water*—is needed for all body processes.

FACTORS AFFECTING EATING AND NUTRITION

- *Age*. Many GI changes occur with aging.
- *Culture*. Culture influences dietary practices, food choices, and food preparation.
- *Religion*. Selecting, preparing, and eating food often involve religious practices. A person may follow all, some, or none of the dietary practices of his or her faith.
- *Finances*. People with limited incomes often buy the cheaper carbohydrate foods. Their diets often lack protein and certain vitamins and minerals.
- *Appetite*. Illness, drugs, anxiety, pain, and depression can cause loss of appetite (anorexia). Unpleasant sights, thoughts, and smells are other causes.
- *Personal choice*. Food likes and dislikes are influenced by foods served in the home. Usually food likes expand with age and social experiences.
- *Body reactions*. People usually avoid foods that cause allergic reactions. They also avoid foods that cause nausea, vomiting, diarrhea, indigestion, gas, or headaches.
- *Illness*. Appetite usually decreases during illness and recovery from injuries. However, nutritional needs increase.
- *Drugs*. Drugs can cause loss of appetite, confusion, nausea, constipation, impaired taste, or changes in GI function. They can cause inflammation of the mouth, throat, esophagus, and stomach.
- *Chewing problems*. Mouth, teeth, and gum problems can affect chewing. Examples include oral pain, dry or sore mouth, gum disease (Chapter 18), and dentures that fit poorly. Broken, decayed, or missing teeth also affect chewing, especially the meat group.
- *Swallowing problems*. Many health problems can affect swallowing. They include stroke, pain, confusion, dry mouth, and diseases of the mouth, throat, and esophagus.
- *Disability*. Disease or injury can affect the hands, wrists, and arms. Assistive devices let the person eat independently.
- *Impaired cognitive function*. Impaired cognitive function may affect the person's ability to use eating utensils. And it may affect eating, chewing, and swallowing.

OBRA DIETARY REQUIREMENTS

- OBRA has requirements for food served in nursing centers.
  - Each person's nutritional and dietary needs are met.
  - The person's diet is well-balanced. It is nourishing and tastes good. Food is well seasoned.
  - Food is appetizing. It has an appealing aroma and is attractive.
  - Foods vary in color and texture.
  - Hot food is served hot. Cold food is served cold.
  - Food is served promptly.
  - Food is prepared to meet each person's needs. Some people need food cut, ground, or chopped. Others have special diets ordered by the doctor.
  - Other foods are offered to residents who refuse the food served. Substituted food must have a similar nutritional value to the first foods served.

- Each person receives at least three meals a day. A bedtime snack is offered.
- The center provides needed assistive devices and utensils.

SPECIAL DIETS

The Sodium-Controlled Diet
- Sodium causes the body to retain water.
- A sodium-controlled diet decreases the amount of sodium in the body. The diet involves:
  - Omitting high-sodium foods. Review Box 23-2, High-Sodium Foods, in the textbook.
  - Not adding salt to food at the table.
  - Limiting the amount of salt used in cooking.
  - Diet planning

Diabetes Meal Plan
- A diabetes meal plan is for people with diabetes. It involves the person's food preferences and calories needed. It also involves eating meals and snacks at regular times.
- Serve the person's meals and snacks on time to maintain a certain blood sugar level.
- Always check what was eaten. Tell the nurse what the person did and did not eat. If not all food was eaten, a between-meal nourishment is needed. The nurse tells you what to give. Tell the nurse about changes in the person's eating habits.

The Dysphagia Diet
- **Dysphagia** means difficulty swallowing. Food thickness is changed to meet the person's needs. Review Box 23-3, Dysphagia, in the textbook.
- You may need to feed a person with dysphagia. To promote the person's comfort:
  - Know the signs and symptoms of dysphagia. Review Box 23-3, Dysphagia, in the textbook.
  - Feed the person according to the care plan and swallow guide.
  - Follow aspiration precautions. Review Box 23-4, Aspiration Precautions, in the textbook. Aspiration is breathing fluid, food, vomitus, or an object into the lungs.
  - Report changes in how the person eats.
  - Observe for signs and symptoms of aspiration: choking, coughing, or difficulty breathing during or after meals, and abnormal breathing or respiratory sounds. Report these observations at once.

MEETING FOOD NEEDS

Preparing for Meals
- Preparing residents for meals promotes their comfort.
  - Assist with elimination needs.
  - Provide oral hygiene. Make sure dentures are in place.
  - Make sure eyeglasses and hearing aids are in place.
  - Make sure incontinent persons are clean and dry.
  - Position the person in a comfortable position.
  - Assist with hand washing.

Serving Meals
- Food is served in containers that keep foods at the correct temperature. Hot food is kept hot. Cold food is kept cold.
- Prompt serving keeps food at the correct temperature.

Feeding the Person
- Serve food and fluid in the order the person prefers. Offer fluids during the meal.
- Use teaspoons to feed the person. The teaspoon should only be one-third ($^1/_3$) full.
- Persons who need to be fed are often angry, humiliated, and embarrassed. Some are depressed, resentful, or refuse to eat. Let them do what they can. If strong enough, let them hold milk or juice cups. Never let them hold hot drinks.
- Always tell the visually impaired person what is on the tray. Describe what you are offering. For persons who feed themselves, use the numbers on the clock for the location of foods.
- Many people pray before eating. Allow time and privacy for prayer.
- Meals provide social contact with others. Engage the person in pleasant conversation. Also, sit facing the person. Allow time for chewing and swallowing.
- Report and record:
  - The amount and kind of food eaten
  - Complaints of nausea or dysphagia
  - Signs and symptoms of dysphagia
  - Signs and symptoms of aspiration
  - The person will eat better if not rushed.
  - Wipe the person's hands, face, and mouth as needed during the meal.

Between-Meal Snacks
- Many special diets involve between-meal snacks. These snacks are served upon arrival on the nursing unit. Follow the same considerations and procedures for serving meal trays and feeding persons.

Calorie Counts
- Calorie records are kept for some people. On a flow sheet, note what the person ate and how much. A nurse or dietitian converts these portions into calories.

CHAPTER 23 REVIEW QUESTIONS
Circle the BEST answer.
1. A person is on a sodium-controlled diet. Which statement is *true*?
   a. High-sodium foods are allowed.
   b. Salt is added at the table.
   c. Pretzels and potato chips are a good snack.
   d. The amount of salt used in cooking is limited.

2. A person is a diabetic. You should do the following *except*
   a. Serve his meals and snacks late
   b. Always check his tray to see what he ate
   c. Tell the nurse what he ate and did not eat
   d. Provide a between-meal snack as the nurse directs

3. A person has dysphagia. You should do the following *except*
   a. Report choking and coughing during a meal at once
   b. Report difficulty in breathing during a meal at the end of the shift
   c. Report changes in how the person eats
   d. Follow aspiration precautions

4. When feeding a person, you do the following *except*
   a. Use a teaspoon to feed the person
   b. Offer fluids during the meal
   c. Let the person do as much as possible
   d. Stand so that you can feed 2 people at once

5. A person is visually impaired. You do the following *except*
   a. Tell the person what is on the tray
   b. Use the numbers on a clock to tell the person the location of food
   c. If feeding the person, describe what you are offering
   d. Let the person guess what is served

Answers to Chapter 23 questions are on p. 450.

CHAPTER 24 FLUID NEEDS
FLUID BALANCE
- Fluid balance is needed for health. The amount of fluid taken in (**intake**) and the amount of fluid lost (**output**) must be equal. When fluid intake exceeds fluid output, body tissues swell with water (**edema**).
- **Dehydration** is a decrease in the amount of water in body tissues. Fluid output exceeds intake. Common causes are poor fluid intake, vomiting, diarrhea, bleeding, excess sweating, and increased urine production.

Normal Fluid Requirements
- An adult needs 1500 milliliters (mL) of water daily to survive. About 2000 to 2500 mL of fluid per day is needed for normal fluid balance. Water requirements increase with hot weather, exercise, fever, illness, and excess fluid loss.
- Older persons may have a decreased sense of thirst. Their bodies need water, but they may not feel thirsty. Offer fluids according to the care plan.

Special Fluid Orders
- The doctor may order the amount of fluid a person can have in 24 hours. Intake and output (I&O) records are kept.

- *Encourage fluids.* The person drinks an increased amount of fluid.
- *Restrict fluids.* Fluids are limited to a certain amount.
- *Nothing by mouth (NPO).* The person cannot eat or drink anything.
- *Thickened liquids.* All liquids are thickened, including water. Thickness depends on the person's ability to swallow.

Providing Drinking Water
- Patients and residents need fresh drinking water each shift. Follow the agency's procedure for providing fresh water.
- Water mugs can spread microbes. To prevent the spread of microbes:
  - Make sure the mug is labeled with the person's name and room and bed number.
  - Do not touch the rim or inside of the mug or lid.
  - Do not let the ice scoop touch the mug, lid, or straw.
  - Place the ice scoop in the holder or on a towel, not in the ice container or dispenser.
  - Make sure the person's mug is clean and free of cracks and chips.

INTAKE AND OUTPUT
- Intake is the amount of fluid taken in.
- Output is the amount of fluid lost.
- Intake and output (I&O) records are kept. They are used to evaluate fluid balance and kidney function.
- All fluids taken by mouth are measured and recorded—water, milk, and so forth. So are foods that melt at room temperature—ice cream, sherbet, custard, pudding, gelatin, and Popsicles.
- Output includes urine, vomitus, diarrhea, and wound drainage.

MEASURING INTAKE AND OUTPUT
- To measure intake and output, you need to know:
  - 1 ounce (oz) equals 30 mL
  - A pint is about 500 mL
  - A quart is about 1000 mL
  - The serving sizes of bowls, dishes, cups, pitchers, glasses, and other containers
- An I&O record is kept at the bedside. Record I&O measurements in the correct column. Amounts are totaled at the end of the shift. The totals are recorded in the person's chart. They are also shared during the end-of-shift report.
- The urinal, commode, bedpan, or specimen pan is used for voiding. Remind the person not to void in the toilet. Also remind the person not to put toilet tissue into the receptacle.

CHAPTER 24 REVIEW QUESTIONS

Circle the BEST answer.

1. Common causes of dehydration include all of the following *except*
   a. Diarrhea
   b. Fever
   c. Constipation
   d. Bleeding
2. Older persons have a decreased sense of thirst.
   a. True
   b. False
3. Your person is served 1 cup of milk and 1 cup of tea. The person drinks all the fluids. How much will you document as intake?
   a. 480 mL
   b. 60 mL
   c. 240 mL
   d. 500 mL
4. A person is on intake and output. He just ate ice cream. This is recorded as intake.
   a. True
   b. False
5. A person drank a pint of milk at lunch. You know he drank
   a. 250 mL of milk
   b. 350 mL of milk
   c. 500 mL of milk
   d. 750 mL of milk
6. The soup bowl holds 6 ounces. A person ate all of the soup. You record his intake as
   a. 50 mL
   b. 120 mL
   c. 180 mL
   d. 200 mL
7. How often is fresh drinking water provided?
   a. Every 4 hours
   b. Every shift
   c. Every day
   d. Every week

Answers to Chapter 24 questions are on p. 450.

CHAPTER 25 MEASUREMENTS

VITAL SIGNS

- Accuracy is essential when you measure, record, and report vital signs. If unsure of your measurements, promptly ask the nurse to take them again. Unless otherwise ordered, take vital signs with the person at rest—lying or sitting.
- Report the following at once.
  - Any vital sign that is changed from a prior measurement
  - Vital signs above or below the normal range

Body Temperature

- Body temperature is the amount of heat in the body.
- Thermometers are used to measure temperature. It is measured using the Fahrenheit (F) and centigrade or centigrade (C) scales.

- Temperature sites are the mouth, rectum, axilla (underarm), tympanic membrane (ear), and temporal artery (forehead).
- Review Box 25-2, Temperature Sites, in the textbook.
- Normal range for body temperatures depends on the site.
  - Oral: 97.6°F to 99.6°F
  - Rectal: 98.6°F to 100.6°F
  - Axillary: 96.6°F to 98.6°F
  - Tympanic membrane: 98.6°F
  - Temporal artery: 99.6°F
- Older persons have lower body temperatures than younger persons.

TEMPERATURE SITES

- Temperature sites are the mouth, rectum, axilla (underarm), tympanic membrane (ear), and temporal artery (forehead). Review Box 25-2, Temperature Sites, in the textbook. Each site has a normal range. See Table 25-1, Normal Body Temperatures, in the textbook.
- Fever means an elevated body temperature. Always report temperatures that are above or below the normal range.

TAKING TEMPERATURES

- The nurse and care plan tell you:
  - When to take the person's temperature
  - What site to use
  - What thermometer to use
- Review Delegation Guidelines: Taking Temperatures in the textbook.
- Review Promoting Safety and Comfort: Taking Temperatures in the textbook.

ELECTRONIC THERMOMETERS

- Tympanic membrane thermometers are gently inserted into the ear. The temperature is measured in 1 to 3 seconds. These thermometers are not used if there is ear drainage.
- Temporal artery thermometers measure body temperature at the temporal artery in the forehead. These thermometers measure body temperature in 3 to 4 seconds. Follow the manufacturer's instructions for using, cleaning, and storing the device.

GLASS THERMOMETERS

- Long- or slender-tip thermometers are used for oral and axillary temperatures. So are thermometers with stubby and pear-shaped tips. Rectal thermometers have stubby tips.
- Glass thermometers are color-coded.
  - Blue—oral and axillary thermometers
  - Red—rectal thermometers

- If a mercury-glass thermometer breaks, tell the nurse at once. Do not touch the mercury. The agency must follow special procedures for handling all hazardous materials.
- When using a glass thermometer:
  - Use the person's thermometer.
  - Use a rectal thermometer only for rectal temperatures.
  - Rinse the thermometer under cold, running water if it was soaking in a disinfectant. Dry it from the stem to the bulb end with tissues.
  - Discard the thermometer if broken, cracked, or chipped.
  - Shake down the thermometer to below 94°F or 34°C before using it.
  - Clean and store the thermometer following center policy.
  - Use plastic covers following center policy.
  - Practice medical asepsis.
  - Follow Standard Precautions and the Bloodborne Pathogen Standard.

Pulse

- The pulse is the beat of the heart felt at an artery as a wave of blood passes through the artery.

PULSE RATE

- The pulse rate is the number of heartbeats or pulses felt or heard in 1 minute.
- The adult pulse rate is between 60 and 100 beats per minute. Report these abnormal rates to the nurse at once:
  - *Tachycardia*—the heart rate is more than 100 beats per minute.
  - *Bradycardia*—the heart rate is less than 60 beats per minute.

RHYTHM AND FORCE OF THE PULSE

- The rhythm of the pulse should be regular. Report and record an irregular pulse rhythm.
- Report and record if the pulse force is strong, full, bounding, weak, thready, or feeble.

TAKING PULSES

- The radial pulse is used for routine vital signs. Do not use your thumb to take a pulse. Count the pulse for 30 seconds and multiply by 2 if the agency policy permits. If the pulse is irregular, count it for 1 minute. Report and record if the pulse is regular or irregular, strong or weak.
- The apical pulse is on the left side of the chest slightly below the nipple. This pulse is taken with a stethoscope. Count the apical pulse for 1 minute.

Respirations

- Respiration means breathing air into and out of the lungs.
- The healthy adult has 12 to 20 respirations per minute. Respirations are normally quiet, effortless, and regular. Both sides of the chest rise and fall equally.
- Count respirations when the person is at rest. Count respirations right after taking a pulse.
- Count respirations for 30 seconds and multiply the number by 2 if the agency policy permits. If an abnormal pattern is noted, count the respirations for 1 minute.
- Report and record:
  - The respiratory rate
  - Equality and depth of respirations
  - If the respirations were regular or irregular
  - If the person has pain or difficulty breathing
  - Any respiratory noises
  - An abnormal respiratory pattern

Blood Pressure

- Blood pressure (BP) is the amount of force exerted against the walls of an artery by the blood. You measure blood pressure in the brachial artery.

NORMAL AND ABNORMAL BLOOD PRESSURES

- Blood pressure has normal ranges.
  - *Systolic pressure* (upper number)—less than 120 mm Hg
  - *Diastolic pressure* (lower number)—less than 80 mm Hg
- **Hypertension**—blood pressure measurements that remain above a systolic pressure of 140 mm Hg or a diastolic pressure of 90 mm Hg. Report any systolic measurement above 120 mm Hg. Also report a diastolic pressure above 80 mm Hg.
- **Hypotension**—when the systolic blood pressure is below 90 mm Hg and the diastolic pressure is below 60 mm Hg. Report a systolic pressure below 90 mm Hg. Also report a diastolic pressure below 60 mm Hg.
  - Review Box 25-5, Measuring Blood Pressure—Guidelines, in the textbook.

PAIN

- Pain is personal. It differs for each person. If a person complains of pain or discomfort, the person has pain or discomfort. You must believe the person.

Signs and Symptoms

- You cannot see, hear, touch, or smell the person's pain. Rely on what the person tells you. Promptly report any information you collect about pain. Use the person's exact words when reporting and recording pain. The nurse needs the following information.

- *Location*. Where is the pain?
- *Onset and duration*. When did the pain start? How long has it lasted?
- *Intensity*. Ask the person to rate the pain. Use a pain scale.
- *Description*. Ask the person to describe the pain.
- *Factors causing pain*. Ask what the person was doing before the pain started and when it started.
- *Factors affecting pain*. Ask what makes the pain better and what makes it worse.
- *Vital signs*. Increases often occur with acute pain. They may be normal with chronic pain.
- *Other signs and symptoms*. Dizziness, nausea, vomiting, weakness, numbness, and tingling.
- Review Box 25-6, Pain—Signs and Symptoms, in the textbook.

WEIGHT AND HEIGHT

- Weight and height are measured on admission to the agency. Then the person is weighed daily, weekly, or monthly. This is done to measure weight gain or loss.
- When weighing a person, follow the manufacturer's instructions and agency procedures for using the scales. Follow these guidelines when measuring weight and height.
  - The person wears only a gown or pajamas. No footwear is worn.
  - A dry incontinence product is worn.
  - The person voids before being weighed.
  - Weigh the person at the same time of day. Before breakfast is the best time.
  - Use the same scale for daily, weekly, and monthly weights.
  - Balance the scale at zero before weighing the person.

CHAPTER 25 REVIEW QUESTIONS

Circle the BEST answer.

1. Which statement about taking a rectal temperature is *false?*
   a. The bulb end of the thermometer needs to be lubricated.
   b. The thermometer is held in place for 5 minutes.
   c. Privacy is important.
   d. The normal range is 98.6°F to 100.6°F.
2. Which pulse rate should you report at once?
   a. A pulse rate of 52 beats per minute
   b. A pulse rate of 60 beats per minute
   c. A pulse rate of 76 beats per minute
   d. A pulse rate of 100 beats per minute
3. Which statement is *false?*
   a. An irregular pulse is counted for 1 minute.
   b. You may use your thumb to take a radial pulse rate.
   c. The radial pulse is usually used to count a pulse rate.
   d. Tachycardia is a fast pulse rate.

4. Which blood pressure should you report?
   a. 120/80 mm Hg
   b. 88/62 mm Hg
   c. 110/70 mm Hg
   d. 92/68 mm Hg
5. A person complains of pain. You will do the following except
   a. Ask where the pain is
   b. Ask when the pain started
   c. Ask what the intensity of the pain is on a scale of 1 to 10
   d. Ask why he or she is complaining about pain
6. Which statement is *false?*
   a. Have the person void before being weighed.
   b. Weigh the person at the same time of day.
   c. Balance the scale at zero before weighing the person
   d. Have the person wear shoes when being weighed.

Answers to Chapter 25 questions are on p. 450.

CHAPTER 26 COLLECTING SPECIMENS

- Specimens *(samples)* are collected and tested to prevent, detect, and treat disease.
- Urine specimens are collected for urine tests. The random urine specimen is used for a routine urinalysis (u/a). No special measures are needed. The midstream specimen is also called a *clean-voided specimen* or *clean-catch specimen*. The perineal area is cleaned first to reduce the number of microbes in the urethral area. The person starts to void into a device. Then the person stops the urine stream and a sterile specimen container is positioned. The person voids into the container until the specimen is obtained. All urine voided during 24 hours is collected for a 24-hour urine specimen. To prevent microbe growth, the urine is chilled on ice or refrigerated.
- Reagent strips (test strips) have sections that change color when reacting with urine.
- Stools are studied for fat, microbes, worms, blood, and other abnormal contents. Urine must not contaminate the stool specimen.
- *Mucus from the respiratory system is called sputum when expectorated (expelled) through the mouth. Sputum specimens are studied for blood, microbes, and abnormal cells. Sputum is coughed up from the bronchi and trachea.*
- Blood glucose testing is used for persons with diabetes. The skin is punctured and a drop of blood is collected and tested.

CHAPTER 26 REVIEW QUESTIONS

Circle the BEST answer.

1. Specimen are collected and tested for all of the following *except*
   a. Prevent diseases
   b. Treat diseases
   c. Detect diseases
   d. Diagnose diseases

2. A random urine specimen is used for
   a. A routine urinalysis
   b. 24-hour specimen
   c. Midstream specimen
   d. Diagnose UTI
3. When collecting a stool specimen, urine must not contaminate the sample.
   a. True
   b. False
4. Sputum samples are best collected at night.
   a. True
   b. False

Answers to Chapter 26 questions are on p. 450.

CHAPTER 27 EXERCISE AND ACTIVITY NEEDS
BEDREST
- The doctor may order bedrest to treat a health problem.
- Bedrest is ordered to:
  - Reduce physical activity
  - Reduce pain
  - Encourage rest
  - Regain strength
  - Promote healing

Complications from Bedrest
- Pressure ulcers, constipation, and fecal impactions can result. Urinary tract infections and renal calculi (kidney stones) can occur. So can blood clots and pneumonia.
- The musculo-skeletal system is affected by lack of exercise and activity. You help prevent the following to maintain normal movement.
  - A **contracture** is the lack of joint mobility caused by abnormal shortening of a muscle. Common sites are the fingers, wrists, elbows, toes, ankles, knees, and hips. The site is deformed and stiff.
  - **Atrophy** is the decrease in size or the wasting away of tissue. Tissues shrink in size.
- **Orthostatic hypotension (postural hypotension)** is abnormally low blood pressure when the person suddenly stands up. The person is dizzy and weak and has spots before the eyes. Fainting can occur. Slowly changing position is key to prevent orthostatic hypotension.
- Good nursing care prevents complications from bedrest. Good alignment, range-of-motion exercises, and frequent position changes are important measures. These are part of the care plan.

Positioning
- Supportive devices are often used to support and maintain the person in a certain position.
  - *Bed-boards*—are placed under the mattress to prevent the mattress from sagging.
  - *Foot-boards*—are placed at the foot of mattresses to prevent plantar flexion that can lead to footdrop.

In plantar flexion, the foot is bent. Footdrop is when the foot falls down at the ankle (permanent plantar flexion).
  - *Trochanter rolls*—prevent the hips and legs from turning outward (external rotation).
  - *Hip abduction wedges*—keep the hips abducted (apart).
  - *Hand rolls or hand grips*—prevent contractures of the thumb, fingers, and wrist.
  - *Splints*—keep the elbows, wrists, thumbs, fingers, ankles, and knees in normal position.
  - *Bed cradles*—keep the weight of top linens off the feet and toes.

Exercise
- Exercise helps prevent contractures, muscle atrophy, and other complications from bedrest.

RANGE-OF-MOTION EXERCISES
- The movement of a joint to the extent possible without causing pain is the range of motion of the joint.
- **Range-of-motion (ROM)** exercises involve moving the joints through their complete range of motion without causing pain. They are usually done at least two times a day.
- *Active ROM*—exercises are done by the person.
- *Passive ROM*—you move the joints through their range of motion.
- *Active-assistive ROM*—the person does the exercises with some help.
- Review Box 27-1, Range-of-Motion Exercises, in the textbook.
- Range-of-motion exercises can cause injury if not done properly. Practice these rules.
  - Exercise only the joints the nurse tells you to exercise.
  - Expose only the body part being exercised.
  - Use good body mechanics.
  - Support the part being exercised.
  - Move the joint slowly, smoothly, and gently.
  - Do not force a joint beyond its present range of motion.
  - Do not force a joint to the point of pain.
  - Ask the person if he or she has pain or discomfort.
  - Perform ROM exercises to the neck only if allowed by your agency and if the nurse instructs you to do so.

AMBULATION
- **Ambulation** is the act of walking.
- Follow the care plan when helping a person walk. Use a gait (transfer) belt if the person is weak or unsteady. The person also uses hand rails along the wall. Always check the person for orthostatic hypotension.

- When you help the person walk, walk to the side and slightly behind the person on the person's weak side. Encourage the person to use the hand rail on his or her strong side.

Walking Aids

- Crutches are used when the person cannot use one leg or when one or both legs need to gain strength. Check the crutch tips. They must not be worn down, torn, or wet. Check crutches for flaws. Tighten all bolts. Have the person wear flat street shoes with non-skid soles.
- A cane is held on the strong side of the body. The cane tip is about 6 to 10 inches to the side of the foot. It is about 6 to 10 inches in front of the foot on the strong side. The grip is level with the hip. To walk:
  - Step A: The cane is moved forward 6 to 10 inches.
  - Step B: The weak leg (opposite the cane) is moved forward even with the cane.
  - Step C: The strong leg is moved forward and ahead of the cane and the weak leg.
- A walker gives more support than a cane. Wheeled walkers are common. They have wheels on the front legs and rubber tips on the back legs. The person pushes the walker about 6 to 8 inches in front of his or her feet.
- Braces support weak body parts, prevent or correct deformities, or prevent joint movement. A brace is applied over the ankle, knee, or back. Skin and bony points under braces are kept clean and dry. Report redness or signs of skin breakdown at once. The nurse assesses the skin under braces every shift. Also report complaints of pain or discomfort. The care plan tells you when to apply and remove a brace.

CHAPTER 27 REVIEW QUESTIONS

Circle the BEST answer.

1. To prevent orthostatic hypotension, you should
   a. Move a person from the lying position to the sitting position quickly
   b. Move a person from the sitting position to the standing position quickly
   c. Move a person from the lying or sitting position to a standing position slowly
   d. Keep the person in bed
2. Exercise helps prevent contractures and muscle atrophy.
   a. True
   b. False
3. When performing ROM exercises, you should force a joint to the point of pain.
   a. True
   b. False
4. A person's left leg is weaker than his right. The person holds the cane on his right side.
   a. True
   b. False

Answers to Chapter 27 questions are on p. 450.

CHAPTER 28 WOUND CARE

- A **wound** is a break in the skin or mucous membrane.
- The wound is a portal of entry for microbes. Infection is a major threat. Wound care involves preventing infection and further injury to the wound and nearby tissues.

SKIN TEARS

- A **skin tear** is a break or rip in the outer layer of the skin.
- Skin tears are caused by friction, shearing, pulling, or pressure on the skin. Bumping a hand, arm, or leg on any hard surface can cause a skin tear. Beds, bed rails, chairs, wheelchair footplates, and tables are dangers. So is holding the person's arm or leg too tight, removing tape or adhesives, bathing, dressing, and other tasks. Buttons, zippers, jewelry, or long or jagged fingernails or toenails can also cause skin tears.
- Skin tears are painful. They are portals of entry for microbes. Infection is a risk. Tell the nurse at once if you cause or find a skin tear.
- Review Box 28-1, Preventing Skin Tears, in the textbook.

CIRCULATORY ULCERS

- An ulcer is a shallow or deep crater-like sore of the skin or mucous membrane.
- *Circulatory ulcers (vascular ulcers)* are open sores on the lower legs or feet. They are caused by decreased blood flow through the arteries or veins.
- Review Box 28-2, Preventing Circulatory Ulcers, in the textbook.
- *Venous ulcers (stasis ulcers)* are open sores on the lower legs or feet. They are caused by poor blood flow through the veins. The heels and inner aspect of the ankles are common sites for venous ulcers.
- *Arterial ulcers* are open wounds on the lower legs or feet caused by poor arterial blood flow. They are found between the toes, on top of the toes, and on the outer side of the ankle.
- A *diabetic foot ulcer* is an open wound on the foot caused by complications from diabetes. When nerves are affected, the person can lose complete or partial sensation in a foot or leg. The person may not feel pain, heat, or cold. Therefore the person may not feel a cut, blister, burn, or other trauma to the foot. Infection and a large sore can develop. When blood flow to the foot decreases, tissues and cells do not get needed oxygen and nutrients. Sores heal poorly. Tissue death (gangrene) can occur.

Prevention and Treatment

- Check the person's feet and legs every day. Report any sign of a problem to the nurse at once. Follow the care plan to prevent and treat circulatory ulcers.

ELASTIC STOCKINGS

- Elastic stockings exert pressure on the veins. The pressure promotes venous blood return to the heart. The stockings help prevent blood clots in the leg veins.
- Elastic stockings also are called AE stockings (anti-embolic or anti-emboli). They also are called TED hose. TED means thromboembolic disease.
- The nurse measures the person for the correct size of elastic stockings. Most stockings have an opening near the toes that is used to check circulation, skin color, and skin temperature.
- The person usually has two pairs of stockings. One pair is washed; the other pair is worn.
- Stockings should not have twists, creases, or wrinkles after you apply them. Twists can affect circulation. Creases and wrinkles can cause skin breakdown.
- Loose stocking do not promote venous blood return to the heart. Stockings that are too tight can affect circulation. Tell the nurse if the stockings are too loose or tight.

Heat Applications

- When heat is applied to the skin, blood vessels dilate. *Dilate* means to expand or open wider.
- Heat relieves pain, relaxes muscles, promotes healing, reduces tissue swelling, and decreases joint stiffness.

COMPLICATIONS

- High temperatures can cause burns. Report pain, excessive redness, and blisters at once. Also observe for pale skin. When heat is applied too long, blood vessels constrict. Blood flow decreases. Tissue damage occurs.
- Metal implants pose risks. Pacemakers and joint replacements are made of metal. Do not apply heat to an implant area.
- Heat is not applied to a pregnant woman's abdomen. The heat can affect fetal growth.

Cold Applications

- When cold is applied to the skin, blood vessels constrict, or narrow.
- Cold applications reduce pain, prevent swelling, and decrease circulation and bleeding.

COMPLICATIONS

- Complications include pain, burns, blisters, and poor circulation. Burns and blisters occur from intense cold. They also occur when dry cold is in direct contact with the skin.

Applying Heat and Cold

- Protect the person from injury during heat and cold applications. Review Box 28-6, Applying Heat and Cold, in the textbook.

CHAPTER 28 REVIEW QUESTIONS

Circle the BEST answer.
1. The following can cause a skin tear *except*
   a. Friction and shearing
   b. Holding a person's arm or leg too tight
   c. Rings, watches, bracelets
   d. Trimmed, short nails
2. A person is diabetic. Which statement is *false?*
   a. The person may not feel pain in her feet.
   b. The person may not feel heat or cold in her feet.
   c. You need to check her feet weekly for foot problems.
   d. The person is at risk for diabetic foot ulcers.
3. Which statement about elastic stockings is *false?*
   a. Elastic stockings are also called antiembolic stockings.
   b. Elastic stockings should be wrinkle free after being applied.
   c. A person usually has two pairs of elastic stockings.
   d. Elastic stockings are applied after a person gets out of bed.
4. Which statement about elastic stockings is *true?*
   a. Elastic stockings should be loose to promote venous blood return to the heart.
   b. Stockings should not have twists, creases, or wrinkles after you apply them.
   c. The doctor measures the person for the correct size of elastic stockings.
   d. The person should have only one pair of stockings.
5. Complications from a heat application include the following *except*
   a. Excessive redness
   b. Blisters
   c. Pale skin
   d. Cyanotic (bluish) nail beds
6. When applying heat or cold, you should do the following *except*
   a. Ask the nurse what the temperature of the application should be
   b. Cover dry heat or cold applications before applying them
   c. Observe the skin every 2 hours
   d. Know how long to leave the application in place

Answers to Chapter 28 questions are on p. 451.

CHAPTER 29 PRESSURE INJURIES

- A **pressure injury** is a localized injury to the skin and/or underlying tissue, usually over a bony prominence—the back of the head, shoulder blades, elbows, hips, spine, sacrum, knees, ankles, heels, and toes. It is the result of pressure or pressure in combination with shear—when layers of skin rub against each other—or friction—the rubbing of one surface against another.
- *Decubitus ulcer, bed sore,* and *pressure sore* are other terms for pressure ulcer.

- Pressure, shearing, and friction are common causes of skin breakdown and pressure ulcers. Risk factors include breaks in the skin, poor circulation to an area, moisture, dry skin, and irritation by urine and feces.

PERSONS AT RISK

- Persons at risk for pressure ulcers are those who:
  - Are confined to a bed or chair.
  - Need some or total help moving.
  - Are agitated or have involuntary muscle movements.
  - Have urinary or fecal incontinence.
  - Are exposed to moisture.
  - Have poor nutrition.
  - Have poor fluid balance.
  - Have lowered mental awareness.
  - Have problems sensing pain or pressure.
  - Have circulatory problems.
  - Are obese or very thin.
  - Have a healed pressure ulcer.
  - Take drugs that affect wound healing.
  - Refuse some care and treatment measures.
  - Have health problems such as kidney failure, thyroid disease, or diabetes.
  - Smoke.

PRESSURE INJURY STAGES

- In persons with light skin, a red area is the first sign of a pressure ulcer. In persons with dark skin, the skin may have no color change or may appear red, blue, or purple. The area may feel warm or cool. The person may complain of pain, burning, tingling, or itching in the area.
- Box 29-2, Pressure Injury Stages, in the textbook describes pressure injury stages.
- Figures 29-6 through 29-17 in the textbook show the stages of pressure injuries.

PREVENTION AND TREATMENT

- Preventing pressure injuries is much easier than trying to heal them. Review Box 29-3, Preventing Pressure Injuries, in the textbook.
- Pressure ulcers usually occur over bony prominences (pressure points). These areas bear the weight of the body in certain positions. According to the CMS, the sacrum is the most common site for a pressure ulcer. Other sites include:
  - Heels and ears.
  - A urinary catheter can cause pressure and friction on the meatus.
  - Tubes, casts, braces, and other devices can cause pressure on arms, hands, legs, and feet.
  - For people who are obese, pressure ulcers can occur in areas where skin has contact with skin: between abdominal folds, the legs, the buttocks, the thighs, and under the breasts.

- The person at risk for pressure ulcers may be placed on a foam, air, alternating air, gel, or water mattress.
- Protective devices are often used to prevent and treat pressure ulcers and skin breakdown. Protective devices include:
  - Bed cradle
  - Heel and elbow protectors
  - Heel and foot elevators
  - Gel or fluid-filled pads and cushions
  - Egg crate–type pads
  - Special beds
  - Other equipment—pillows, trochanter rolls, foot-boards, and other positioning devices.
- Dressings—if a pressure ulcer has drainage, a dressing that absorbs drainage is used. The dressing absorbs slough, or dead tissue that is shed for the skin.

COMPLICATIONS

- Infection is the most common complication.
- Osteomyelitis is a risk if the pressure ulcer is over a bony prominence. Inflammation of the bone and bone marrow occur.

CHAPTER 29 REVIEW QUESTIONS

Circle the BEST answer.
1. You may expect to find a pressure injury at all of the following sites *except*
   a. Back of the head
   b. Ears
   c. Top of the thigh
   d. Toes
2. Which of the following is not a protective device used to prevent and treat pressure injuries?
   a. Heel elevator
   b. Bed cradle
   c. Drawsheet
   d. Elbow protector
3. In obese people, pressure injuries can occur between abdominal folds.
   a. True
   b. False
4. Pressure injuries usually occur over a bony prominence.
   a. True
   b. False
Answers to Chapter 29 questions are on p. 451.

CHAPTER 30 OXYGEN NEEDS
ALTERED RESPIRATORY FUNCTION

- Hypoxia means that cells do not have enough oxygen.
- Restlessness, dizziness, and disorientation are signs of hypoxia.

- Review Box 30-1, Altered Respiratory Function, in the textbook. Report signs and symptoms of hypoxia to the nurse at once. Hypoxia is life-threatening.

Abnormal Respirations

- Adults normally have 12 to 20 respirations per minute. They are quiet, effortless, and regular. Both sides of the chest rise and fall equally. Report these observations at once:
  - **Tachypnea**—rapid breathing. Respirations are 20 or more per minute.
  - **Bradypnea**—slow breathing. Respirations are fewer than 12 per minute.
  - **Apnea**—lack or absence of breathing.
  - **Hypoventilation**—breathing (ventilation) is slow, shallow, and sometimes irregular.
  - **Hyperventilation**—breathing (ventilation) is rapid and deeper than normal.
  - **Dyspnea**—difficult, labored, or painful breathing.
  - **Cheyne-Stokes respirations**—respirations gradually increase in rate and depth. Then they become shallow and slow. Breathing may stop for 10 to 20 seconds.
  - **Orthopnea**—breathing deeply and comfortably only when sitting.
  - **Kussmaul respirations**—very deep and rapid respirations.

MEETING OXYGEN NEEDS

Positioning

- Breathing is usually easier in semi-Fowler's and Fowler's positions. Persons with difficulty breathing often prefer the **orthopneic position** (sitting up and leaning over a table to breathe). Position changes are needed at least every 2 hours. Follow the care plan.

Deep Breathing and Coughing

- Deep breathing moves air into most parts of the lungs. Coughing removes mucus. Deep breathing and coughing are usually done every 1 to 2 hours while the person is awake. They help prevent pneumonia and atelectasis (the collapse of a portion of the lung).

ASSISTING WITH OXYGEN THERAPY

Oxygen Devices

- *Nasal cannula.* The prongs are inserted into the nostrils. A band goes behind the ears and under the chin to keep the device in place. A nasal cannula allows eating and drinking. Tight prongs can irritate the nose. Pressure on the ears and cheekbones is possible.
- *Simple face mask.* It covers the nose and mouth. The mask has small holes in the sides. Talking and eating are hard to do with a mask. Listen carefully. Moisture can build up under the mask. Keep the face clean and dry. Masks are removed for eating. Usually oxygen is given by cannula during meals.

Oxygen Flow Rates

- The flow rate is the amount of oxygen given. It is measured in liters per minute (L/min).
- The doctor orders 1 to 15 L/min.
- The nurse and care plan tell you the person's flow rate.
- When giving care and checking the person, always check the flow rate. Tell the nurse at once if it is too high or too low. A nurse or respiratory therapist will adjust the flow rate.

Oxygen Safety

- Review Box 30-2, Oxygen Safety, in your textbook.
- You do not give oxygen. You assist the nurse in providing safe care.
- Always check the oxygen level when you are with or near persons using oxygen systems that contain a limited amount of oxygen. Oxygen tanks and liquid oxygen systems are examples. Report a low oxygen level to the nurse at once.
- Follow the rules for fire and the use of oxygen in Chapter 10.
- Never remove the oxygen device. However, turn off the oxygen flow if there is a fire.
- Make sure the oxygen device is secure but not tight.
- Check for signs of irritation from the oxygen device—behind the ears, under the nose, and around the face.
- Keep the face clean and dry when a mask is used.
- Never shut off the oxygen flow.
- Do not adjust the flow rate unless allowed by your state and agency.
- Tell the nurse at once if the flow rate is too high or too low.
- Tell the nurse at once if the humidifier is not bubbling.
- Secure tubing to the person's garment. Follow agency policy.
- Make sure there are no kinks in the tubing.
- Make sure the person does not lie on any part of the tubing.
- Report signs of hypoxia, respiratory distress, or abnormal breathing to the nurse at once.
- Give oral hygiene as directed. Follow the care plan.
- Make sure the oxygen device is clean and free of mucus.
- Make sure the oxygen tank is secure in its holder.

CHAPTER 30 REVIEW QUESTIONS

Circle the BEST answer.
1. Which statement is *false*?
   a. Restlessness, dizziness, and disorientation are signs of hypoxia.
   b. Hypoxia is life-threatening.
   c. Report signs and symptoms of hypoxia at the end of the shift.
   d. Anything that affects respiratory function can cause hypoxia.

2. Adults normally have
   a. 8 to 10 respirations per minute
   b. 12 to 20 respirations per minute
   c. 10 to 12 respirations per minute
   d. 20 to 24 respirations per minute
3. Dyspnea is
   a. Difficult, labored, or painful breathing
   b. Slow breathing with fewer than 12 respirations per minute
   c. Rapid breathing with 24 or more respirations per minute
   d. Lack or absence of breathing
4. Which statement about positioning is *false?*
   a. Breathing is usually easier in semi-Fowler's or Fowler's position.
   b. Persons with difficulty breathing often prefer the orthopneic position.
   c. Position changes are needed at least every 4 hours.
   d. Follow the person's care plan for positioning preferences.
5. A person has a nasal cannula. Which statement is *false?*
   a. You will leave the nasal cannula on while the person is eating.
   b. You will watch the nose area for irritation.
   c. You will watch the ears and cheekbones for skin breakdown.
   d. You will take the nasal cannula off while the person is eating.

Answers to Chapter 30 questions are on p. 451.

CHAPTER 31 REHABILITATION NEEDS

- A **disability** is any lost, absent, or impaired physical or mental function.
- **Rehabilitation** is the process of restoring the person to his or her highest possible level of physical, psychological, social, and economic function. The goal is to improve abilities. This promotes function at the highest level of independence.
- Restorative nursing care is care that helps the person regain health, strength, and independence. A restorative aide is a nursing assistant with special training in restorative nursing and rehabilitation skills.

REHABILITATION AND THE WHOLE PERSON

- Rehabilitation takes longer in older persons. Changes from aging affect healing, mobility, vision, hearing, and other functions. Chronic health problems can slow recovery.

Physical Aspects

- Rehabilitation starts when the person first seeks health care. Complications, such as contractures and pressure ulcers, are prevented.

- *Self-care.* Self-care for activities of daily living (ADL) is a major goal. ADLs are the activities usually done during a normal day in a person's life. The health team evaluates the need for self-help devices.
- *Elimination.* Bowel or bladder training may be needed. Fecal impaction, constipation, and fecal incontinence are prevented.
- *Mobility.* The person may need crutches, a walker, a cane, a brace, a wheelchair, or a prosthesis. A prosthesis is an artificial replacement for a missing body part.
- *Nutrition.* The person may need a dysphagia diet or enteral nutrition.
- *Communication.* Aphasia may occur from a stroke. Aphasia is the total or partial loss of the ability to use or understand language. Speech therapy and communication devices are helpful.

Psychological and Social Aspects

- A disability can affect function and appearance. Self-esteem and relationships may suffer. The person may feel unwhole, useless, unattractive, unclean, or undesirable. The person may deny the disability. The person may expect therapy to correct the problem. He or she may be depressed, angry, and hostile.
- Successful rehabilitation depends on the person's attitude. The person must accept his or her limits and be motivated. The focus is on abilities and strengths. Despair and frustration are common. Progress may be slow. Old fears and emotions may recur.
- Remind persons of their progress. They need help accepting disabilities and limits. Give support, reassurance, and encouragement. Spiritual support helps some people. Psychological and social needs are part of the care plan.

THE REHABILITATION TEAM

- Rehabilitation is a team effort. The person is the key member. The health team and family help the person set goals and plan care. The focus is on regaining function and independence.

Your Role

- Every part of your job focuses on promoting the person's independence. Preventing decline in function also is a goal. Review Box 31-1, Assisting with Rehabilitation Needs, in the textbook.

REHABILITATION PROGRAMS AND SERVICES

- Common rehabilitation programs include:
  - Cardiac rehabilitation—for heart disorders
  - Brain injury rehabilitation—for nervous system disorders including traumatic brain injury

- Spinal cord rehabilitation—for spinal cord injuries
- Stroke rehabilitation—after a stroke
- Respiratory rehabilitation—for respiratory system disorders, after lung surgery, or for respiratory complications from other health problems
- Musculo-skeletal rehabilitation—for fractures, joint replacement surgery, and other musculo-skeletal problems
- Rehabilitation for complex medical and surgical conditions—for wound care, diabetes, burns, and other complex problems
- The process often continues after hospital discharge. The person may need home care or care in a nursing center or rehabilitation agency.

QUALITY OF LIFE

- To promote quality of life:
  - *Protect the right to privacy.* The person relearns old or practices new skills in private. Others do not need to see mistakes, falls, spills, clumsiness, anger, or tears.
  - *Encourage personal choice.* This gives the person control.
  - *Protect the right to be free from abuse and mistreatment.* Sometimes improvement is not seen for weeks. Repeated explanations and demonstrations may have little or no results. You and other staff and family may become upset and short-tempered. However, no one can shout, scream, or yell at the person. Nor can they call the person names or hit or strike the person. Unkind remarks are not allowed. Report signs of abuse or mistreatment.
  - *Learn to deal with your anger and frustration.* The person does not choose loss of function. If the process upsets you, discuss your feelings with the nurse.
  - *Encourage activities.* Provide support and reassurance to the person with the disability. Remind the person that others with disabilities can give support and understanding.
  - *Provide a safe setting.* The setting must meet the person's needs. The over-bed table, bedside stand, and call light are moved to the person's strong side.
  - *Show patience, understanding, and sensitivity.* The person may be upset and discouraged. Give support, encouragement, and praise when needed. Stress the person's abilities and strengths. Do not give pity or sympathy.

CHAPTER 31 REVIEW QUESTIONS

Circle the BEST answer.
1. Successful rehabilitation depends on the person's attitude.
   a. True
   b. False
2. A person with a disability may be depressed, angry, and hostile.
   a. True
   b. False
3. A person needs rehabilitation. You should do the following *except*
   a. Let the person relearn old skills in private
   b. Let the person practice new skills in private
   c. Encourage the person to make choices
   d. Shout at the person
4. You saw a family member hit and scream at a person. You need to report your observations to the nurse.
   a. True
   b. False
5. A person has a weak left arm. You will
   a. Place the call light on his left side
   b. Place the call light on his right side
   c. Give him sympathy
   d. Give him pity

Answers to Chapter 31 questions are on p. 451.

CHAPTER 32 HEARING, SPEECH, AND VISION PROBLEMS

HEARING LOSS

- Hearing loss is not being able to hear the normal range of sounds associated with normal hearing. Deafness is the most severe form of hearing loss.
- Obvious signs and symptoms of hearing loss include:
  - Speaking too loudly
  - Leaning forward to hear
  - Turning and cupping the better ear toward the speaker
  - Answering questions or responding inappropriately
  - Asking for words to be repeated
  - Asking others to speak louder or to speak more slowly and clearly
  - Having trouble hearing over the phone
  - Having problems following conversations when two or more people are talking
  - Turning up the TV, radio, or music volume so loud that others complain
- Persons with hearing loss may wear hearing aids or lip-read (speech-read). They watch facial expressions, gestures, and body language. Some people learn American Sign Language (ASL). Others may have hearing assistance dogs.
- Review Box 32-2, Measures to Promote Hearing, in the textbook.
- Hearing aids are battery operated. If the device does not seem to work properly:
  - Check if the hearing aid is on. It has an on and off switch.
  - Check the battery position.
  - Insert a new battery if needed.
  - Clean the hearing aid. Follow the nurse's directions and the manufacturer's instructions.

- Hearing aids are turned off when not in use. The battery is removed.
- Handle and care for hearing aids properly. If lost or damaged, report it to the nurse at once.

EYE DISORDERS

- *Glaucoma*. Glaucoma results when fluid builds up in the eye and causes pressure on the optic nerve. The optic nerve is damaged. Vision loss with eventual blindness occurs. Drugs and surgery can control glaucoma and prevent further damage to the optic nerve. Prior damage cannot be reversed.
- *Cataract*. Cataract is a clouding of the lens in the eye. Signs and symptoms include cloudy, blurry, or dimmed vision. Colors seem faded. Persons may also be sensitive to light and glares or see halos around lights. Poor vision at night and double vision in one eye are other symptoms. Surgery is the only treatment. Review the list of post-operative care measures in Box 32-5, Cataract Surgery—Post-Operative Care, in the textbook.
- Age-related macular degeneration (AMD) blurs central vision.
- Diabetic retinopathy is a complication of diabetes. Tiny blood vessels in the retina are damaged. It is a leading cause of blindness. The person needs to control diabetes, blood pressure, and cholesterol. Laser surgery may help.

Impaired Vision and Blindness

- Birth defects, injuries, and eye diseases are among the many causes of impaired vision and blindness. They also are complications of some diseases.
- Rehabilitation programs help the person adjust to the vision loss and learn to be independent. The person learns to use visual and adaptive devices, Braille, long canes, and guide dogs.
- Review Box 32-6, Caring for Blind and Visually Impaired Persons, in the textbook.

Corrective Lenses

- Clean eyeglasses daily and as needed.
- Protect eyeglasses from loss or damage. When not worn, put them in their case.
- Contact lenses are cleaned, removed, and stored according to the manufacturer's instructions.

CHAPTER 32 REVIEW QUESTIONS

Circle the BEST answer.
1. Signs and symptoms of hearing loss include all of the following *except*
   a. Speaking too loudly
   b. Leaning forward to hear
   c. Answering questions appropriately
   d. Turning up the TV

2. To promote hearing, you
   a. Speak in a loud tone
   b. Maintain eye contact
   c. Chew gum while talking
   d. Wear a mask
3. Cataracts cause
   a. Blurry vision
   b. Clear vision
   c. Pain in the eyes
   d. Single vision
4. Eyeglasses are to be stored in their case in the top drawer of the bedside stand when not in use.
   a. True
   b. False

Answers to Chapter 32 questions are on p. 451.

CHAPTER 33 COMMON HEALTH PROBLEMS

CANCER

- Cancer is the second leading cause of death in the United States.
- Review Box 33-1, Cancer—General Signs and Symptoms, in the textbook.
- Surgery, radiation therapy, and chemotherapy are the most common treatments.
- Persons with cancer have many needs. They include:
  - Pain relief or control
  - Rest and exercise
  - Fluids and nutrition
  - Preventing skin breakdown
  - Preventing bowel problems (constipation, diarrhea)
  - Dealing with treatment side effects
  - Psychological and social needs
  - Spiritual needs
  - Sexual needs
- Anger, fear, and depression are common. Some surgeries are disfiguring. The person may feel unwhole, unattractive, or unclean. The person and family need support.
- Talk to the person. Do not avoid the person because you are uncomfortable. Use touch and listening to show that you care.
- Spiritual needs are important. A spiritual leader may provide comfort.

MUSCULO-SKELETAL DISORDERS

Arthritis

- Arthritis means joint inflammation.
- *Osteoarthritis (degenerative joint disease)*. The fingers, spine (neck and lower back), and weight-bearing joints (hips, knees, and feet) are often affected. Treatment involves pain relief, heat and cold applications, exercise, rest and joint care, weight control, and a healthy life-style. Falls are prevented. Help is

given with ADLs as needed. Toilet seat risers are helpful when hips and knees are affected. So are chairs with higher seats and armrests. Some people need joint replacement surgery.

- *Rheumatoid arthritis.* Rheumatoid arthritis (RA) causes joint pain, swelling, stiffness, and loss of function. Joints are tender, warm, and swollen. Fatigue and fever are common. The person does not feel well. The person's care plan may include rest balanced with exercise, proper positioning, joint care, weight control, measures to reduce stress, and measures to prevent falls. Drugs are given for pain relief and inflammation. Heat and cold applications may be ordered. Some persons need joint replacement surgery. Emotional support is needed. Persons with RA need to stay as active as possible. Give encouragement and praise. Listen when the person needs to talk.

Osteoporosis

- With osteoporosis, the bone becomes porous and brittle. Bones are fragile and break easily. Spine, hip, wrist, and rib fractures are common.
- Older people are at risk. The risk increases for women after menopause. Lack of estrogen and low levels of dietary calcium cause bone changes. All ethnic groups are at risk. Other risk factors include a family history of the disease, being thin or having a small frame, eating disorders, tobacco use, alcoholism, lack of exercise, bedrest, and immobility. Exercise and activity are needed for bone strength. Bone must bear weight to form properly. If not, calcium is lost from the bone and it becomes porous and brittle.
- Fractures are a major threat. Prevention is important. Doctors often order calcium and vitamin supplements. Estrogen is ordered for some women. Other preventive measures include:
  - Exercising weight-bearing joints
  - No smoking
  - Limiting alcohol and caffeine
  - Back supports or corsets for good posture
  - Walking aids if needed
  - Safety measures to prevent falls and accidents
  - Good body mechanics
  - Safe moving, transferring, turning, and positioning procedures

NERVOUS SYSTEM DISORDERS

Stroke

- Stroke is also called a brain attack or cerebrovascular accident (CVA). It is the third leading cause of death in the United States. Review Box 33-6, Stroke—Warning Signs, in the textbook.
- The effects of stroke include:
  - Loss of face, hand, arm, leg, or body control.
  - **Hemiplegia**—paralysis on one side of the body.

- Changing emotions (crying easily or mood swings, sometimes for no reason).
- Difficulty swallowing (dysphagia).
- Aphasia or slowed or slurred speech. Aphasia is the total or partial loss of the ability to use or understand language.
- Changes in sight, touch, movement, and thought.
- Impaired memory.
- Urinary frequency, urgency, or incontinence.
- Loss of bowel control or constipation.
- Depression and frustration.
- The health team helps the person regain the highest possible level of function. Review Box 33-7, Stroke Care Measures, in the textbook.

Aphasia

- **Aphasia** is the total or partial loss of the ability to use or understand language.
- *Expressive aphasia* relates to difficulty expressing or sending out thoughts. Thinking is clear. The person knows what to say but has difficulty or cannot speak the words.
- *Receptive aphasia* relates to difficulty understanding language. The person has trouble understanding what is said or read. People and common objects are not recognized.

Parkinson's Disease

- Parkinson's disease is a slow, progressive disorder with no cure. Persons over the age of 50 are at risk. Signs and symptoms become worse over time. They include:
  - *Tremors*—often start in the hand. Pill-rolling movements—rubbing the thumb and index finger—may occur. The person may have trembling in the hands, arms, legs, jaw, and face.
  - *Rigid, stiff muscles*—in the arms, legs, neck, and trunk.
  - *Slow movements*—the person has a slow, shuffling gait.
  - *Stooped posture and impaired balance*—it is hard to walk. Falls are a risk.
  - *Mask-like expression*—the person cannot blink and smile. A fixed stare is common.
- Other signs and symptoms that develop over time include swallowing and chewing problems, constipation, and bladder problems. Sleep problems, depression, and emotional changes (fear, insecurity) can occur. So can memory loss and slow thinking. The person may have slurred, monotone, and soft speech. Some people talk too fast or repeat what they say.
- Drugs are ordered to treat and control the disease. Exercise and physical therapy improve strength, posture, balance, and mobility. Therapy is needed for speech and swallowing problems. The person may need help with eating and self-care. Safety measures are needed to prevent falls and injury.

Multiple Sclerosis

- Multiple sclerosis (MS) is a chronic disease. The myelin (which covers nerve fibers) in the brain and spinal cord is destroyed. Nerve impulses are not sent to and from the brain in a normal manner. Functions are impaired or lost. There is no cure.
- Symptoms usually start between the ages of 20 and 40. Signs and symptoms depend on the damaged area. They may include vision problems, muscle weakness in the arms and legs, balance problems that affect standing and walking. Tingling, prickling, or numb sensations may occur. Also, partial or complete paralysis and pain may occur. In addition, there may be speech problems, tremors, dizziness, concentration, attention, memory, and judgment problems, as well as depression, bowel and bladder problems, problems with sexual function, hearing loss, and fatigue.
- Persons with MS are kept active as long as possible and as independent as possible. Skin care, hygiene, and range-of-motion exercises are important. So are turning, positioning, and deep breathing and coughing. Bowel and bladder elimination is promoted. Injuries and complications from bedrest are prevented.

Amyotrophic Lateral Sclerosis

- Amyotrophic lateral sclerosis (ALS) is a disease that attacks the nerve cells that control voluntary muscles. It is rapidly progressive and fatal. Most common in men, it usually strikes between 40 and 60 years of age. Most die 3 to 5 years after onset.
- Motor nerve cells in the brain, brainstem, and spinal cord are affected. These cells stop sending messages to the muscles. The muscles weaken, waste away (atrophy), and twitch. Over time, the brain cannot start voluntary movements or control them. The person cannot move the arms, legs, and body. Eventually respiratory muscles fail. The disease usually does not affect the mind. Sight, smell, taste, hearing, and touch are not affected. Usually bowel and bladder functions remain intact.
- ALS has no cure. Some drugs can slow the disease and improve symptoms. The person is kept active and independent to the extent possible. The care plan reflects the person's changing needs.

Spinal Cord Injury

- Spinal cord injuries can seriously damage the nervous system. Common causes are stab or gunshot wounds, motor vehicle crashes, falls, and sports injuries. Paralysis (loss of muscle function, sensation, or both) can result.
- The higher the level of injury, the more functions lost:
  - *Lumbar injuries*—sensory and muscle function in the legs is lost. The person has **paraplegia**—paralysis and loss of sensory function in legs and lower trunk.
  - *Thoracic injuries*—sensory and muscle function below the chest is lost. The person has paraplegia.
  - *Cervical injuries*—sensory and muscle function of the arms, legs, and trunk is lost. Paralysis in the arms, legs, and trunk is called **quadriplegia** or **tetraplegia.**
- Review Box 33-8, Paralysis—Care Measures, in the textbook.

CARDIOVASCULAR DISORDERS

Hypertension

- With *hypertension* (high blood pressure), the resting blood pressure is too high. The systolic pressure is 140 mm Hg or higher. Or the diastolic pressure is 90 mm Hg or higher. Such measurements must occur several times.
- Narrowed blood vessels are a common cause. Kidney disorders, head injuries, some pregnancy problems, and adrenal gland tumors are causes. Hypertension can lead to stroke, hardening of the arteries, heart attack, heart failure, kidney failure, and blindness.
- Life-style changes can lower blood pressure. Certain drugs lower blood pressure.

Coronary Artery Disease

- Coronary arteries supply the heart with blood. In coronary artery disease (CAD), the coronary arteries become hardened and narrow. The heart muscle gets less blood and oxygen. CAD also is called *coronary heart disease* and *heart disease*.
- The most common cause is atherosclerosis. Plaque—made up of cholesterol, fat, and other substances—collects on artery walls. The narrowed arteries block blood flow. Blood clots can form along the plaque and block blood flow.
- The major complications of CAD are angina, myocardial infarction (heart attack), irregular heartbeats, and sudden death.
- CAD can be treated. Treatment goals are to:
  - Relieve symptoms.
  - Slow or stop atherosclerosis.
  - Lower the risk of blood clots.
  - Widen or bypass clogged arteries.
  - Reduce cardiac events.
- CAD requires life-style changes. Drugs may be used to decrease the heart's workload, relieve symptoms, prevent a heart attack or sudden death, or delay the need for procedures that open or bypass diseased arteries.

Angina

- Angina is chest pain. It is from reduced blood flow and oxygen to part of the heart muscle. Chest pain is described as tightness, pressure, squeezing, or burning in the chest. Pain can occur in the shoulders, arms, neck, jaw, or back. The person may be pale, feel faint, and perspire. Dyspnea is common. Nausea, fatigue, and weakness may occur. Some persons complain of "gas" or indigestion.

- Rest often relieves symptoms in 3 to 15 minutes. Chest pain lasting longer than a few minutes and not relieved by rest and nitroglycerin may signal heart attack. The person needs emergency care.

Myocardial Infarction

- Myocardial infarction (MI) also is called *heart attack, acute myocardial infarction (AMI),* and *acute coronary syndrome (ACS).*
- Blood flow to the heart muscle is suddenly blocked. Part of the heart muscle dies. MI is an emergency. Sudden cardiac death *(sudden cardiac arrest)* can occur.
- Review Box 33-10, Myocardial Infarction—Signs and Symptoms, in the textbook.
- The person may need medical or surgical procedures to open or bypass the diseased artery. Cardiac rehabilitation is needed.

Heart Failure

- Heart failure or congestive heart failure (CHF) occurs when the heart is weakened and cannot pump normally. Blood backs up. Tissue congestion occurs.
- Drugs are given to strengthen the heart. They also reduce the amount of fluid in the body. A sodium-controlled diet is ordered. Oxygen is given. Semi-Fowler's position is preferred for breathing. I&O, daily weight, elastic stockings, and range-of-motion exercises are part of the care plan.

RESPIRATORY DISORDERS

Chronic Obstructive Pulmonary Disease

- Two disorders are grouped under chronic obstructive pulmonary disease (COPD). They are chronic bronchitis and emphysema. These disorders obstruct air flow. Lung function is gradually lost.
- *Chronic bronchitis.* Bronchitis means inflammation of the bronchi. Chronic bronchitis occurs after repeated episodes of bronchitis. Smoking is the major cause. Smoker's cough in the morning is often the first symptom of chronic bronchitis. Over time, the cough becomes more frequent. The person has difficulty breathing and tires easily. The person must stop smoking. Oxygen therapy and breathing exercises are often ordered. If a respiratory tract infection occurs, the person needs prompt treatment.
- *Emphysema.* In emphysema, the alveoli enlarge and become less elastic. They do not expand and shrink normally when breathing in and out. Trapped air is not exhaled. Smoking is the most common cause. The person has shortness of breath and a cough. Sputum may contain pus. Fatigue is common. The person works hard to breathe in and out. Breathing is easier when the

person sits upright and slightly forward. The person must stop smoking. Respiratory therapy, breathing exercises, oxygen, and drug therapy are ordered.

Asthma

- In asthma, the airway becomes inflamed and narrow. Extra mucus is produced. Dyspnea results. Wheezing and coughing are common. So are pain and tightening in the chest. Asthma usually is triggered by allergies. Other triggers include air pollutants and irritants, smoking and secondhand smoke, respiratory tract infections, exertion, and cold air. Asthma is treated with drugs. Severe attacks may require emergency care.

Influenza

- Influenza (flu) is a respiratory infection caused by viruses. Pneumonia is a common complication. Signs and symptoms include high fever for 3 to 4 days, headache, general aches and pains, fatigue and weakness, chest discomfort, cough, stuffy nose, sneezing, and sore throat. Treatment involves fluids and rest. Follow Standard Precautions. The flu vaccine is the best prevention.

Pneumonia

- Pneumonia is an inflammation and infection of lung tissue. Bacteria, viruses, and other microbes are causes.
- High fever, chills, painful cough, chest pain on breathing, and rapid pulse occur. Shortness of breath and rapid breathing also occur. Cyanosis may be present. Sputum is thick and white, green, yellow, or rust-colored. Other signs and symptoms are nausea, vomiting, headache, tiredness, and muscle aches.
- Drugs are ordered for infection and pain. Fluid intake is increased. Intravenous therapy (IV) and oxygen may be needed. Semi-Fowler's position eases breathing. Rest is important. Standard Precautions are followed. Transmission-Based Precautions are used depending on the cause.

Tuberculosis

- Tuberculosis (TB) is a bacterial infection in the lungs. TB is spread by airborne droplets with coughing, sneezing, speaking, singing, or laughing. Those who have close, frequent contact with an infected person are at risk. TB is more likely to occur in close, crowded areas. Age, poor nutrition, and HIV infection are other risk factors.
- Signs and symptoms are tiredness, loss of appetite, weight loss, fever, and night sweats. Cough and sputum production increase over time. Sputum may contain blood. Chest pain occurs.
- Drugs for TB are given. Standard Precautions and Transmission-Based Precautions are needed. The person must cover the mouth and nose with tissues when

sneezing, coughing, or producing sputum. Tissues are flushed down the toilet, placed in a BIOHAZARD bag, or placed in a paper bag and burned. Hand washing after contact with sputum is essential.

DIGESTIVE DISORDERS

Vomiting

- These measures are needed.
  - Follow Standard Precautions and the Bloodborne Pathogen Standard.
  - Turn the person's head well to one side. This prevents aspiration.
  - Place a kidney basin under the person's chin.
  - Move vomitus away from the person.
  - Provide oral hygiene.
  - Observe vomitus for color, odor, and undigested food. If it looks like coffee grounds, it contains undigested blood. This signals bleeding. Report your observations.
  - Measure, report, and record the amount of vomitus. Also record the amount on the I&O record.
  - Save a specimen for laboratory study.
  - Dispose of vomitus after the nurse observes it.
  - Eliminate odors.
  - Provide for comfort.

Diverticular Disease

- Small pouches can develop in the colon. The pouches bulge outward through weak spots in the colon. Each pouch is called a *diverticulum*. *Diverticulosis* is the condition of having these pouches. The pouches can become infected or inflamed—*diverticulitis*. Age, a low-fiber diet, and constipation are risk factors. Fever, nausea and vomiting, chills, and cramping are likely. Bloating, rectal bleeding, frequent urination, and pain while voiding can occur.

Hepatitis

- Hepatitis is an inflammation of the liver. It can be mild or cause death. Signs and symptoms are listed in Box 33-12, Hepatitis—Signs and Symptoms, in the textbook. Some people do not have symptoms.
- There are five major types of hepatitis virus: hepatitis A, spread by the fecal-oral route; hepatitis B, spread through contact with infected blood and body fluids; hepatitis C, spread by infected blood; hepatitis D and hepatitis E (uncommon in the United States), spread through contaminated food or water.
- Treatment involves rest, a healthy diet, fluids, and no alcohol.
- Protect yourself and others. Follow Standard Precautions and the Bloodborne Pathogen Standard. Isolation precautions are ordered as necessary. Assist the person with hygiene and hand washing as needed.

URINARY SYSTEM DISORDERS

Urinary Tract Infections (UTIs)

- UTIs are common. Catheterization, urological exams, intercourse, poor perineal hygiene, immobility, and poor fluid intake are common causes.

Kidney Stones

- Kidney stones (calculi) are hard deposits in the kidney. Bedrest, immobility, and poor fluid intake are risk factors.
- Stones vary in size from grains of sand to golf-ball size. The person needs to drink 2000 to 3000 mL a day to help stones pass from the body.

Kidney Failure

- In kidney failure (renal failure) the kidneys do not function or are severely impaired. Waste products are not removed from the blood. Fluid is retained. Heart failure and hypertension easily result.
- Acute kidney failure is sudden. Blood flow to the kidneys is severely decreased. Causes include severe injury or bleeding, heart attack, heart failure, burns, infection, and severe allergic reactions.
- With chronic kidney failure the kidneys cannot meet the body's needs. Hypertension and diabetes are common causes. Infections, urinary tract obstructions, and tumors are other causes.

Prostate Enlargement

- The prostate grows larger as a man grows older. This is called benign prostatic hyperplasia (BPH). The enlarged prostate presses against the urethra. This obstructs urine flow through the urethra. Bladder function is gradually lost. Most men in their 60s and older have some symptoms of BPH. Common problems are:
  - Weak urine stream
  - Frequent voiding of small amounts of urine
  - Urgency and leaking or dribbling of urine
  - Frequent voiding at night
  - Urinary retention

REPRODUCTIVE DISORDERS

Sexually Transmitted Diseases

- A sexually transmitted disease (STD) is spread by oral, vaginal, or anal sex. Some people do not have signs and symptoms or are not aware of an infection. Others know but do not seek treatment because of embarrassment. Standard Precautions and the Bloodborne Pathogen Standard are followed.

ENDOCRINE DISORDERS

Diabetes

- In this disorder the body cannot produce or use insulin properly. Insulin is needed for glucose to move from the blood into the cells. Sugar builds up in the blood. Cells do not have enough sugar for energy and cannot function. There are three types of diabetes.

- *Type 1 diabetes*. Occurs most often in children. The pancreas produces little or no insulin.
- *Type 2 diabetes*. This type is more common in older persons but is becoming more common in children, teens, and young adults. The pancreas secretes insulin but the body cannot use it well.
- *Gestational diabetes*. Develops during pregnancy.

- Diabetes must be controlled to prevent complications. Complications include blindness, renal failure, nerve damage, and damage to the gums and teeth. Heart and blood vessel diseases are very serious problems. They can lead to stroke, heart attack, and slow healing. Foot and leg wounds and ulcers are very serious.
- Good foot care is needed. Corns, blisters, calluses, and other foot problems can lead to an infection and amputation.
- Blood glucose is monitored daily or three or four times a day for:
  - *Hypoglycemia*—low sugar in the blood
  - *Hyperglycemia*—high sugar in the blood
- Review Table 33-1, Hypoglycemia and Hyperglycemia, in the textbook for the causes, signs, and symptoms of hypoglycemia and hyperglycemia. Both can lead to death if not corrected. You must call for the nurse at once.

IMMUNE SYSTEM DISORDERS

- The immune system protects the body from microbes, cancer cells, and other harmful substances. It defends against threats inside and outside the body.
- Autoimmune disorders can occur. The immune system attacks the body's own normal cells, tissues, or organs. Most are chronic. Common disorders include:
  - Graves' disease
  - Lupus
  - Multiple sclerosis
  - Rheumatoid arthritis
  - Type 1 diabetes

Acquired Immunodeficiency Syndrome

- Acquired immunodeficiency syndrome (AIDS) is caused by the human immunodeficiency virus (HIV). It destroys the body's ability to fight infections and certain cancers. The virus is spread through body fluids—blood, semen, vaginal secretions, and breast milk. HIV is not spread by saliva, tears, sweat, sneezing, coughing, insects, or casual contact.
- Persons with AIDS are at risk for pneumonia, tuberculosis, Kaposi's sarcoma (a cancer), and nervous system damage.

- To protect yourself and others from the virus, follow Standard Precautions and the Bloodborne Pathogen Standard.
- Review Box 33-16, Caring for the Person with AIDS, in the textbook for care procedures.
- Older persons also get AIDS. They get and spread HIV through sexual contact and IV drug use. Aging and some diseases can mask the signs and symptoms of AIDS. Older persons are less likely to be tested for HIV/AIDS.

SKIN DISORDERS

- There are many types of skin disorders, such as alopecia, hirsutism, dandruff, lice, scabies, skin tears, pressure ulcers, and burns. Shingles is caused by the same virus that causes chicken pox. The person has a rash with fluid-filled blisters on one side of the body. Burning or tingling pain, numbness, and itching can occur. Persons with weakened immune systems, cancer treatments, transplant surgeries, and stress and who have had chicken pox are at risk. The doctor orders anti-viral drugs and drugs for pain relief. Lesions are infectious until they crust over. A vaccine is available to prevent shingles.

CHAPTER 33 REVIEW QUESTIONS

Circle the BEST answer.

1. A person with cancer may need all the following *except*
   a. Pain relief or control
   b. Avoidance by you
   c. Fluids and nutrition
   d. Psychological support
2. The person had a stroke. Care includes all the following except
   a. Place the call light on the person's strong side
   b. Reposition the person every 2 hours
   c. Perform ROM exercises as ordered
   d. Place objects on the affected side
3. The person with hemiplegia
   a. Is paralyzed on one side of the body
   b. Has both arms paralyzed
   c. Has both legs paralyzed
   d. Has all extremities paralyzed
4. The person with multiple sclerosis should be kept active as long as possible.
   a. True
   b. False
5. The person has paralysis in the legs and lower trunk. This is called
   a. Quadriplegia
   b. Paraplegia
   c. Hemiplegia
   d. Tetraplegia
6. Fever is a common symptom of osteoarthritis.
   a. True
   b. False

7. Which statement about angina is *false?*
   a. Angina is chest pain.
   b. The person may be pale and perspire.
   c. Rest often relieves the symptoms.
   d. You do not report angina to the nurse.
8. A person has heart failure. You do all the following *except*
   a. Measure intake and output
   b. Measure weight daily
   c. Promote a diet that is high in salt
   d. Restrict fluids as ordered
9. Which position is usually best for the person with pneumonia?
   a. Semi-Fowler's
   b. Prone
   c. Supine
   d. Trendelenburg's
10. A bacterial infection in the lungs is
    a. Asthma
    b. Bronchitis
    c. Tuberculosis
    d. Emphysema
11. Which statement is *false?*
    a. Older persons are at high risk for urinary tract infections.
    b. Skin irritation and infection can occur if urine leaks onto the skin
    c. Benign prostatic hypertrophy may cause urinary problems in women.
    d. Some people may not be aware of having a sexually transmitted disease.
12. An STD is spread by oral, vaginal, or anal sex.
    a. True
    b. False
13. A person with an STD always has signs and symptoms.
    a. True
    b. False
14. A person is vomiting. You should do all the following *except*
    a. Follow Standard Precautions and the Bloodborne Pathogen Standard
    b. Keep the person supine
    c. Provide oral hygiene
    d. Observe vomitus for color, odor, and undigested food
15. A person with diabetes is trembling and sweating and feels faint. You
    a. Tell the nurse immediately
    b. Tell the nurse at the end of the shift
    c. Tell another nursing assistant
    d. Ignore the symptoms
16. All of the following are signs and symptoms of hepatitis *except*
    a. Itching
    b. Diarrhea
    c. Skin rash
    d. Increased appetite

17. Which statement about HIV is *false?*
    a. HIV is spread through body fluids.
    b. Standard Precautions and the Bloodborne Pathogen Standard are followed.
    c. Older persons cannot get and spread HIV.
    d. Older persons are less likely to be tested for HIV/AIDS.
18. The immune system defends against threats inside and outside the body.
    a. True
    b. False

Answers to Chapter 33 questions are on p. 451.

CHAPTER 34 MENTAL HEALTH DISORDERS

- The whole person has physical, social, psychological, and spiritual parts. Each part affects the other.
- *Mental* relates to the mind.
- **Mental health** means the person copes with and adjusts to everyday stresses in ways accepted by society.
- Stress is the response or change in the body caused by any emotional, physical, social, or economic factor.
- **Mental health disorder** is a disturbance in the ability to cope with or adjust to stress. Behavior and function are impaired. Mental illness and psychiatric disorder also mean mental health disorder. Causes of mental health disorders include:
  - Not being able to cope or adjust to stress
  - Chemical imbalances
  - Genetics
  - Physical, biological, or psychological factors
  - Drug or substance abuse
  - Social and cultural factors

ANXIETY DISORDERS

- **Anxiety** is a vague, uneasy feeling in response to stress. The person may not know why or the cause. The person senses danger or harm—real or imagined. Some anxiety is normal. Review Box 34-1, Anxiety—Signs and Symptoms, in the textbook.
- Coping and defense mechanisms are used to relieve anxiety. Defense mechanisms are unconscious reactions that block unpleasant or threatening feelings. In mental health disorders, they are used poorly. Review Box 34-2, Defense Mechanisms, in the textbook.
- Some common anxiety disorders include panic disorder, phobias, obsessive-compulsive disorder, post-traumatic stress disorder, and generalized anxiety disorder. Generalized anxiety disorder is when the person has at least 6 months of extreme anxiety. Worry can prevent the person from normal function.
  - *Panic disorder.* **Panic** is an intense and sudden feeling of fear, anxiety, terror, or dread. Onset is

sudden with no obvious reason. The person cannot function. Signs and symptoms of anxiety are severe.

- *Phobias.* **Phobia** means an intense fear. The person has an intense fear of an object, situation, or activity that has little or no actual danger. The person avoids what is feared. When faced with the fear, the person has high anxiety and cannot function.
- *Obsessive-compulsive disorder (OCD).* An **obsession** is a recurrent, unwanted thought, idea, or image. **Compulsion** is repeating an act over and over again. The act may not make sense but the person has much anxiety if the act is not done.
- *Post-traumatic stress disorder (PTSD).* PTSD occurs after a terrifying event. The event involved physical harm or the threat of physical harm. Review Box 34-3, Post-Traumatic Stress Disorder—Signs and Symptoms, in the textbook. Flashbacks are common. A **flashback** is reliving the trauma in thoughts during the day and in nightmares during sleep. The person may believe that the trauma is happening all over again. Signs and symptoms usually develop about 3 months after the harmful event. Or they may emerge years later. PTSD can develop at any age.

SCHIZOPHRENIA

- *Schizophrenia* means split mind. It is a severe, chronic, disabling brain disorder that involves:
  - **Psychosis**—a state of severe mental impairment. The person does not view the real or unreal correctly.
  - **Delusion**—a false belief.
  - **Hallucination**—seeing, hearing, smelling, or feeling something that is not real.
  - **Paranoia**—a disorder of the mind. The person has false beliefs (delusions). He or she is suspicious about a person or situation.
  - **Delusion of grandeur**—an exaggerated belief about one's importance, wealth, power, or talents.
  - **Delusion of persecution**—the false belief that one is being mistreated, abused, or harassed.
- The person with schizophrenia has problems relating to others. He or she may be paranoid. Paranoia is a disorder of the mind. The person has false beliefs (delusions) and suspicion about a person or situation. The person may have difficulty organizing thoughts. Responses are inappropriate. Communication is disturbed. The person may withdraw. Some people regress to an earlier time or condition. Some persons with schizophrenia attempt suicide.

MOOD DISORDERS

- Mood disorders involve feelings, emotions, and moods.

Bipolar Disorder

- Bipolar means two poles or ends.
- The person with bipolar disorder has severe extremes in mood, energy, and ability to function. There are emotional lows (depression) and emotional highs (mania). This disorder is also called manic-depressive illness. This disorder must be managed throughout life. Review Box 34-4, Bipolar Disorder—Signs and Symptoms, in the textbook. Bipolar disorder can damage relationships and affect school or work performance. Some people are suicidal.

Depression

- Depression involves the body, mood, and thoughts. Symptoms affect work, study, sleep, eating, and other activities. The person is very sad.
- Depression is common in older persons. They have many losses—death of family and friends, loss of health, loss of body functions, loss of independence. Some medical conditions and drug side effects can cause symptoms of depression. Review Box 34-5, Depression in Older Persons—Warning Signs, in the textbook. Depression in older persons is often overlooked or a wrong diagnosis is made.

PERSONALITY DISORDERS

- Personality disorders involve rigid and maladaptive behaviors. Because of behavior, persons with personality disorders cannot function well in society.
- The person with *antisocial personality disorder* has a long-term pattern of thinking and behaviors that violates the rights of others. He or she has no regard for right and wrong.
- The person with *borderline personality disorder* (BPD) has unstable moods, behaviors, and relationships often involving extreme reactions; unstable self-image; impulsive, dangerous, and suicidal behaviors; intense anger or anger control problems; paranoid thoughts; and feelings of emptiness or boredom.

SUBSTANCE ABUSE AND ADDICTION

- Substance abuse or addiction occurs when a person over-uses or depends on alcohol or drugs. Physical and mental health are affected. So is the welfare of others. The substances involved affect the nervous system either by depressing or stimulating it.

Alcoholism

- Alcohol affects alertness, judgment, coordination, and reaction time. Over time, heavy drinking damages the brain, central nervous system, liver, heart, kidneys, and stomach. It causes changes in the heart and blood vessels. It also can cause forgetfulness and confusion.

Alcoholism is a chronic disease. There is no cure. However, alcoholism can be treated. Counseling and drugs are used to help the person stop drinking. The person must avoid all alcohol to avoid a relapse.
- Alcohol effects vary with age. Even small amounts can make older persons feel "high." Older persons are at risk for falls, vehicle crashes, and other injuries from drinking. Mixing alcohol with some drugs can be harmful or fatal. Alcohol also makes some health problems worse.

SUICIDE

- **Suicide** means to kill oneself.
- Suicide is most often linked to depression, alcohol or substance abuse, or stressful events. Review Box 34-7, Suicide Risk Factors, in the textbook.
- If a person mentions or talks about suicide, take the person seriously. Call for the nurse at once. Do not leave the person alone.
- Suicide contagion is exposure to suicidal behaviors within one's family, one's peer group, or media reports of suicide.

CARE AND TREATMENT

- Treatment of mental health disorders involves having the person explore his or her thoughts and feelings. This is done through psychotherapy and behavior, group, occupational, art, and family therapies. Often drugs are ordered.
- The care plan reflects the person's needs. The physical, safety and security, and emotional needs of the person must be met.
- Communication is important. Be alert to nonverbal communication.

CHAPTER 34 REVIEW QUESTIONS

Circle the BEST answer.

1. A person may not know why anxiety occurs.
   a. True
   b. False
2. Panic is an intense and sudden feeling of fear, anxiety, terror, or dread.
   a. True
   b. False
3. A person with an obsessive-compulsive disorder has a ritual that is repeated over and over again.
   a. True
   b. False
4. A person talks about suicide. You must do the following *except*
   a. Call the nurse at once
   b. Stay with the person
   c. Leave the person alone
   d. Take the person seriously

5. Which statement is *false*?
   a. Communication is important when caring for a person with a mental health disorder.
   b. You should be alert to nonverbal communication when caring for a person with a mental health disorder.
   c. The care plan reflects the needs of the person.
   d. The focus is only on the person's emotional needs.

Answers to Chapter 34 questions are on p. 451.

CHAPTER 35 CONFUSION AND DEMENTIA

- Changes in the brain and nervous system occur with aging. Review Box 35-1, Nervous System Changes From Aging, in the textbook.
- Changes in the brain can affect **cognitive function**—memory, thinking, reasoning, ability to understand, judgment, and behavior.

CONFUSION

- Confusion is a mental state of being disoriented to person, time, place, situation, or identity.
- Confusion has many causes. Diseases, infections, hearing and vision loss, brain injury, and drug side effects are some causes. Reduced blood flow to the brain affects memory, daily activities, and behaviors. Acute confusion (delirium) may occur. Delirium is a state of sudden severe confusion and rapid changes in brain function.
- When caring for the confused person:
  - Follow the person's care plan.
  - Provide for safety.
  - Face the person and speak clearly.
  - Call the person by name every time you are in contact with him or her.
  - State your name. Show your name tag.
  - Give the date and time each morning. Repeat as needed during the day and evening.
  - Explain what you are going to do and why.
  - Give clear, simple directions and answers to questions.
  - Ask clear, simple questions. Give the person time to respond.
  - Keep calendars and clocks with large numbers in the person's room. Remind the person of holidays, birthdays, and other events.
  - Have the person wear eyeglasses and hearing aids as needed.
  - Use touch to communicate.
  - Place familiar objects and pictures within the person's view.
  - Provide newspapers, magazines, TV, and radio. Read to the person if appropriate.
  - Discuss current events with the person.
  - Maintain the day-night cycle.
  - Provide a calm, relaxed, and peaceful setting.

- Follow the person's routine.
- Break tasks into small steps when helping the person.
- Do not rearrange furniture or the person's belongings.
- Encourage the person to take part in self-care.
- Be consistent.

DEMENTIA

- **Dementia** is the loss of cognitive function that interferes with routine personal, social, and occupational activities.
- Dementia is not a normal part of aging. Most older people do not have dementia. Pseudodementia means false dementia. There are signs and symptoms of dementia but no changes in the brain.
- Some early warning signs include problems with language, dressing, cooking, personality changes, poor or decreased judgment, and driving, as well as getting lost in familiar places and misplacing items.
- Permanent dementias result from changes in the brain.
- Alzheimer's disease is the most common type of permanent dementia.

ALZHEIMER'S DISEASE

- Alzheimer's disease (AD) is a brain disease. Memory, thinking, reasoning, judgment, language, behavior, mood, and personality are affected.

Signs of AD
- The classic sign of AD is gradual loss of short-term memory. Warning signs include:
  - Asking the same questions over and over again.
  - Repeating the same story—word for word, again and again.
  - The person forgets activities that were once done regularly with ease.
  - Losing the ability to pay bills or balance a checkbook.
  - Getting lost in familiar places. Or misplacing household objects.
  - Neglecting to bathe or wearing the same clothes over and over again. Meanwhile, the person insists that a bath was taken or that clothes were changed.
  - Relying on someone else to make decisions or answer questions that he or she would have handled.
- Review Box 35-5, Alzheimer's Disease—Signs, in the textbook for other signs of AD.

Behaviors
- The following behaviors are common with AD.
  - *Wandering*. Persons with AD are not oriented to person, place, and time. They may wander away from home and not find their way back. Leaving an agency without staff knowledge is called elopement. The person cannot tell what is safe or dangerous.
  - *Sundowning*. With sundowning, signs, symptoms, and behaviors of AD increase during hours of darkness. As daylight ends, confusion, restlessness, anxiety, agitation, and other symptoms increase. It may continue throughout the night.
  - *Hallucinations*. The person with AD may see, hear, smell, or feel things that are not real.
  - *Delusions*. People with AD may think they are some other person. A person may believe that the caregiver is someone else.
  - *Catastrophic reactions*. The person reacts as if there is a disaster or tragedy. The person may scream, cry, or be agitated or combative.
  - *Agitation and restlessness*. The person may pace, hit, or yell. The person may be unable to sleep.
  - *Aggression and combativeness*. These behaviors include hitting, pinching, grabbing, biting, or swearing.
  - *Screaming*. Persons with AD may scream to communicate.
  - *Abnormal sexual behaviors*. Sexual behaviors may involve the wrong person, the wrong time, and the wrong place. Persons with AD cannot control behavior.
  - *Repetitive behaviors*. Persons with AD repeat the same motions, words, or questions over and over again.
  - *Rummaging and hiding things*. The person may search for things by moving things around, turning things over, or looking through something such as a drawer or closet. The person my hide things, throw things away, or lose something.

CARE OF PERSONS WITH AD AND OTHER DEMENTIAS

- People with AD do not choose to be forgetful, incontinent, agitated, or rude. Nor do they choose to have other behaviors, signs, and symptoms of the disease. The disease causes the behaviors.
- Safety, hygiene, nutrition and fluids, elimination, and activity needs must be met. So must comfort and sleep needs. Review Box 35-9, Care of Persons with AD and Other Dementias, in the textbook.
- The person can have other health problems and injuries. However, the person may not be aware of pain, fever, constipation, incontinence, or other signs and symptoms. Carefully observe the person. Report any change in the person's usual behavior to the nurse.
- Infection is a risk. Provide good skin care, oral hygiene, and perineal care after bowel and bladder elimination.
- Supervised activities meet the person's needs and cognitive abilities.

- Impaired communication is a common problem. Avoid giving orders, wanting the truth, and correcting the person's errors. Review Box 35-8, Communication—Persons with AD or Other Dementias, in the textbook.
- Always look for dangers in the person's room and in the hallways, lounges, dining areas, and other areas on the nursing unit. Remove the danger if you can.
- Every staff member must be alert to persons who wander. Such persons are allowed to wander in safe areas.

The Family
- The family may have physical, emotional, social, and financial stresses. The family often feels hopeless. No matter what is done, the person only gets worse. Anger and resentment may result. Guilt feelings are common.
- The family is an important part of the health team. They may help plan the person's care. For many persons, family members provide comfort. The family also needs support and understanding from the health team.

CHAPTER 35 REVIEW QUESTIONS

Circle the BEST answer.

1. Cognitive function involves all of the following *except*
   a. Memory and thinking
   b. Reasoning and understanding
   c. Personality and mood
   d. Judgment and behavior
2. When caring for a confused person, you do the following *except*
   a. Provide for safety
   b. Maintain the day-night schedule
   c. Keep calendars and clocks in the person's room
   d. Ask difficult-to-understand questions and give complex directions
3. Which statement about dementia is *false?*
   a. Dementia is a normal part of aging.
   b. The person may have changes in personality.
   c. Alzheimer's disease is the most common type of dementia.
   d. The person may have changes in behavior.
4. When caring for persons with AD, you do the following *except*
   a. Provide good skin care
   b. Talk to them in a calm voice
   c. Observe them closely for unusual behavior
   d. Allow personal choice in wandering

Answers to Chapter 35 questions are on p. 451.

CHAPTER 36 EMERGENCY CARE
EMERGENCY CARE

- First aid is the emergency care given to an ill or injured person before medical help arrives.

- Rules for emergency care include:
  - Know your limits. Do not do more than you are able.
  - Stay calm.
  - Know where to find emergency supplies.
  - Follow Standard Precautions and the Bloodborne Pathogen Standard to the extent possible.
  - Check for life-threatening problems. Check for breathing, a pulse, and bleeding.
  - Keep the person lying down or as you found him or her.
  - Move the person only if the setting is unsafe. If the scene is not safe enough for you to approach, wait for help to arrive.
  - Perform necessary emergency measures.
  - Call for help or have someone activate the Emergency Medical Services (EMS) system.
  - Do not remove clothes unless necessary.
  - Keep the person warm. Cover the person with a blanket, coat, or sweater.
  - Reassure the person. Explain what is happening and that help was called.
  - Do not give the person fluids.
  - Keep onlookers away. They invade privacy.
- Review Box 36-1, Emergency Care Rules, in the textbook for more information.

BASIC LIFE SUPPORT FOR ADULTS
- Sudden cardiac arrest (SCA) or cardiac arrest is when the heart stops suddenly and without warning. There are three major signs of SCA:
  - No response
  - No breathing or no normal breathing
  - No pulse
- Cardiopulmonary resuscitation (CPR) must be started at once when a person has SCA.
- CPR supports breathing and circulation. It provides blood and oxygen to the heart, brain, and other organs until advanced emergency care is given. CPR is done if the person does not respond, is not breathing, and has no pulse.

CPR INVOLVES:
- *Chest compressions*—the heart, brain, and other organs must receive blood. Chest compressions force blood through the circulatory system.
- *Airway*—the airway must be open and clear of obstructions. The head tilt–chin lift method opens the airway.
- *Breathing*—the person must get oxygen. Air is not inhaled when breathing stops. The person is given breaths. A rescuer inflates the person's lungs.
- *Defibrillation*—ventricular fibrillation (VF, V-fib) is an abnormal heart rhythm. Rather than beating in a regular rhythm, the heart shakes and quivers.

The heart does not pump blood. The heart, brain, and other organs do not receive blood and oxygen. A *defibrillator* is used to deliver a shock to the heart. This allows the return of a regular heart rhythm. Defibrillation as soon as possible after the onset of VF (V-fib) increases the person's chance of survival.

- *Hemorrhage.* Hemorrhage is the excessive loss of blood in a short time. If bleeding is not stopped, the person will die. Hemorrhage is internal or external. You cannot see internal hemorrhage. Pain, shock, vomiting blood, coughing up blood, and loss of consciousness signal internal hemorrhage. Keep the person warm, flat, and quiet until help arrives and do not give fluids. External bleeding is usually seen. To control bleeding:
  - Follow the rules in Box 36-1, Emergency Care Rules, in the textbook.
  - Do not remove any objects that have pierced or stabbed the person.
  - Place a sterile dressing directly over the wound. Or use any clean material.
  - Apply firm pressure directly over the bleeding site. Do not release pressure until the bleeding stops.
  - Do not remove the dressing or material.
  - Bind the wound when bleeding stops.

FAINTING

- **Fainting** is the sudden loss of consciousness from an inadequate blood supply to the brain. Common causes are hunger, fatigue, fear, pain, standing in one position for a long time, and being in a warm, crowded room.
- Warning signals are dizziness, perspiration, and blackness before the eyes. The person looks pale. The pulse is weak. Respirations are shallow if consciousness is lost. Emergency care includes:
  - Have the person sit or lie down before fainting occurs.
  - If sitting, the person bends forward and places the head between the knees.
  - If the person is lying down, raise the legs.
  - Loosen tight clothing.
  - Keep the person lying down if fainting has occurred. Raise the legs.
  - Do not let the person get up until symptoms have subsided for about 5 minutes.
  - Help the person to a sitting position after recovery from fainting.
- *Shock.* Shock results when organs and tissues do not get enough blood. Blood loss, heart attack, burns, and severe infection are causes. Signs and symptoms include low or falling blood pressure; rapid and weak pulse; rapid respirations; cold, moist, and pale skin; thirst; restlessness; confusion; and loss of consciousness as shock worsens. Keep the person lying down. If the person does not have injuries

from trauma, raise the feet 6 to 12 inches. Maintain an open airway and control bleeding. Begin CPR if cardiac arrest occurs.
- *Stroke.* Stroke (cerebrovascular accident) occurs when the brain is suddenly deprived of its blood supply. A stroke may be caused by a thrombus, an embolus, or hemorrhage if a blood vessel in the brain ruptures. Signs of stroke vary. Loss of consciousness or semi-consciousness, rapid pulse, labored respirations, high blood pressure, facial drooping, and hemiplegia (paralysis on one side of the body) are signs of a stroke. Confusion, numbness, slurred speech, aphasia, loss of vision, sudden and severe headache, dizziness, unsteadiness, and falling are also signs and symptoms. For emergency care, follow the rules in Box 36-1 in the textbook.

SEIZURES

- Seizures (convulsions) are violent and sudden contractions or tremors of muscle groups. Movements are uncontrolled. The person may lose consciousness. The major types of seizures are:
  - Partial seizure
  - Generalized tonic-clonic seizure (grand mal seizure)
  - Generalized absence (petit mal) seizure
- Causes include brain abnormality, head injury, high fever, brain tumors, poisoning, nervous system disorders or infections, or lack of blood flow to the brain.
- You cannot stop a seizure. However, you can protect the person from injury.
  - Follow the rules in Box 36-1 in the textbook.
  - Do not leave the person alone.
  - Lower the person to the floor.
  - Note the time the seizure started.
  - Place something soft under the person's head.
  - Loosen tight jewelry and clothing around the person's neck.
  - Turn the person onto his or her side. Make sure the head is turned to the side.
  - Do not put any object or your fingers between the person's teeth.
  - Do not try to stop the seizure or control the person's movements.
  - Move furniture, equipment, and sharp objects away from the person.
  - Note the time when the seizure ends.
  - Make sure the mouth is clear of food, fluids, and saliva after the seizure.
  - Provide basic life support if the person is not breathing after the seizure.

BURNS

- Burns can severely disable a person. They can also cause death. Some common causes of burns include:
  - Scalds from hot liquids

- Electrical injuries
- Falling asleep while smoking
- Sunburn
- Chemicals
- For emergency care of burns, follow the rules in Box 36-1 in the textbook. Remove the person from the fire or burn source. Apply cold or cool water until pain is relieved. Do not apply ice directly to the burn. Do not remove burned clothing. Cover burns with sterile, cool, moist coverings. Do not put oil, butter, salve, or ointments on the burns. Keep blisters intact. Cover the person with a blanket or coat to prevent heat loss.

CHAPTER 36 REVIEW QUESTIONS

Circle the BEST answer.

1. During an emergency, you do all of the following *except*
   a. Perform only procedures you have been trained to do
   b. Keep the person lying down or as you found him or her
   c. Let the person become cold
   d. Reassure the person and explain what is happening
2. During an emergency, you keep onlookers away.
   a. True
   b. False
3. During a seizure, you do the following *except*
   a. Turn the person's body to the side
   b. Place your fingers in the person's mouth
   c. Note the time the seizure started and ended
   d. Turn the person's head to the side
4. Which statement about fainting is *false*?
   a. If standing, have the person sit down before fainting occurs.
   b. If sitting, have the person bend forward and place his head between his knees before fainting occurs.
   c. Tighten the person's clothing.
   d. Raise the legs if the person is lying down.

Answers to Chapter 36 questions are on p. 451.

CHAPTER 37 END-OF-LIFE CARE

- End-of-life care describes the support and care given during the time surrounding death.
- An illness or injury from which the person will not likely recover is a terminal illness. Terminally ill persons can choose palliative care or hospice care.
- Palliative care involves relieving or reducing the intensity of uncomfortable symptoms without producing a cure. Hospice care focuses on the physical, emotional, social, and spiritual needs of dying persons and their families. Pain relief and comfort are stressed.

ATTITUDES ABOUT DEATH

- Attitudes about death often change as a person grows older and with changing circumstances.

Cultural and Spiritual Needs

- Practices and attitudes about death differ among cultures.
- Attitudes about death are closely related to religion. Many religions practice rites and rituals during the dying process and at the time of death. Reincarnation is the belief that the spirit or soul is reborn in another human body or in another form of life.

Age

- Adults fear pain and suffering, dying alone, and the invasion of privacy. They also fear loneliness and separation from loved ones. Adults often resent death because it affects plans, hopes, dreams, and ambitions.
- Older persons usually have fewer fears than younger adults. Some welcome death as freedom from pain, suffering, and disability. Death also means reunion with those who have died. Like younger adults, they often fear dying alone.

THE STAGES OF DYING

- Dr. Kübler-Ross described five stages of dying. They are also called the "stages of grief." They are:
  - *Stage 1: Denial.* The person refuses to believe he or she is going to die.
  - *Stage 2: Anger.* There is anger and rage, often at family, friends, and the health team.
  - *Stage 3: Bargaining.* Often the person bargains with God or a higher power for more time.
  - *Stage 4: Depression.* The person is sad and mourns things that were lost and the future loss of life.
  - *Stage 5: Acceptance.* The person is calm and at peace. The person accepts death. This stage may last for many months or years. Reaching the acceptance stage does not mean death is near.
- Dying persons do not always pass through all five stages. A person may never get beyond a certain stage. Some move back and forth between stages.

COMFORT NEEDS

- Comfort is a basic part of end-of-life care. It involves physical, mental and emotional, and spiritual needs. Comfort goals are to:
  - Prevent or relieve suffering to the extent possible
  - Respect and follow end-of-life wishes
- Dying persons may want to talk about their fears, worries, and anxieties. You need to listen and use touch.
  - *Listening.* Let the person express feelings and emotions in his or her own way. Do not worry about saying the wrong thing or finding the right words. You do not need to say anything.
  - *Touch.* Touch shows caring and concern. Sometimes the person does not want to talk but needs you nearby. Silence, along with touch, is a meaningful way to communicate.

- Some people may want to see a spiritual leader. Or they may want to take part in religious practices.

Physical Needs
- Dying may take a few minutes, hours, days, or weeks.
- As the person weakens, basic needs are met. The person may depend on others for basic needs and activities of daily living. Every effort is made to promote physical and psychological comfort. The person is allowed to die in peace and with dignity.

PAIN

- Some dying persons do not have pain. Others may have severe pain. Always report signs and symptoms of pain at once. Pain management is important. The nurse can give pain-relief drugs. Preventing and controlling pain is easier than relieving pain. Skin care, personal and oral hygiene, back massages, frequent position changes, good alignment, and supportive devices promote comfort.

BREATHING PROBLEMS

- Shortness of breath and difficulty breathing (dyspnea) are common end-of-life problems. Semi-Fowler's position and oxygen are helpful.
- Noisy breathing (death rattle) is common as death nears. This is due to mucus collecting in the airway. The side-lying position, suctioning by the nurse, and drugs to reduce the amount of mucus may help.

VISION, HEARING, AND SPEECH

- Vision blurs and gradually fails. Explain what you are doing to the person or in the room. Provide good eye care.
- Hearing is one of the last functions lost. Always assume that the person can hear. Speak in a normal voice. Offer words of comfort.
- Speech becomes harder. Anticipate the person's needs. Do not ask questions that need long answers. Despite speech problems, you must talk to the person.

MOUTH, NOSE, AND SKIN

- Frequent oral hygiene is given as death nears. Oral hygiene is needed if mucus collects in the mouth and the person cannot swallow.
- Crusting and irritation of the nostrils can occur. Carefully clean the nose.
- Circulation fails and body temperature rises as death nears. Sweating increases.

- Skin care, bathing, and preventing pressure ulcers are necessary. Change linens and gowns whenever needed. Observe for signs of cold and prevent drafts.

NUTRITION

- Nausea, vomiting, and loss of appetite are common at the end of life. The doctor can order drugs for nausea and vomiting.
- Some persons are too tired or too weak to eat. You may need to feed them.
- As death nears, loss of appetite is common. The person may choose not to eat or drink. Do not force the person to eat or drink. Report refusal to eat or drink to the nurse.

ELIMINATION

- Urinary and fecal incontinence may occur. Give perineal care as needed. Constipation and urinary retention are common.

THE PERSON'S ROOM

- The person's room should be comfortable and pleasant. It should be well lit and well ventilated. Remove unnecessary equipment.
- Mementos, pictures, cards, flowers, and religious items provide comfort. The person and family arrange the room as they wish.

THE FAMILY

- This is a hard time for family. The family goes through stages like the dying person. Be available, courteous, and considerate.
- The person and family need time together. However, you cannot neglect care because the family is present. Most agencies let family members help give care.

LEGAL ISSUES

- *Advance directives.* An advance directive is a document stating a person's wishes about health care when that person cannot make his or her own decisions. The following are examples:
  - *Living wills.* A living will is a document about measures that support or maintain life when death is likely. A living will may instruct doctors not to start measures that prolong dying or to remove measures that prolong dying.
  - *Durable power of attorney for health care.* This gives the power to make health care decisions to

another person. When a person cannot make health care decisions, the person with durable power of attorney can do so. That person is often called a health care proxy.

- *"Do Not Resuscitate" (DNR) order*. This means the person will not be resuscitated. The person is allowed to die with peace and dignity. The doctor writes the DNR order after consulting with the person and family.
- You may not agree with care and resuscitation decisions. However, you must follow the person's or family's wishes and the doctor's orders. These may be against your personal, religious, and cultural values. If so, discuss the matter with the nurse. An assignment change may be needed.

SIGNS OF DEATH

- There are signs that death is near.
  - Movement, muscle tone, and sensation are lost.
  - Abdominal distention, fecal incontinence, nausea, and vomiting are common.
  - Body temperature rises. The person feels cool, looks pale, and perspires heavily.
  - The pulse is fast or slow, weak, and irregular. Blood pressure starts to fall.
  - Slow or rapid and shallow respirations are observed. Mucus collects in the airway. This causes the death rattle that is heard.
  - Pain decreases as the person loses consciousness. Some people are conscious until the moment of death.
  - The signs of death include no pulse, no respirations, and no blood pressure. The pupils are dilated and fixed.

CARE OF THE BODY AFTER DEATH

- Care of the body after death is called post-mortem care.
- Post-mortem care is done to maintain a good appearance of the body. Within 2 to 4 hours after death, rigor mortis develops. Rigor mortis is the stiffness or rigidity of skeletal muscles that occurs after death. The body is positioned in normal alignment before rigor mortis sets in.
- Moving the body when giving post-mortem care can cause remaining air in the lungs, stomach, and intestines to be expelled. When air is expelled, sounds are produced.
- When giving post-mortem care, follow Standard Precautions and the Bloodborne Pathogen Standard.
- Review Delegation Guidelines: Care of the Body After Death, Promoting Safety and Comfort: Care of

the Body After Death, and procedure: Assisting With Post-Mortem Care in the textbook.

CHAPTER 37 REVIEW QUESTIONS

Circle the BEST answer.

1. Which statement is *false*?
   a. Adults fear dying alone.
   b. Older persons usually have fewer fears about dying than younger adults.
   c. Adults often resent death.
   d. All adults welcome death.
2. Persons in the denial stage of dying
   a. Are angry
   b. Bargain with God
   c. Refuse to believe that they are dying
   d. Are calm and at peace
3. When caring for a person who is dying, you should do the following *except*
   a. Listen to the person
   b. Talk about your feelings about death
   c. Provide privacy during spiritual moments
   d. Use touch to show care and concern
4. When caring for a dying person, you provide all of the following *except*
   a. Eye care
   b. Oral hygiene
   c. Good skin care
   d. Physical exercise
5. When giving postmortem care, you should wear gloves.
   a. True
   b. False

Answers to Chapter 37 questions are on p. 451.

CHAPTER 38 GETTING A JOB
GETTING A JOB

- Find out about jobs and places to apply for work through newspapers, employment agencies, nursing agencies, yellow pages, people you know, the Internet, school placement counselors, and your clinical experience site.
- Employers look for dependable, skilled applicants with values and attitudes that fit the agency.
- The employer checks the nursing assistant registry and requests proof that you completed a nursing assistant training and competency evaluation program.
- You get a job application from human resources or on-line.
- You attend an interview at which the employer evaluates you and you learn about the agency. You must be on time, well groomed, polite, and professional and give complete and honest answers to questions.
- Share your skills list.

CHAPTER 38 REVIEW QUESTIONS

Circle the BEST answer.
1. Agencies want staff who are dependable, well-groomed, and have needed job skills.
   a. True
   b. False
2. Which of the following interview question is not allowed by the EEOC?
   a. Why do you want to work here?
   b. What did you like least about your last job?
   c. Why should I hire you?
   d. How many sick days did you use last year?

3. After the interview it is advisable to send a thank-you note within
   a. 2 days
   b. 1 day
   c. 1 week
   d. 2 weeks

Answers to Chapter 38 questions are on p. 451.

This test contains 75 questions. For each question, circle the BEST answer.

1. A nurse asks you to give a person his drug when he is done in the bathroom. Your response to the nurse is
   A. "I will give the drug for you."
   B. "I will ask the other nursing assistant to give the drug."
   C. "I am sorry, but I cannot give that drug. I will let you know when he is out of the bathroom."
   D. "I refuse to give that drug."

2. An ethical person
   A. Does not judge others
   B. Avoids persons whose standards and values are different from his or hers
   C. Is prejudiced and biased
   D. Causes harm to another person

3. You smell alcohol on the breath of a co-worker. You
   A. Ignore the situation
   B. Tell the co-worker to get counseling
   C. Take a break and drink some alcohol, too
   D. Tell the nurse at once

4. A person's call light goes unanswered. He gets out of bed and falls. His leg is broken. This is
   A. Neglect
   B. Emotional abuse
   C. Physical abuse
   D. Malpractice

5. Your mom asks you about a person on your unit. How should you respond?
   A. "She is walking better now that she is receiving physical therapy."
   B. "I'm sorry, but I cannot talk about her. It is unprofessional and violates her privacy and confidentiality."
   C. "Don't tell anyone I told you, but she is getting worse."
   D. "She has been very sad recently and needs visitors."

6. You are going off duty. The nursing assistant coming on duty is on the unit with you. A person puts her call light on. Your response is
   A. "I'm ready to go. I will let you answer that light."
   B. "I've been here all day, so I am not answering that light."
   C. "No one helped me answer lights when I came on duty."
   D. "I will answer that light so that you can get organized for the shift."

7. When recording in the medical record, you
   A. Write in pencil
   B. Spell words incorrectly
   C. Use only agency-approved abbreviations
   D. Record what your co-worker did

8. You are answering the phone in the nurses' station. You
   A. Answer in a rushed manner
   B. Give a courteous greeting
   C. End the conversation and hang up without saying good-bye
   D. Give confidential information about a resident to the caller

9. A person who was admitted to the nursing center yesterday does not feel safe. You
   A. Are rude as you care for the person
   B. Ignore the person's requests for information
   C. Show the person around the nursing center
   D. Act rushed as you care for the person

10. A person is angry and is shouting at you. You should
    A. Yell back at the person
    B. Stay calm and professional
    C. Put the person in a room away from others
    D. Call the family

11. When speaking with another person, you
    A. Use medical terms that may not be familiar to the person
    B. Mumble your words as you talk
    C. Ask several questions at a time
    D. Speak clearly and distinctly

12. To use a transfer or gait belt safely, you should
    A. Ignore the manufacturer's instructions
    B. Leave the excess strap dangling
    C. Apply the belt over bare skin
    D. Apply the belt under the breasts

13. When you are listening to a person, you
    A. Look around the room
    B. Sit with your arms crossed
    C. Act rushed and not interested in what the person is saying
    D. Have good eye contact with the person

14. When caring for a person who is comatose, you
    A. Make jokes about how sick the person is
    B. Care for the person without talking to him or her
    C. Explain what you are doing to him or her
    D. Discuss your problems with the other nursing assistant in the room with you

15. You need to give care to a person when a visitor is present. You
    A. Politely ask the visitor to leave the room
    B. Do the care in the presence of the visitor
    C. Expose the person's body in front of the visitor
    D. Rudely tell the visitor where to wait while you care for the person

16. A person tells you he wants to talk with a minister. You
    A. Ignore the request
    B. Tell the nurse
    C. Ask what the person wants to discuss with the minister
    D. Tell the person there is no need to talk with a minister

17. When you care for a person who has a restraint, you
    A. Observe the person every 15 minutes
    B. Remove the restraint and reposition the person every 4 hours
    C. Apply the restraint tightly
    D. Apply the restraint incorrectly

18. As a person ages
    A. The skin becomes less dry
    B. Muscle strength increases
    C. Reflexes are faster
    D. Bladder muscles weaken

19. A person you are caring for touches your buttocks several times. You
    A. Tell the person you like being touched
    B. Ask the person not to touch you again
    C. Tell the person's daughter
    D. Tell the person's girlfriend

20. You are transporting a person in a wheelchair. You
    A. Pull the chair backward
    B. Let the person's feet touch the floor
    C. Push the chair forward
    D. Rest the footplates on the person's leg

21. You cannot read the person's name on the identification (ID) bracelet. You
    A. Tell the nurse so that a new bracelet can be made
    B. Ignore the fact that you cannot read the name
    C. Ask another nursing assistant to identify the person
    D. Tell the family the person needs a new ID bracelet

22. The universal sign of choking is
    A. Holding your breath
    B. Clutching at the throat
    C. Having difficulty breathing
    D. Coughing

23. A person is on a diabetic diet. You
    A. Serve the person's meals late
    B. Let the person eat whenever he or she is hungry
    C. Sometimes check the tray to see what was eaten
    D. Tell the nurse about changes in the person's eating habits

24. With mild airway obstruction
    A. The person is usually unconscious
    B. The person cannot speak
    C. Forceful coughing often does not remove the object
    D. Forceful coughing often can remove the object

25. To relieve severe airway obstruction in a conscious adult, you do
    A. Abdominal thrusts
    B. Back thrusts
    C. Chest compressions
    D. A finger sweep

26. Faulty electrical equipment
    A. Can be used in a nursing center
    B. Should be given to the nurse
    C. Should be taken home by you for repair
    D. Should be used only with alert persons

27. A warning label has been removed from a hazardous substance container. You
    A. May use the substance if you know what is in the container
    B. Leave the container where it is
    C. Take the container to the nurse and explain the problem
    D. Tell another nursing assistant about the missing label

28. A person's beliefs and values are different from your views. What should you do?
    A. Refuse to care for the person
    B. Delegate care to another nursing assistant
    C. Tell the nurse about your concerns
    D. Tell the person how you feel

29. You find a person smoking in the nursing center. You should
    A. Ignore the situation
    B. Tell the person to leave
    C. Tell another nursing assistant
    D. Ask the person to put out the cigarette and show him or her where smoking is permitted

30. During a fire, the first thing you do is
    A. Rescue persons in immediate danger
    B. Sound the nearest fire alarm
    C. Close doors and windows to confine the fire
    D. Extinguish the fire

31. A person with Alzheimer's disease has increased restlessness and confusion as daylight ends. You
    A. Try to reason with the person
    B. Ask the person to tell you what is bothering him or her
    C. Provide a calm, quiet setting late in the day
    D. Complete his or her treatments and activities late in the day

32. To prevent suffocation, you should
    A. Make sure dentures fit loosely
    B. Cut food into large pieces
    C. Make sure the person can chew and swallow the food served
    D. Ignore loose teeth or dentures

33. When using a wheelchair, you should
    A. Lock both wheels before you transfer a person to and from the wheelchair
    B. Lock only one wheel before you transfer a person to and from the wheelchair
    C. Let the person's feet touch the floor when the chair is moving
    D. Let the person stand on the footplates
34. A person begins to fall while you are walking him or her. You should
    A. Try to prevent the fall
    B. Ease the person to the floor
    C. Yell at the person for falling
    D. Tell the nurse at the end of the shift
35. A person has a restraint on. You know that
    A. Restraints are used for staff convenience
    B. Death from strangulation is a risk factor when using a restraint
    C. Restraints may be used to punish a person
    D. A written nurse's order is required for a restraint
36. Before feeding a person, you
    A. Tell the other nursing assistant
    B. Go to the restroom
    C. Wash your hands
    D. Tell the nurse
37. When wearing gloves, you remember to
    A. Wear them several times before discarding them
    B. Wear the same ones from room to room
    C. Wear gloves with a tear or puncture
    D. Change gloves when they become contaminated with urine
38. When washing your hands, you
    A. Use hot water
    B. Let your uniform touch the sink
    C. Keep your watch at your wrist
    D. Keep your hands and forearms lower than your elbows
39. You need to move a box from the floor to the counter in the utility room. You
    A. Bend from your waist to pick up the box
    B. Hold the box away from your body as you pick it up
    C. Bend your knees and squat to lift the box
    D. Stand with your feet close together as you pick up the box
40. The nurse asks you to place a person in Fowler's position. You
    A. Put the bed flat
    B. Raise the head of the bed between 45 and 60 degrees
    C. Raise the head of the bed between 80 and 90 degrees
    D. Raise the head of the bed 15 degrees
41. You accidentally scratch a person. This could be
    A. Neglect
    B. Negligence
    C. Malpractice
    D. Physical abuse

42. You positioned a person in a chair. For good body alignment, you
    A. Have the person's back and buttocks against the back of the chair
    B. Leave the person's feet unsupported
    C. Have the backs of the person's knees touch the edge of the chair
    D. Have the person sit on the edge of the chair
43. You need to transfer a person with a weak left leg from the bed to the wheelchair. You
    A. Help the person on his or her left side
    B. Help the person on his or her right side
    C. Keep the person in bed
    D. Ask the person what side moves first
44. A person tries to scratch and kick you. You should
    A. Protect yourself from harm
    B. Argue with the person
    C. Become angry with the person
    D. Ignore the person
45. When moving a person up in bed
    A. Window coverings may be left open so that people can look in
    B. Body parts may be exposed
    C. Ask the person to help
    D. Ask the person to lie still
46. For comfort, most older persons prefer
    A. Rooms that are cold
    B. Restrooms that smell of urine
    C. Loud talking and laughter in the nurses' station
    D. Lighting that meets their needs
47. Call lights are
    A. Placed on the person's strong side
    B. Answered when time permits
    C. Kept on the bedside table
    D. Kept on the person's weak side
48. A nurse asks you to inspect a person's closet. You
    A. Tell the nurse you cannot do this
    B. Inspect the closet when the person is in the dining room
    C. Ask the person if you can inspect his or her closet
    D. Tell the nurse to inspect the closet
49. When changing bed linens, you
    A. Hold the linen close to your uniform
    B. Shake the sheet when putting it on the bed
    C. Take only needed linen into the person's room
    D. Put dirty linen on the floor
50. To use a fire extinguisher, you
    A. Keep the safety pin in the extinguisher
    B. Direct the hose or nozzle at the top of the fire
    C. Squeeze the lever to start the stream
    D. Sweep the stream at the top of the fire
51. When doing mouth care for an unconscious person, you
    A. Do not need to wear gloves
    B. Give mouth care at least every 2 hours
    C. Place the person in a supine position
    D. Keep the mouth open with your fingers

52. A person is angry because he did not get to the activity room on time because a co-worker did not come to work. How should you respond to him?
    A. "It's not my fault. A co-worker called off today and we are short-staffed."
    B. "I'm sorry you were late for activities. I will try to plan better."
    C. "I am doing the best I can."
    D. "I'm just too busy."
53. You are asked to clean a person's dentures. You
    A. Use hot water
    B. Hold the dentures firmly and line the basin with a towel
    C. Wrap the dentures in tissues after cleaning
    D. Store the dentures in a denture cup with the person's room number on it
54. When bathing a person, you notice a rash that was not there before. You
    A. Do nothing
    B. Tell the person
    C. Tell the nurse and record it in the medical record
    D. Tell the person's daughter
55. When washing a person's eyes, you
    A. Use soap
    B. Clean the eye near you first
    C. Wipe from the inner to the outer aspect of the eye
    D. Wipe from the outer aspect to the inner aspect of the eye
56. When giving a back massage, you
    A. Use cold lotion
    B. Use light strokes
    C. Massage reddened bony areas
    D. Look for bruises and breaks in the skin
57. You need to give perineal care to a female. You
    A. Separate the labia and clean downward from front to back
    B. Separate the labia and clean upward from back to front
    C. Wear gloves only if there is drainage
    D. Only use water
58. When giving a person a tub bath or shower, you
    A. Do not give the person a call light
    B. Turn the hot water on first, then the cold water
    C. Stay within hearing distance if the person can be left alone
    D. Direct water toward the person while adjusting the water temperature
59. A person is on an anticoagulant. You
    A. Use a safety razor
    B. Use an electric razor
    C. Let him grow a beard
    D. Let him choose which type of razor to use
60. A person with a weak left arm wants to remove his or her sweater. You
    A. Let the person do it without any assistance
    B. Help the person remove the sweater from his or her right arm first
    C. Help the person remove the sweater from his or her left arm first
    D. Tell the person to keep the sweater on

61. When talking with a person, you should call the person
    A. "Honey"
    B. By his or her first name
    C. By his or her title—Mr. or Mrs. or Miss
    D. "Grandpa" or "Grandma"
62. A person has an indwelling catheter. You
    A. Let the person lie on the tubing
    B. Disconnect the catheter from the drainage tubing every 8 hours
    C. Secure the catheter to the lower leg
    D. Measure and record the amount of urine in the drainage bag
63. A person needs to eat a diet that contains carbohydrates. Carbohydrates
    A. Are needed for tissue repair and growth
    B. Provide energy and fiber for bowel elimination
    C. Add flavor to food and help the body use certain vitamins
    D. Are needed for nerve and muscle function
64. You are taking a rectal temperature with a glass thermometer. You
    A. Insert the thermometer before lubricating it
    B. Leave the privacy curtain open
    C. Leave the thermometer in place for 10 minutes
    D. Hold the thermometer in place
65. A person has a blood pressure (BP) of 86/58 mm Hg. You
    A. Report the BP to the nurse at once
    B. Record the BP but do not tell the nurse
    C. Ask the unit secretary to tell the nurse
    D. Retake the BP in 30 minutes before telling the nurse
66. On which person would you take an oral temperature?
    A. An unconscious person
    B. The person receiving oxygen
    C. The person who breathes through his or her mouth
    D. A conscious person
67. When caring for a person who is blind or visually impaired, you
    A. Offer the person your arm and have the person walk a half step behind you
    B. Do as much for the person as possible
    C. Shout at the person when talking with him or her
    D. Touch the person before indicating your presence
68. You are caring for a person with dementia. You
    A. Misplace the person's clothes
    B. Choose the activities the person attends
    C. Send personal items home
    D. Let the family make choices if the person cannot
69. When providing rehabilitation and restorative care for a person, you
    A. Can shout or scream at the person
    B. Can hit or strike the person
    C. Can call the person names
    D. Discuss your anger with the nurse

70. While bathing a person, you
    A. Keep doors and windows open
    B. Wash from the dirtiest areas to the cleanest areas
    C. Encourage the person to help as much as possible
    D. Rub the skin dry
71. When a person is dying
    A. Assume that the person can hear you
    B. Oral care is done every 5 hours
    C. Skin care is done weekly
    D. Reposition the person every 3 hours
72. A person is on intake and output. You
    A. Measure only liquids such as water and juice
    B. Measure ice cream and gelatin as part of intake
    C. Measure IV fluids
    D. Measure tube feedings
73. A person has been on bedrest. You need to have the person walk. What will you do first?
    A. Help the person move quickly.
    B. Have the person dangle before getting out of bed.
    C. Have the person sit in a chair.
    D. Walk with the person as soon as he or she gets out of bed.

74. Your ring accidentally causes a skin tear on an elderly person. You
    A. Tell yourself to be more careful the next time
    B. Tell the nurse at once
    C. Do nothing
    D. Hope no one finds out
75. To protect a person's privacy, you should
    A. Keep all information about the person confidential
    B. Discuss the person's treatment with another nursing assistant in the lunch room
    C. Open the person's mail
    D. Keep the privacy curtain open when providing care to the person

PRACTICE EXAMINATION 2

This test contains 75 questions. For each question, circle the BEST answer.

1. You can refuse to do a delegated task when
   A. You are too busy
   B. You do not like the task
   C. The task is not in your job description
   D. It is the end of the shift

2. Mr. Smith does not want life-saving measures. You
   A. Explain to Mr. Smith why he should have life-saving measures
   B. Respect his decision
   C. Explain to Mr. Smith's family why life-saving measures are needed
   D. Tell your friend about Mr. Smith's decision

3. You are walking by a resident's room. You hear a nurse shouting at a person. This is
   A. Battery
   B. Malpractice
   C. Verbal abuse
   D. Neglect

4. When communicating with a foreign-speaking person, you
   A. Speak loudly or shout
   B. Use medical terms the person may not understand
   C. Use words the person seems to understand
   D. Speak quickly and mumble

5. To protect a person from getting burned, you
   A. Allow smoking in bed
   B. Turn hot water on first, then cold water
   C. Assist the person with drinking or eating hot food
   D. Let the person sleep with a heating pad

6. To prevent equipment accidents, you should
   A. Use two-pronged plugs on all electrical devices
   B. Follow the manufacturer's instructions
   C. Wipe up spills when you have time
   D. Use unfamiliar equipment without training

7. To prevent a person from falling, you should
   A. Ignore call lights
   B. Use throw rugs on the floor
   C. Keep the bed in a high position
   D. Use grab bars in showers

8. You need to wash your hands
   A. Before you document a procedure
   B. After you remove gloves
   C. After you talk with a person
   D. After you talk with a co-worker

9. You need to move a person weighing 250 pounds in bed. You
   A. Do the procedure alone
   B. Keep the privacy curtain open
   C. Ask the person to lie still
   D. Ask for assistance from at least two other staff members

10. When transferring a person from a bed to a wheelchair, you never
    A. Ask a co-worker to help you
    B. Use a transfer or gait belt
    C. Have the person put his or her arms around your neck
    D. Lock the wheels on the wheelchair

11. When making a bed, you
    A. Keep the bed in the low position
    B. Wear gloves when removing linen
    C. Raise the head of the bed
    D. Raise the foot of the bed

12. To give perineal care to a male, you
    A. Use a circular motion and work toward the meatus
    B. Use a circular motion and start at the meatus and work outward
    C. Wear gloves only if there is drainage
    D. Use only water

13. A person with a weak left arm wants to put his or her sweater on. You
    A. Let the person do it without any assistance
    B. Help the person put the sweater on his or her right arm first
    C. Help the person put the sweater on his or her left arm first
    D. Tell the person to keep the sweater off

14. A person has an indwelling catheter. You
    A. Let the drainage bag touch the floor
    B. Keep the drainage bag higher than the bladder
    C. Hang the drainage bag on a bed rail
    D. Have the drainage bag hang from the bed frame or chair

15. A person needs to eat a diet that contains protein. Protein
    A. Is needed for tissue repair and growth
    B. Provides energy and fiber for bowel elimination
    C. Adds flavor to food and helps the body use certain vitamins
    D. Is needed for nerve and muscle function

16. Older persons
    A. Have an increased sense of thirst
    B. Need less water than younger persons
    C. May not feel thirsty
    D. Seldom need to have water offered to them

17. A person is NPO. You
    A. Post a sign in the bathroom
    B. Keep the water pitcher filled at the bedside
    C. Remove the water pitcher and glass from the room
    D. Provide oral hygiene every day

18. A person drank 3 oz of milk at lunch. He or she drank
    A. 30 mL
    B. 60 mL
    C. 90 mL
    D. 120 mL
19. When feeding a person, you
    A. Offer fluids at the end of the meal
    B. Use forks
    C. Do not talk to the person
    D. Allow time for chewing and swallowing
20. You need to perform range of motion (ROM) exercises to a person's right shoulder. You
    A. Force the joint beyond its present ROM
    B. Move the joint quickly
    C. Force the joint to the point of pain
    D. Support the part being exercised
21. A person has a weak left leg. The person should
    A. Hold the cane in his or her left hand
    B. Hold the cane in his or her right hand
    C. Hold the cane in either hand
    D. Use a walker
22. To promote comfort and relieve pain, you
    A. Keep wrinkles in the bed linens
    B. Position the person in good alignment
    C. Talk loudly to the person
    D. Use sudden and jarring movements of the bed or chair
23. A person is receiving oxygen through a nasal cannula. You
    A. Turn the oxygen higher when he or she is short of breath
    B. Fill the humidifier when it is not bubbling
    C. Check behind the ears and under the nose for signs of irritation
    D. Remove the cannula when the person goes to the dining room
24. You accidentally dropped a mercury-glass thermometer. You
    A. Tell the nurse at once
    B. Put the mercury in your pocket
    C. Pick up the pieces of glass with your hands
    D. Touch the mercury
25. When taking a person's pulse, you
    A. Use the brachial pulse
    B. Take the pulse for 30 seconds if it is irregular
    C. Tell the nurse if the pulse is less than 60 beats per minute
    D. Use your thumb to take a pulse
26. You are counting respirations on a person. You
    A. Tell the person you are counting his or her respirations
    B. Count for 1 minute if an abnormal breathing pattern is noted
    C. Report a rate of 16 respirations per minute to the nurse at once
    D. Count for 30 seconds if an abnormal breathing pattern is noted
27. You are taking blood pressures on people assigned to you. An older person has a blood pressure (BP) of 158/96 mm Hg. You
    A. Report the BP to the nurse at once
    B. Finish taking all the blood pressures before telling the nurse
    C. Retake the BP in 30 minutes before telling the nurse
    D. Ask the unit secretary to tell the nurse about the BP
28. When would you take a rectal temperature?
    A. The person has diarrhea.
    B. The person is confused.
    C. The person is unconscious.
    D. The person is agitated.
29. A person has been admitted to the nursing center recently. You
    A. Look through his or her belongings
    B. Ignore his or her questions
    C. Speak in a gentle, calm voice
    D. Enter the person's room without knocking
30. When taking a person's height and weight, you
    A. Let the person wear shoes
    B. Have the person void before being weighed
    C. Weigh the person at different times of the day
    D. Balance the scale every 6 months
31. A person is bedfast. To prevent pressure injuries, you
    A. Reposition the person at least every 3 hours
    B. Massage reddened areas
    C. Let heels and ankles touch the bed
    D. Keep the skin free of moisture from urine, stools, or perspiration
32. A person has a hearing problem. When talking with the person, you
    A. Keep the TV or radio on
    B. Shout
    C. Face the person
    D. Speak quickly
33. When caring for a person who is blind or visually impaired, you
    A. Place furniture and equipment where the person walks
    B. Keep the lights off
    C. Explain the location of food and beverages
    D. Rearrange furniture and equipment
34. You are caring for a person with dementia. You
    A. Share information about the person's care
    B. Share information about the person's condition
    C. Protect confidential information
    D. Expose the person's body when you provide care
35. When caring for a confused person, you
    A. Call the person "Honey"
    B. Do not need to explain what you are doing
    C. Ask clear, simple questions
    D. Remove the calendar from the person's room

36. A person with Alzheimer's disease likes to wander. You
    A. Keep the person in his or her room
    B. Restrain the person
    C. Argue with the person who wants to leave
    D. Exercise the person as ordered
37. Restorative nursing programs
    A. Help maintain the lowest level of function
    B. Promote self-care measures
    C. Focus on the disability, not the person
    D. Help the person lose strength and independence
38. When caring for a person with a disability, you
    A. Focus on his or her limitations
    B. Expect progress in a rehabilitation program to be fast
    C. Remind the person of his or her progress in the rehabilitation program
    D. Deny the disability
39. After a person dies, you
    A. Can expose his or her body unnecessarily
    B. Can discuss the person's diagnosis with your family
    C. Can talk about the family's reactions to your friends
    D. Respect the person's right to privacy
40. You enter a person's room and find a fire in the wastebasket. Your first action is to
    A. Remove the person from the room
    B. Close the door
    C. Call for help
    D. Activate the fire alarm
41. You leave a person lying in urine and he or she develops a bedsore. This is
    A. Fraud
    B. Neglect
    C. Assault
    D. Battery
42. A nurse asks you to place a drug and a sterile dressing on a small foot wound. You
    A. Agree to do the task
    B. Ask another nursing assistant to do the task
    C. Politely tell the nurse you cannot do that task
    D. Report the nurse to the director of nursing
43. You observe that a person's urine is foul-smelling and dark amber. Your first action is to
    A. Tell the other nursing assistant
    B. Tell the person
    C. Tell the nurse
    D. Record the observation
44. A daughter asks you for water for her mom. Your response is
    A. "I am not caring for your mom. I will get her nursing assistant for you."
    B. "I do not have time to do that."
    C. "That's not my job."
    D. "I will be happy to do that."

45. A person has a restraint on. You
    A. Observe the person for breathing and circulation complications every 30 minutes
    B. Know that unnecessary restraint is false imprisonment
    C. Use the most restrictive type of restraint
    D. Know that restraints decrease confusion and agitation
46. The nurse asks you to place a person in the supine position. You
    A. Elevate the head of the bed 45 degrees
    B. Elevate the foot of the bed 15 degrees
    C. Place the person on his or her back with the bed flat
    D. Place the person on his or her abdomen
47. The most important way to prevent or avoid spreading infection is to
    A. Wash hands
    B. Cover your nose when coughing
    C. Use disposable gloves
    D. Wear a mask
48. You are eating lunch and a nursing assistant begins to gossip about another person. You
    A. Join the conversation and talk about the person
    B. Remove yourself from the group
    C. Tell your roommate about the gossip you heard at lunch
    D. Tell another nursing assistant about the gossip you heard
49. When moving a person up in bed, you should
    A. Raise the head of the bed
    B. Ask the person to keep his or her legs straight
    C. Cause friction and shearing
    D. Ask a co-worker to help you
50. A person is on a sodium-controlled diet. This means
    A. Canned vegetables are omitted from his or her diet
    B. Salt may be added to food at the table
    C. Large amounts of salt are used in cooking
    D. Ham is eaten regularly
51. Elastic stockings
    A. Are applied after a person gets out of bed
    B. Should not have wrinkles or creases after being applied
    C. Come in one size only
    D. Are forced on the person
52. While walking, the person begins to fall. You
    A. Call for help
    B. Reach for a chair
    C. Ease the person to the floor
    D. Ask a visitor to help
53. Before bathing a person, you should
    A. Offer the bedpan or urinal
    B. Partially undress the person
    C. Raise the head of the bed
    D. Open the privacy curtain

54. When taking a rectal temperature with a glass thermometer, you insert the thermometer
    A. 1 inch
    B. 1.5 inches
    C. 2 inches
    D. 2.5 inches
55. Touch
    A. Is a form of nonverbal communication
    B. Is a form of verbal communication
    C. Means the same thing to everyone
    D. Should be used for all persons
56. You may share information about a person's care and condition to
    A. The staff caring for the person
    B. The person's daughter
    C. Your family members
    D. The volunteer in the gift shop
57. A person tells you he or she has pain upon urination. You
    A. Tell the nurse
    B. Let the nurse document this information
    C. Ask the person to tell you if it happens again
    D. Tell the person's son
58. A person's culture and religion are different from yours. You
    A. Laugh about the person's customs
    B. Tell your family about the person's customs
    C. Ask the person to explain his or her beliefs and practices to you
    D. Tell the person his or her beliefs and customs are silly
59. You need to wear gloves when you
    A. Do range-of-motion exercises
    B. Feed a person
    C. Give perineal care
    D. Walk a person
60. An older person is normally alert. Today he or she is confused. What should you do?
    A. Ask the person why he or she is confused
    B. Ignore the confusion
    C. Check to see if the person is confused later in the day
    D. Tell the nurse
61. While walking with a person, he tells you he feels faint. What do you do first?
    A. Have the person sit down.
    B. Call for the nurse.
    C. Open the window.
    D. Ask the person to take a deep breath.
62. You are asked to encourage fluids for a person. You
    A. Increase the person's fluid intake
    B. Decrease the person's fluid intake
    C. Limit fluids to meal times
    D. Keep fluids where the person cannot reach them

63. Communication fails when you
    A. Use words the other person understands
    B. Talk too much
    C. Let others express their feelings and concerns
    D. Talk about a topic that is uncomfortable
64. During bathing, a person may
    A. Decide what products to use
    B. Be exposed in the shower room
    C. Have visitors present without his or her permission
    D. Have no personal choices
65. People in late adulthood need to
    A. Adjust to increased income
    B. Adjust to their health being better
    C. Develop new friends and relationships
    D. Adjust to increased strength
66. When measuring blood pressure, you should do the following except
    A. Apply the cuff to a bare upper arm
    B. Turn off the TV
    C. Locate the brachial artery
    D. Use the arm with an IV infusion
67. You find clean linen on the floor in a person's room. You
    A. Use the linen to make the bed
    B. Return the linen to the linen cart
    C. Put the linen in the laundry
    D. Tell the nurse
68. When doing mouth care on an unconscious person, you
    A. Use a large amount of fluid
    B. Position the person on his or her side
    C. Do the task without telling the person what you are doing
    D. Insert his or her dentures when done
69. When brushing or combing a person's hair, you
    A. Cut matted or tangled hair
    B. Encourage the person to do as much as possible
    C. Style the hair as you want
    D. Perform the task weekly
70. When providing nail and foot care, you
    A. Cut fingernails with scissors
    B. Trim toenails for a diabetic person
    C. Trim toenails for a person with poor circulation
    D. Check between the toes for cracks and sores
71. An indwelling catheter becomes disconnected from the drainage system. You
    A. Reconnect the tubing to the catheter quickly without gloves
    B. Tell the nurse at once
    C. Get a new drainage system
    D. Touch the ends of the catheter
72. Urinary drainage bags are
    A. Hung on the bed rail
    B. Emptied and measured at the end of each shift
    C. Kept on the floor
    D. Kept higher than the person's bladder

73. A person needs a condom catheter applied. You remember to
    A. Apply it to a penis that is red and irritated
    B. Use adhesive tape to secure the catheter
    C. Use elastic tape to secure the catheter
    D. Act in an unprofessional manner
74. For comfort during bowel elimination
    A. Have the person use the bedpan rather than the bathroom or commode if possible
    B. Permit visitors to stay
    C. Keep the door and privacy curtain open
    D. Leave the person alone if possible
75. You are transferring a person with a weak right side from the wheelchair to the bed. You
    A. Place the wheelchair on the left side of the bed
    B. Place the wheelchair on the right side of the bed
    C. Keep the person in the wheelchair
    D. Ask the person what side moves first

SKILLS EVALUATION REVIEW

Each state has its own policies and procedures for the skills test. The following information is an overview of what to expect.

- To pass the skills evaluation, you will need to perform all five skills correctly.
- A nurse evaluates your performance of certain skills. Having someone watch as you work is not a new experience. Your instructor evaluated your performance during your training program. While you are working, your supervisor evaluates your skills.
- Mannequins and people are used as "patients" or "residents," depending on the skills you are performing.
- If you make a mistake, tell the evaluator what you did wrong. Then perform the skill correctly. Do not panic.
- Take whatever equipment you normally take to or use at work. Wear a watch with a second hand. You may need it to measure vital signs and check how much time you have left.

BEFORE AND DURING THE PROCEDURE

- Hand washing is evaluated at the beginning of the skills test. You are expected to know when to wash your hands. Therefore you may not be told to do so. Follow the rules for hand hygiene during the test.
- Before entering a person's room, knock on the door. Greet the person by name and introduce yourself before beginning a procedure. Check the identification (ID) or the photo ID to make certain you are giving care to the right person.
- Explain what you are going to do before beginning the procedure and as needed throughout the procedure.
- Always follow the rules of medical asepsis. For example, remove gloves and dispose of them properly. Keep clean linen separated from dirty linen.
- Always protect the person's rights throughout the skills test.
- Communicate with the person as you give care. Focus on the person's needs and interests. Always treat the person with respect. Do not talk about yourself or your personal problems.
- Provide privacy. This involves pulling the privacy curtain around the bed, closing doors, and asking visitors to leave the room.
- Promote safety for the person. For example, lock the wheelchair when you transfer a person to and from it. Place the bed in the lowest horizontal position when the person must get out of bed or when you are done giving care.

- Make sure the signaling device is within the person's reach. Attaching it to the bed or bed rail does not mean the person can reach it.
- Use good body mechanics. Raise the bed and overbed table to a good working height.
- Provide for comfort.
  - Make sure the person and linens are clean and dry. The person may have become incontinent during the procedure.
  - Change or straighten bed linens as needed.
  - Position the person for comfort and in good alignment.
  - Provide pillows as directed by the nurse and the care plan.
  - Raise the head of the bed as the person prefers and as allowed by the nurse and the care plan.
  - Provide for warmth. The person may need an extra blanket, a lap blanket, a sweater, socks, and so on.
  - Adjust lighting to meet the person's needs.
  - Make sure eyeglasses, hearing aids, and other devices are in place as needed.
  - Ask the person if he or she is comfortable.
  - Ask the person if there is anything else you can do for him or her.
  - Make sure the person is covered for warmth and privacy.

SKILLS

Ask your instructor to tell you which of the following skills are tested in your state. Place a checkmark in the box in front of each tested skill so that it will be easy for you to reference. The skills marked with an asterisk (*) are used with permission of National Council of State Boards of Nursing (NCSBN). These skills are offered as a study guide to you. The word "client" refers to the resident or person receiving care. You are responsible for following the most current standards, practices, and guidelines of your state.

The steps in boldface type are critical element steps. Critical element steps must be done correctly to pass the skill. If you miss a critical element step, you will not pass the skills evaluation. For example, you are to transfer a client from the bed to a wheelchair. You will fail if you do not lock the wheels on the wheelchair before transferring the person. An automatic failure is one that could potentially cause harm to a person. Your state may mark critical element steps in another way—with underline or italics. If your state has one, review the candidate's handbook.

☐ *HAND HYGIENE (HAND WASHING) (CHAPTER 13)

1. Addresses client by name and introduces self to client by name
2. Turns on water at sink
3. Wets hands and wrists thoroughly
4. Applies soap to hands
5. **Lathers all surfaces of wrists, hands, and fingers, producing friction for at least 20 (twenty) seconds, keeping hands lower than the elbows and the fingertips down.**
6. Cleans fingernails by rubbing fingertips against palms of the opposite hand
7. **Rinses all surfaces of wrists, hands, and fingers, keeping hands lower than the elbows and the fingertips down**
8. Uses clean, dry paper towel/towels to dry all surfaces of hands, wrists, and fingers and then disposes of paper towel/towels into waste container
9. Uses clean, dry paper towel/towels to turn off faucet and then disposes of paper towel/towels into waste container or uses knee/foot control to turn off faucet
10. Does not touch inside of sink at any time

☐ *APPLIES ONE KNEE-HIGH ELASTIC STOCKING (CHAPTER 28)

1. Explains procedure, speaking clearly, slowly, and directly, maintaining face-to-face contact whenever possible
2. Privacy is provided with a curtain, screen, or door
3. The person is in supine position (lying down in bed) while stocking is applied
4. Turns stocking inside-out, at least to the heel
5. Places foot of stocking over toes, foot, and heel
6. Pulls top of stocking over foot, heel, and leg
7. Moves foot and leg gently and naturally, avoiding force and overextension of limb and joints
8. **Finishes procedure with no twists or wrinkles and heel of stocking (if present) is over heel and opening in toe area (if present) is either over or under toe area**
9. Signaling device is within reach and bed is in low position
10. After completing skill, performs hand hygiene

☐ *ASSISTS TO AMBULATE USING A TRANSFER BELT (CHAPTER 27)

1. Explains procedure, speaking clearly, slowly, and directly, maintaining face-to-face contact whenever possible
2. **Before assisting to stand, client is wearing shoes**
3. Before assisting to stand, bed is at a safe level
4. Before assisting to stand, checks and/or locks bed wheels
5. **Before assisting to stand, client is assisted to sitting position with feet flat on the floor**
6. Before assisting to stand, applies transfer belt securely at the waist over clothing/gown
7. Before assisting to stand, provides instructions to enable the person to assist in standing including prearranged signal to alert client to begin standing
8. Stands facing client positioning self to ensure safety of candidate and client during transfer. Counts to three (or says other prearranged signal) to alert the person to begin standing
9. On signal, gradually assists client to stand by grasping transfer belt on both sides with an upward grasp (candidate's hands are in upward position), maintaining stability of the person's legs
10. Walks slightly behind and to one side of client for a distance of ten (10) feet, while holding onto the belt
11. After ambulation, assists client to bed and removes transfer belt
12. Signaling device is within reach and bed is in low position
13. After completing skill, performs hand hygiene

☐ *ASSISTS WITH USE OF BEDPAN (CHAPTER 20)

1. Explains procedure speaking clearly, slowly, and directly, maintaining face-to-face contact whenever possible
2. Privacy is provided with a curtain, screen, or door
3. Before placing bedpan, lowers head of bed
4. Puts on clean gloves before handling bedpan
5. **Places bedpan correctly under client's buttocks**
6. Removes and disposes of gloves (without contaminating self) into waste container and performs hand hygiene
7. After positioning client on bedpan and removing gloves, raises head of bed
8. Toilet tissue is within reach
9. Hand wipe is within reach and client is instructed to clean hands with hand wipe when finished
10. Signaling device is within reach and client is asked to signal when finished
11. Puts on clean gloves before removing bedpan
12. Head of bed is lowered before bedpan is removed
13. Avoids overexposure of client
14. Empties and rinses bedpan and pours rinse into toilet
15. After rinsing bedpan, places bedpan in designated dirty supply area
16. After placing bedpan in designated dirty supply area, removes and disposes of gloves (without contaminating self) into waste container and performs hand hygiene
17. Signaling device is within reach and bed is in low position

*Reproduced and used with permission from the *Nurse Assistant Candidate Handbook* from National Council of State Boards of Nursing (NCSBN), Chicago, Ill, © 2016.

☐ ***CLEANS UPPER OR LOWER DENTURE (CHAPTER 18)**

1. Puts on clean gloves before handling denture
2. Bottom of sink is lined and/or sink is partially filled with water before denture is held over sink
3. Rinses denture in moderate temperature running water before brushing them
4. Applies toothpaste to toothbrush
5. Brushes surfaces of denture
6. Rinses surfaces of denture under moderate temperature running water
7. Before placing denture into cup, rinses denture cup and lid
8. Places denture in denture cup with moderate temperature water/solution and places lid on cup
9. Rinses toothbrush and places in designated toothbrush basin/container
10. Maintains clean technique with placement of toothbrush and denture
11. Sink liner is removed and disposed of appropriately and/or sink is drained
12. After rinsing equipment and disposing of sink liner, removes and disposes of gloves (without contaminating self) into waste container and performs hand hygiene

☐ ***COUNTS AND RECORDS RADIAL PULSE (CHAPTER 25)****

1. Explains procedure, speaking clearly, slowly, and directly, maintaining face-to-face contact whenever possible
2. Places fingertips on thumb side of client's wrist to locate radial pulse
3. Counts beats for 1 full minute
4. Signaling device is within reach
5. Before recording, performs hand hygiene
6. **After obtaining pulse by palpating in radial artery position, records pulse rate within plus or minus four beats of evaluator's reading**

☐ ***COUNTS AND RECORDS RESPIRATIONS (CHAPTER 25)†**

1. Explains procedure (for testing purposes), speaking clearly, slowly, and directly, maintaining face-to-face contact whenever possible
2. Counts respirations for 1 full minute
3. Signaling device is within reach
4. Performs hand hygiene
5. **Records respiration rate within plus or minus two breaths of evaluator's reading**

☐ ***DONNING AND REMOVING PPE (GOWN AND GLOVES) (CHAPTER 13)**

1. Picks up gown and unfolds
2. Facing the back opening of the gown places arms through each sleeve
3. Fastens the neck opening
4. Secures gown at waist making sure that back of clothing is covered by gown (as much as possible)
5. Puts on gloves
6. Cuffs of gloves overlap cuffs of gown
7. **Before removing gown, with one gloved hand, grasps the other glove at the palm, removes glove**
8. **Slips fingers from ungloved hand underneath cuff of remaining glove at wrist, and removes glove turning it inside out as it is removed**
9. Disposes of gloves into designated waste container without contaminating self
10. After removing gloves, unfastens gown at neck and waist
11. After removing gloves, removes gown without touching outside of gown
12. While removing gown, holds gown away from body without touching the floor, turns gown inward and keeps it inside out
13. Disposes of gown in designated container without contaminating self
14. After completing skill, performs hand hygiene

☐ ***DRESSES THE PERSON WITH AFFECTED (WEAK) RIGHT ARM (CHAPTER 19)**

1. Explains procedure, speaking clearly, slowly, and directly, maintaining face-to-face contact whenever possible
2. Privacy is provided with a curtain, screen, or door
3. Asks which shirt he or she would like to wear and dresses him or her in shirt of choice
4. While avoiding overexposure of client, removes gown from the unaffected side first, then removes gown from the affected side and disposes of gown into soiled linen container
5. **Assists to put the right (affected/weak) arm through the right sleeve of the shirt before placing garment on left (unaffected) arm**
6. While putting on shirt, moves body gently and naturally, avoiding force and overextension of limbs and joints
7. Finishes with clothing in place
8. Signaling device is within reach and bed is in low position
9. After completing skill, performs hand hygiene

---

*Reproduced and used with permission from the *Nurse Assistant Candidate Handbook* from National Council of State Boards of Nursing (NCSBN), Chicago, Ill, © 2016.
**Count for 1 full minute.
†Count for 1 full minute. For testing purposes you may explain to the client that you will be counting the respirations.

□ *FEEDS CLIENT WHO CANNOT FEED SELF (CHAPTER 23)

1. Explains procedure to client, speaking clearly, slowly, and directly, maintaining face-to-face contact whenever possible
2. Before feeding, looks at name card on tray and asks client to state name
3. **Before feeding client, client is in an upright sitting position (75–90 degrees)**
4. Places tray where the food can be easily seen by client
5. Candidate cleans the client's hands with hand wipe before beginning feeding
6. Candidate sits facing client during feeding
7. Tells client what foods are on tray and asks what client would like to eat first
8. Using spoon, offers client one bite of each type of food on tray, telling client the content of each spoonful
9. Offers beverage at least once during meal
10. Candidate asks client if they are ready for next bite of food or sip of beverage
11. At end of meal, candidate cleans client's mouth and hands with wipes
12. Removes food tray and places tray in designated dirty supply area
13. Signaling device is within client's reach
14. After completing skill, performs hand hygiene

□ *GIVES MODIFIED BED BATH (FACE AND ONE ARM, HAND, AND UNDERARM) (CHAPTER 18)

1. Explains procedure, speaking clearly, slowly, and directly, maintaining face-to-face contact whenever possible
2. Privacy is provided with a curtain, screen, or door
3. Removes gown and places in soiled linen container, while avoiding overexposure of the client
4. Before washing, checks water temperature for safety and comfort and asks client to verify comfort of water
5. Puts on clean gloves before washing client
6. **Beginning with eyes, washes eyes with wet washcloth (no soap), using a different area of the washcloth for each stroke, washing inner aspect to outer aspect, then proceeds to wash face**
7. Dries face with towel
8. Exposes one arm and places towel underneath arm
9. Applies soap to wet washcloth
10. Washes arm, hand, and underarm, keeping rest of body covered
11. Rinses and dries arm, hand, and underarm
12. Moves body gently and naturally, avoiding force and overextension of limbs and joints

13. Puts clean gown on the person
14. Empties, rinses, and dries basin
15. After rinsing and drying basin, places basin in designated dirty supply area
16. Disposes of linen into soiled linen container
17. Avoids contact between candidate clothing and used linens
18. After placing basin in designated dirty supply area, and disposing of used linen, removes and disposes of gloves (without contaminating self) into waste container and washes hands
19. Signaling device is within reach and bed is in low position

□ MAKES AN OCCUPIED BED (CLIENT DOES NOT NEED ASSISTANCE TO TURN) (CHAPTER 17)

1. Explains procedure, speaking clearly, slowly, and directly, maintaining face-to-face contact whenever possible
2. Privacy is provided with a curtain, screen, or door
3. Lowers head of bed before moving the person
4. The person is covered while linens are changed
5. Loosens top linen from the end of the bed
6. Raises side rail on side to which the person will move and the person moves toward raised side rail
7. Loosens bottom used linen on working side and moves bottom used linen toward center of bed
8. Places and tucks in clean bottom linen or fitted bottom sheet on working side and tucks under the person
9. Before going to other side, the person moves back onto clean bottom linen
10. Raises side rail then goes to other side of bed
11. Removes used bottom linen
12. Pulls and tucks in clean bottom linen, finishing with bottom sheet free of wrinkles
13. The person is covered with clean top sheet and bath blanket/used top sheet has been removed
14. Changes pillowcase
15. Linen is centered and tucked at foot of bed
16. Avoids contact between candidate's clothing and used linen
17. Disposes of used linen into soiled linen container and avoids putting linen on floor
18. Signaling device is within reach and bed is in low position
19. Performs hand hygiene

□ *MEASURES AND RECORDS BLOOD PRESSURE (CHAPTER 25)

1. Explains procedure, speaking clearly, slowly, and directly, maintaining face-to-face contact whenever possible

2. Before using stethoscope, wipes bell/diaphragm and earpieces of stethoscope with alcohol
3. Client's arm is positioned with palm up and upper arm is exposed
4. Feels for brachial artery on inner aspect of arm, at bend of elbow
5. Places blood pressure cuff snugly on the client's upper arm with sensor/arrow over brachial artery site
6. Earpieces of stethoscope are in ears and bell/diaphragm is over brachial artery site
7. Candidate inflates cuff between 160 mm Hg to 180 mm Hg. If beat is heard immediately upon cuff deflation, completely deflate cuff. Reinflate cuff to no more than 200 mm Hg
8. Deflates cuff slowly and notes the **first** sound (systolic reading), and **last** sound (diastolic reading) (If rounding needed, measurements are rounded **UP** to the nearest 2 mm of mercury)
9. Removes cuff
10. Signaling device is within reach
11. Before recording, performs hand hygiene
12. **After obtaining reading using BP cuff and stethoscope, records both systolic and diastolic pressures each within plus or minus 8 mm of evaluator's reading**

☐ *MEASURES AND RECORDS URINARY OUTPUT (CHAPTER 24)

1. Puts on clean gloves before handling bedpan
2. Pours the contents of the bedpan into measuring container without spilling or splashing urine outside of container
3. Measures the amount of urine at eye level with container on flat surface
4. After measuring urine, empties contents of measuring container into toilet
5. Rinses measuring container and pours rinse water into toilet
6. Rinses bedpan and pours rinse into toilet
7. After rinsing equipment, and before recording output, removes and disposes of gloves (without contaminating self) into waste container and performs hand hygiene
8. **Records contents of container within plus or minus 25 mL/cc of evaluator's reading**

☐ *MEASURES AND RECORDS WEIGHT OF AMBULATORY CLIENT (CHAPTER 25)

1. Explains procedure, speaking clearly, slowly, and directly, maintaining face-to-face contact whenever possible
2. Client has shoes on before walking to scale
3. Before client steps onto scale, candidate sets scale to zero

4. While client steps onto scale, candidate stands next to scale and assists client, if needed, onto center of the scale; then obtains client's weight
5. While client steps off scale, candidate stands next to scale and assists client, if needed, off scale before recording weight
6. Before recording, performs hand hygiene
7. **Records weight based on indicator on scale. Weight is within plus or minus 2 lbs of evaluator's reading (If weight recorded in kg weight is within plus or minus 0.9 kg of evaluator's reading)**

☐ *PERFORMS MODIFIED PASSIVE RANGE OF MOTION (PROM) FOR ONE KNEE AND ONE ANKLE (CHAPTER 27)

1. Explains procedure, speaking clearly, slowly, and directly, maintaining face-to-face contact whenever possible
2. Privacy is provided with a curtain, screen, or door
3. Instructs client to inform candidate if pain is experienced during exercise
4. Supports leg at knee and ankle while performing range of motion for knee
5. Bends the knee then returns leg to the client's normal position (extension/flexion) (AT LEAST THREE TIMES unless pain is verbalized)
6. Supports foot and ankle close to the bed while performing range of motion for ankle
7. Pushes/pulls foot toward head (dorsiflexion), and pushes/pulls foot down, toes point down (plantar flexion) (AT LEAST THREE TIMES unless pain is verbalized)
8. **While supporting the limb, moves joints gently, slowly, and smoothly through the range of motion, discontinuing exercise if client verbalizes pain**
9. Signaling device is within reach and bed is in low position
10. After completing skill, performs hand hygiene

☐ *PERFORMS PASSIVE RANGE OF MOTION (PROM) FOR ONE SHOULDER (CHAPTER 27)

1. Explains procedure, speaking clearly, slowly, and directly, maintaining face-to-face contact whenever possible
2. Privacy is provided with a curtain, screen, or door
3. Instructs the person to inform candidate if pain is experienced during exercise
4. Supports the person's upper and lower arm while performing range of motion for shoulder
5. **Raises the client's straightened arm from side position upward toward head to ear level and returns arm down to side of body (flexion/extension) (AT LEAST THREE TIMES unless pain is verbalized). Supporting the limb, moves joint gently, slowly, and**

*Reproduced and used with permission from the *Nurse Assistant Candidate Handbook* from National Council of State Boards of Nursing (NCSBN), Chicago, IL, © 2016.

smoothly through the range of motion, discontinuing exercise if client verbalizes pain

6. **Moves client's straightened arm away from the side of body to shoulder level and returns to side of body (abduction/adduction) (AT LEAST THREE TIMES unless pain is verbalized). Supporting the limb, moves joint gently, slowly, and smoothly through the range of motion, discontinuing exercise if client verbalizes pain**

7. Signaling device is within reach and bed is in low position

8. After completing skill, performs hand hygiene

☐ PERFORMS PASSIVE RANGE OF MOTION OF LOWER EXTREMITY (HIP, KNEE, ANKLE) (CHAPTER 27)

1. Washes hands before contact with the person

2. Identifies self to the person by name and addresses client by name; checks the ID bracelet against the assignment sheet

3. Explains procedure to client, speaking clearly, slowly, and directly, maintaining face-to-face contact whenever possible

4. Provides for client's privacy during procedure with curtain, screen, or door

5. Positions the person supine and in good body alignment

6. Supports the person's leg by placing one hand under knee and other hand under ankle

7. Raises the leg (flexion)

8. Straightens the leg (hyperextension)

9. Moves entire leg away from body (abduction) (Performs AT LEAST THREE TIMES unless pain occurs)

10. Moves entire leg toward body (adduction) (Performs AT LEAST THREE TIMES unless pain occurs)

11. Turns the leg inward (internal rotation)

12. Turns the leg outward (external rotation)

13. Bends the person's knee and hip toward the person's trunk (flexion) (Performs AT LEAST THREE TIMES unless pain occurs)

14. Straightens knee and hip (extension) (Performs AT LEAST THREE TIMES unless pain occurs)

15. Places one hand under foot, places other hand under the ankle

16. Bends the ankle (flexion) and straightens the ankle (extension) (Performs AT LEAST THREE TIMES unless pain occurs)

17. Turns the ankle inward (internal rotation) and turns the ankle outward (external rotation) (Performs AT LEAST THREE TIMES unless pain occurs)

18. Provides for comfort

19. Before leaving the person, places signaling device within the person's reach

20. Performs hand hygiene

☐ PERFORMS PASSIVE RANGE OF MOTION OF UPPER EXTREMITY (SHOULDER, ELBOW, WRIST, FINGER) (CHAPTER 27)

1. Washes hands before contact with the person

2. Identifies self to the person by name and addresses the person by name; checks the ID bracelet against the assignment sheet.

3. Explains procedure to the person, speaking clearly, slowly, and directly, maintaining face-to-face contact whenever possible

4. Provides for the person's privacy during procedure with curtain, screen, or door

5. Positions the person supine

6. Grasps the wrist with one hand and grasps the elbow with the other hand

7. Raises the arm straight in front and overhead and then brings arm down to side (flexion/extension) (Performs AT LEAST THREE TIMES unless pain occurs)

8. Moves the person's straightened arm away from the side of the body and moves straightened arm to the side of the body (abduction/adduction) (Performs AT LEAST THREE TIMES unless pain occurs)

9. Flexes and extends (bends and straightens) elbow through range-of-motion exercises (Performs AT LEAST THREE TIMES unless pain occurs)

10. Provides range-of-motion exercises to wrist (Performs AT LEAST THREE TIMES unless pain occurs)

11. Holds the wrist with both hands

12. Bends the hand down (flexion) and straightens the hand (extension)

13. Bends the hand back (hyperextension)

14. Turns the hand toward the thumb (radial flexion) and turns the hand toward the little finger (ulnar flexion)

15. Moves finger and thumb joints through range-of-motion exercises (Performs AT LEAST THREE TIMES unless pain occurs)

16. Spreads the fingers and thumb apart (abduction) and brings the fingers and thumb together (adduction)

17. Straightens the fingers so the fingers, hand, and arm are straight (extension)

18. Places signaling device within the person's reach

19. Performs hand hygiene

☐ MAKES AN UNOCCUPIED (CLOSED) BED (CHAPTER 17)

1. Performs hand hygiene

2. Collects clean linen

3. Places clean linen on a clean surface

4. Raises the bed for good body mechanics

5. Puts on gloves

6. Removes linen without contaminating uniform. Rolls each piece away from self

7. Discards linen into laundry bag and incontinence products and bed protectors in the trash
8. Removes and discards the gloves. Performs hand hygiene
9. Moves the mattress to the head of the bed
10. Applies mattress pad
11. Applies bottom sheet at the top and then foot of the bed, keeping it smooth, tight, and free of wrinkles
12. Places the top sheet and bedspread on the bed, keeping them smooth and free of wrinkles
13. Tucks in top linens at the foot of the bed. Turns the top sheet down over the bedspread; hem-stitching is down. Makes mitered corners so that they are smooth and tight
14. Applies clean pillowcase with extra material under the pillow at the seam end of the pillowcase
15. Attaches signaling device to the bed
16. Lowers the bed to its lowest position. Locks the bed wheels
17. Performs hand hygiene

☐ *POSITIONS ON SIDE (CHAPTER 14)

1. Explains procedure, speaking clearly, slowly, and directly, maintaining face-to-face contact whenever possible
2. Privacy is provided with a curtain, screen, or door
3. Before turning, lowers head of bed
4. Raises side rail on side to which body will be turned
5. Slowly rolls onto side as one unit toward raised side rail
6. Places or adjusts pillow under head for support
7. Candidate positions client so that client is not lying on arm
8. Supports top arm with supportive device
9. Places supportive device behind client's back
10. Places supportive device between legs with top knee flexed; knee and ankle supported
11. Signaling device is within reach and bed is in low position
12. After completing skill, performs hand hygiene

☐ *PROVIDES CATHETER CARE FOR FEMALE (CHAPTER 21)

1. Explains procedure, speaking clearly, slowly, and directly, maintaining face-to-face contact whenever possible
2. Privacy is provided with a curtain, screen, or door
3. Before washing, checks water temperature for safety and comfort and asks the person to verify comfort of water
4. Puts on clean gloves before washing
5. Places linen protector under perineal area before washing
6. Exposes area surrounding catheter while avoiding overexposure of client

7. Applies soap to wet washcloth
8. **While holding catheter at meatus without tugging, cleans at least 4 inches of catheter from meatus, moving in only one direction (i.e., away from meatus), using a clean area of the cloth for each stroke**
9. **While holding catheter at meatus without tugging, rinses at least 4 inches of catheter from meatus, moving only in one direction, away from meatus, using a clean area of the cloth for each stroke**
10. While holding catheter at meatus without tugging, dries at least 4 inches of catheter moving away from meatus
11. Empties, rinses, and dries basin
12. After rinsing and drying basin, places basin in designated dirty supply area
13. Disposes of used linen into soiled linen container and disposes of linen protector appropriately
14. Avoids contact between candidate clothing and used linen
15. After disposing of used linen and cleaning equipment, removes and disposes of gloves (without contaminating self) into waste container and washes hands
16. Signaling device is within reach and bed is in low position

☐ PROVIDES FINGERNAIL CARE ON ONE HAND (CHAPTER 19)

1. Explains procedure, speaking clearly, slowly, and directly, maintaining face-to-face contact whenever possible
2. Before immersing fingernails, checks water temperature for safety and comfort and asks the person to verify comfort of water
3. Basin is in a comfortable position for the person
4. Puts on clean gloves before cleaning fingernails
5. Fingernails are immersed in basin of water
6. Cleans under each fingernail with orangewood stick
7. Wipes orangewood stick on towel after each nail
8. Dries fingernail area
9. Candidate feels each nail and files as needed
10. Disposes of orangewood stick and emery board into waste container (for testing purposes)
11. Empties, rinses, and dries basin
12. After rinsing basin, places basin in designated dirty supply area
13. Disposes of used linen into soiled linen container
14. After cleaning nails and equipment, and disposing of used linen, removes and disposes of gloves (without contaminating self) into waste container and washes hands
15. Signaling device is within reach

☐ *PROVIDES FOOT CARE ON ONE FOOT (CHAPTER 19)

1. Explains procedure, speaking clearly, slowly, and directly, maintaining face-to-face contact whenever possible
2. Privacy is provided with a curtain, screen, or door
3. Before washing, checks water temperature for safety and comfort and asks the person to verify comfort of water
4. Basin is in a comfortable position for client and on protective barrier
5. Puts on clean gloves before washing foot
6. The person's bare foot is placed into the water
7. Applies soap to wet washcloth
8. Lifts foot from water and washes foot (including between the toes)
9. Foot is rinsed (including between the toes)
10. Dries foot (including between the toes)
11. Applies lotion to top and bottom of foot, removing excess (if any) with a towel
12. Supports foot and ankle during procedure
13. Empties, rinses, and dries basin
14. After rinsing and drying basin, places basin in designated dirty supply area
15. Disposes of used linen into soiled linen container
16. After cleaning foot and equipment, and disposing of used linen, removes and disposes of gloves (without contaminating self) into waste container and washes hands
17. Signaling device is within reach

☐ *PROVIDES MOUTH CARE (CHAPTER 18)

1. Explains procedure, speaking clearly, slowly, and directly, maintaining face-to-face contact whenever possible
2. Privacy is provided with a curtain, screen, or door
3. Before providing mouth care, client is in upright sitting position (75–90 degrees)
4. Puts on clean gloves before cleaning mouth
5. Places clothing protector across chest before providing mouth care
6. Secures cup of water and moistens toothbrush
7. Before cleaning mouth, applies toothpaste to moistened toothbrush
8. **Cleans mouth (including tongue and surfaces of teeth) using gentle motions**
9. Maintains clean technique with placement of toothbrush
10. Candidate holds emesis basin to chin while the person rinses mouth
11. Candidate wipes mouth and removes clothing protector
12. After rinsing toothbrush, empty, rinse and dry the basin and place used toothbrush in designated basin/container

13. Places basin and toothbrush in designated dirty supply area
14. Disposes of used linen into soiled linen container
15. After placing basin and toothbrush in designated dirty supply area, and disposing of used linen, removes and disposes of gloves (without contaminating self) into waste container and washes hands
16. Signaling device is within reach and bed is in low position

☐ *PROVIDES PERINEAL CARE (PERI-CARE) FOR FEMALE (CHAPTER 18)

1. Explains procedure, speaking clearly, slowly, and directly, maintaining face-to-face contact whenever possible
2. Privacy is provided with a curtain, screen, or door
3. Before washing, checks water temperature for safety and comfort and asks client to verify comfort of water
4. Puts on clean gloves before washing perineal area
5. Places pad/linen protector under perineal area before washing
6. Exposes perineal area while avoiding overexposure of client
7. Applies soap to wet washcloth
8. **Washes genital area, moving from front to back, while using a clean area of the washcloth for each stroke**
9. **Using clean washcloth, rinses soap from genital area, moving from front to back, while using a clean area of the washcloth for each stroke**
10. Dries genital area moving from front to back with towel
11. **After washing genital area, turns to side, then washes and rinses rectal area moving from front to back using a clean area of washcloth for each stroke. Dries with towel**
12. Repositions client
13. Empties, rinses, and dries basin
14. After rinsing and drying basin, places basin in designated dirty supply area
15. Disposes of used linen into soiled linen container and disposes of linen protector appropriately
16. Avoids contact between candidate clothing and used linen
17. After disposing of used linen, and placing used equipment in designated dirty supply area, removes and disposes of gloves (without contaminating self) into waste container and washes hands
18. Signaling device is within reach and bed is in low position

☐ ***TRANSFERS FROM BED TO WHEELCHAIR USING TRANSFER BELT (CHAPTER 16)**

1. Explains procedure, speaking clearly, slowly, and directly, maintaining face-to-face contact whenever possible
2. Privacy is provided with a curtain, screen, or door
3. Before assisting to stand, wheelchair is positioned along side of bed, at head of bed facing foot or foot of bed facing head
4. Before assisting to stand, footrests are folded up or removed
5. Before assisting to stand, bed is at a safe level
6. **Before assisting to stand, locks wheels on wheelchair**
7. Before assisting to stand, checks and/or locks bed wheels
8. **Before assisting to stand, client is assisted to a sitting position with feet flat on the floor**
9. Before assisting to stand, client is wearing shoes
10. Before assisting to stand, applies transfer belt securely at the waist over clothing/gown
11. Before assisting to stand, provides instructions to enable client to assist in transfer including prearranged signal to alert when to begin standing
12. Stands facing client, positioning self to ensure safety of candidate and the person during transfer. Counts to three (or says other prearranged signal) to alert client to begin standing
13. On signal, gradually assists client to stand by grasping transfer belt on both sides with an upward grasp (candidates hands are in upward position) and maintaining stability of the person's legs
14. Assists client to turn to stand in front of wheelchair with back of client's legs against wheelchair
15. Lowers the person into wheelchair
16. Positions the person with hips touching back of wheelchair and transfer belt is removed
17. Positions feet on footrests
18. Signaling device is within reach
19. After completing skill, performs hand hygiene

☐ **PERFORMS ABDOMINAL THRUSTS (CHAPTER 10)**

1. Asks the person if he or she is choking
2. Stands or kneels behind the person
3. Wraps arms around the person's waist
4. Makes a fist with one hand
5. Places thumb side of fist against the person's abdomen
6. Positions fist in middle above navel and well below the end of the sternum (breastbone)
7. Grasps fist with other hand

8. Presses fist into the person's abdomen with a quick upward thrust
9. Repeats thrusts until object is expelled or client becomes unresponsive

☐ **ASSISTS TO AMBULATE WITH CANE OR WALKER (CHAPTER 27)**

1. Explains procedure, speaking clearly, slowly, and directly, maintaining face-to-face contact whenever possible
2. Locks bed wheels or wheelchair brakes
3. Assists the person to a sitting position on the side of the bed
4. **Before ambulating, puts on and properly fastens non-skid footwear**
5. Makes sure feet are flat on the floor
6. Applies gait belt at the waist over clothing
7. Positions cane or walker correctly. Cane is on the client's strong side
8. Assists the person to stand, using correct body mechanics
9. Stands behind and slightly to the side of the person on the person's weak side
10. Holds the belt at the side and back. If not using a gait belt, has one arm around the back and the other at the elbow to support the person
11. Ambulates client
12. Assists the person to pivot and sit, using correct body mechanics, and removes the gait belt
13. Places signaling device within reach
14. Performs hand hygiene

☐ **CALCULATES FLUID INTAKE (CHAPTER 24)**

1. Observes dinner tray
2. Determines, in milliliters (mL), the amount of fluid in full containers, as well as in unconsumed food items like popsicles
3. Determines, in milliliters (mL), the amount of fluid consumed from each container and food item
4. Determines total fluid consumed in mL
5. Records total fluid consumed on intake and output (I&O) sheet
6. Calculated total is within required range of evaluator's reading

☐ **BRUSHES OR COMBS CLIENT'S HAIR (CHAPTER 19)**

1. Explains procedure, speaking clearly, slowly, and directly, maintaining face-to-face contact whenever possible
2. Collects brush or comb and bath towel and arranges items on bedside stand

*Reproduced and used with permission from the *Nurse Assistant Candidate Handbook* from National Council of State Boards of Nursing (NCSBN), Chicago, IL, © 2016.

3. Positions the person in chair or raised bed with bed rails up if used and client in semi-Fowler's position if allowed
4. Asks the person how he or she wants his or her hair styled
5. Places towel across the person's back and shoulders or across the pillow
6. Combs/brushes hair gently and completely in sections, starting at scalp and brushing toward hair ends
7. Leaves hair neatly brushed, combed, and/or styled as the person prefers
8. Removes towel
9. Removes hair from comb or brush
10. Places signaling device within reach
11. Lowers bed to lowest position
12. Performs hand hygiene

☐ TRANSFERS A CLIENT USING A MECHANICAL LIFT (CHAPTER 16)

1. Asks a co-worker to help
2. Assembles required equipment; performs safety check of slings, straps, hooks, and chains
3. Checks the person's weight to ensure it does not exceed the lift's capacity
4. Explains procedure, speaking clearly, slowly, and directly, maintaining face-to-face contact whenever possible
5. Provides for privacy during procedure with curtain, screen, or door
6. Locks the bed wheels
7. Raises the bed for proper body mechanics
8. Lowers the head of the bed to a level appropriate for the client
9. Stands on one side of the bed; co-worker stands on the other side
10. Lowers the bed rails if up
11. Centers the sling under the client following the manufacturer's instructions
12. Positions the client in semi-Fowler's position
13. Positions a chair to lower the client into it at the head of the bed, even with the head-board and about 1 foot away from the bed
14. Lowers the bed to its lowest position
15. Raises the lift to position it over the person
16. Positions the lift over the person
17. Locks the lift wheels
18. Attaches the sling to the sling hooks
19. Raises head of bed to sitting position
20. Crosses the persons's arms over the chest
21. Raises the lift high enough until the client and sling are free of the bed
22. Instructs co-worker to support the person's legs as candidate moves the lift and the client away from the bed
23. Positions the lift so that the person's back is toward the chair
24. Positions the chair so that candidate can lower person into it
25. Slowly lowers the person into the chair

26. Places the person in comfortable position, in correct body alignment
27. Lowers the lift to unhook the sling hooks and unhooks the sling
28. Removes the sling from under the person unless otherwise indicated
29. Puts footwear on the person and positions feet on floor or wheelchair footplates
30. Covers the person's lap and legs with a lap blanket
31. Positions the chair as the person prefers
32. Places signaling device within reach
33. Performs hand hygiene

☐ PROVIDES MOUTH CARE FOR AN UNCONSCIOUS CLIENT (CHAPTER 18)

1. Collects cleaning agent, swabs, padded tongue blade, water cup, hand towel, kidney basis, lip lubricant, paper towels, and gloves
2. Places paper towels on the overbed table and arranges items on top of them
3. Explains procedure, speaking clearly, slowly, and directly, maintaining face-to-face contact whenever possible
4. Provides for privacy during procedure with curtain, screen, or door
5. Raises the bed
6. Performs hand hygiene
7. Lowers the bed rail near candidate
8. Puts on gloves
9. Positions the person on side with head turned well to one side
10. Places the towel under the person's face
11. Places the kidney basin under the chin
12. Separates upper and lower teeth, using padded tongue blade
13. Uses swabs or toothbrush and toothpaste or other cleaning solution
14. Cleans inside of mouth including the gums, tongue, teeth, and inside of the cheeks
15. Swabs roof of mouth and the lips using moistened clean swab, swabs the mouth to rinse
16. Cleans and dries face
17. Removes the towel and kidney basin
18. Applies lubricant to the lips
19. Removes supplies. Cleans, rinses, dries, and returns equipment to its proper place. Discards disposable items. Wipes off the overbed table with paper towels and discards the paper towels
20. Positions the person for comfort and safety
21. Removes and discards the gloves
22. Lowers the bed to lowest position
23. Places signaling device within the reach
24. Performs hand hygiene

☐ PROVIDES DRINKING WATER (CHAPTER 24)

1. Performs hand hygiene
2. Assembles equipment—ice, scoop, pitcher, mug, straw, paper towels, towel for scoop, cart

3. Covers cart with paper towels and places items on paper towels
4. Takes cart to the person's room
5. Explains procedure to the person, speaking clearly, slowly, and directly, maintaining face-to-face contact whenever possible
6. Uses the scoop to fill the pitcher with ice; does not let the scoop touch the rim or inside of the pitcher
7. Uses the scoop to fill the mug with ice and does not let scoop touch the mug
8. Places scoop on the towel
9. Adds water to pitcher and to mug
10. Places the pitcher, mug, and straw (if used) on the overbed table, within the person's reach
11. Places signaling device within reach
12. Performs hand hygiene

☐ PROVIDES PERINEAL CARE FOR UNCIRCUMCISED MALE (CHAPTER 18)

1. Collects soap, washcloths, bath towel, bath blanket, bath thermometer, wash basin, waterproof pad, gloves, paper towels
2. Covers overbed table with paper towels and arranges items on top of them
3. Explains procedure, speaking clearly, slowly, and directly, maintaining face-to-face contact whenever possible
4. Provides for privacy during procedure with curtain, screen, or door
5. Performs hand hygiene
6. Fills basin with comfortably warm water, measures water temperature, and asks the person to check the water temperature
7. Puts on gloves
8. Elevates bed to working height
9. Covers the person with a bath blanket
10. Positions the person on the back
11. Places waterproof pad under buttocks
12. Retracts the foreskin
13. Gently grasps penis
14. Using a circular motion, cleans the tip by starting at the meatus of the urethra and working outward, using a clean part of the washcloth each time
15. Rinses the area with another washcloth, using the same circular motion
16. Returns the foreskin to its natural position immediately after rinsing
17. Cleans the shaft of the penis with firm, downward strokes and rinses the area
18. Helps the person flex his knees and spread his legs
19. Cleans the scrotum, rinses well, and observes for redness and irritation of the skin folds
20. Pats dry the penis and the scrotum
21. Helps the person turn on side away from the candidate
22. Cleans the rectal area, washing from the scrotum to the anus, rinsing, and drying well
23. Removes the waterproof pad
24. Lowers the bed

25. Removes and discards the gloves
26. Performs hand hygiene
27. Places signaling device within reach

☐ EMPTIES AND RECORDS CONTENT OF URINARY DRAINAGE BAG (CHAPTER 21)

1. Collects a graduate (measuring container), gloves, paper towels, and antiseptic wipes
2. Explains procedure, speaking clearly, slowly, and directly, maintaining face-to-face contact whenever possible
3. Performs hand hygiene
4. Provides for privacy
5. Puts on gloves
6. Places a paper towel on the floor
7. Places the graduate on the paper towel
8. Places the graduate under the collection bag
9. Opens the clamp on the drain
10. Lets all urine drain into the graduate—does not let the drain touch the graduate
11. Cleans the end of the drain with antiseptic wipe
12. Closes and positions the clamp
13. Measures urine
14. Removes and discards the paper towel
15. Empties the contents of the graduate into the toilet and flushes
16. Rinses the graduate and empties the rinse into the toilet
17. Cleans and disinfects the graduate and returns the graduate to its proper place
18. Removes the gloves and discards
19. Performs hand hygiene
20. Records the time and amount of urine on the intake and output (I&O) record
21. Provides for comfort
22. Places the signaling device within reach

☐ APPLIES A VEST RESTRAINT (CHAPTER 12)

1. Obtains the correct type and size of restraint from the nurse
2. Performs hand hygiene
3. Explains procedure, speaking clearly, slowly, and directly, maintaining face-to-face contact whenever possible
4. Provides for privacy during procedure with curtain, screen, or door
5. Makes sure the person is comfortable and in good alignment
6. Assists the person to a sitting position. If in a wheelchair, the person is positioned as far back in the wheelchair as possible
7. Applies the restraint over clothing following the manufacturer's instructions—the "V" part of the vest crosses in front
8. Brings the straps through the slots
9. Makes sure the vest is free of wrinkles in the front and back

10. Positions the straps at a 45-degree angle between the wheelchair seat and sides. If in bed, helps the client lie down
11. Makes sure the client is comfortable and in good alignment
12. Secures the straps to the chair or to the moveable part of the bed frame at waist level
13. Uses the buckle or a quick-release tie that can be released with one pull
14. Makes sure the buckle or tie is out of the person's reach
15. Makes sure the vest is snug—slides an open hand between the restraint and the person
16. Places the signaling device within reach
17. Performs hand hygiene

☐ PERFORMS A BACK RUB (MASSAGE) (CHAPTER 17)

1. Performs hand hygiene
2. Explains procedure, speaking clearly, slowly, and directly, maintaining face-to-face contact whenever possible
3. Provides for privacy during procedure with curtain, screen, or door
4. Raises the bed for good body mechanics
5. Lowers the bed rail near the candidate, if up
6. Positions the person in the prone or side-lying position
7. Exposes the back, shoulders, upper arms, and buttocks (if person gives consent) and covers the rest of the body with a bath blanket
8. If person is in side-lying position, lays bath towel on the bed along the back
9. Warms the lotion
10. Explains that lotion may feel cool and wet
11. Using firm strokes, strokes up from buttocks to shoulders, down over the upper arms, up the upper arms, across the shoulders, and down the back to the buttocks, keeping hands in contact with the person's skin
12. Repeats for at least 3 minutes. Kneads the back by grasping the skin between thumb and fingers and going from buttocks up to shoulders on either side of back
13. Applies lotion to bony areas and massages with circular motions using the tips of the index and middle fingers
14. Does not massage reddened, bony areas
15. Strokes with long, firm movements to end the massage and tells the person when candidate is finished
16. Straightens and secures clothing or sleepwear
17. Returns the person to comfortable and safe position and removes the towel and bath blanket
18. Places the signaling device within reach
19. Lowers the bed to its lowest position
20. Raises or lowers bed rails per care plan, returns lotion to proper place, and follows agency policy for dirty linen.
21. Performs hand hygiene

☐ POSITIONS FOLEY CATHETER (CHAPTER 21)

1. Explains procedure, speaking clearly, slowly, and directly, maintaining face-to-face contact whenever possible
2. Performs hand hygiene
3. Puts on gloves
4. Secures catheter and drainage tubing according to facility procedure to maintain connection
5. Places tubing over leg
6. Positions drainage tubing so that urine flows freely into drainage bag and has no kinks
7. Coils the drainage tubing on the bed and secures it to the bottom linen using a clip, bed sheet clamp, tape, pin with rubber band, or other device as the nurse directs
8. Checks for leaks and checks the site where the catheter connects to the drainage bag
9. Attaches bag to bed frame, below level of bladder
10. Performs hand hygiene

☐ APPLIES COLD PACK OR WARM COMPRESS (CHAPTER 28)

1. Performs hand hygiene
2. Collects commercial pack, pack cover, ties, tape, or rolled gauze (if needed)
3. Explains procedure, speaking clearly, slowly, and directly, maintaining face-to-face contact whenever possible
4. Provides for privacy during procedure with curtain, screen, or door
5. Positions the person for the procedure
6. Places the waterproof pad (if needed) under the body part
7. Covers cold pack or warm compress with towel or other protective cover
8. Properly places cold pack or warm compress on site and notes the time
9. Secures the pack in place with ties, tape, rolled gauze, or Velcro straps
10. Checks the person for complications every 5 minutes
11. Checks the cold pack or warm compress every 5 minutes and changes the application if cooling or warming occurs
12. Removes the application at the specified time— usually after 15 to 20 minutes
13. Provides for comfort
14. Places the signaling device within reach
15. Performs hand hygiene

☐ POSITIONS FOR AN ENEMA (CHAPTER 22)

1. Performs hand hygiene
2. Explains procedure, speaking clearly, slowly, and directly, maintaining face-to-face contact whenever possible
3. Provides for privacy

4. Raises the bed and raises the bed rails if used
5. Positions the person in Sims' position or in a left side-lying position
6. Covers the person with bath blanket and fanfolds linens to the foot of the bed
7. Places a waterproof pad under the buttocks
8. Places the signaling device within reach
9. Performs hand hygiene

☐ PREPARES CLIENT FOR A MEAL (CHAPTER 23)

1. Perform hand hygiene
2. Explains procedure, speaking clearly, slowly, and directly, maintaining face-to-face contact whenever possible
3. Assists with oral hygiene, wearing gloves
4. Assists with elimination, wearing gloves
5. Assists with hand washing, wearing gloves
6. Discards gloves and washes hands
7. *If the person will eat in bed:*
   a. Raises the head of the bed to a comfortable position
   b. Removes items from the overbed table and cleans the overbed table
   c. Adjusts the overbed table in front of the person
8. *If the person will sit in a chair:*
   a. Positions the person in a chair or wheelchair
   b. Removes items from the overbed table and cleans the table
   c. Adjusts the overbed table in front of the person
9. Places the signaling device within reach
10. Perform hand hygiene

☐ TAKES AND RECORDS AXILLARY TEMPERATURE, PULSE, AND RESPIRATIONS (CHAPTER 25)

1. Performs hand hygiene
2. Explains procedure, speaking clearly, slowly, and directly, maintaining face-to-face contact whenever possible
3. Provides for the person's privacy during procedure with curtain, screen, or door
4. Positions the person
5. Inserts probe into a probe cover
6. Turns on digital oral thermometer
7. Helps the person remove arm from gown
8. Dries axilla and places thermometer in the center of the axilla
9. Places the person's arm over the chest
10. Holds thermometer in place for appropriate length of time
11. Removes and reads thermometer
12. Records temperature on pad of paper
13. Discards sheath from thermometer
14. Places fingertips on thumb side of the person's wrist to locate radial pulse
15. Notes if the pulse is strong or weak, regular or irregular

16. Counts beats for 1 full minute
17. Records pulse rate on pad of paper
18. Counts respirations for 1 full minute
19. Counts each chest rise and fall as 1 respiration
20. Records respirations on pad of paper
21. Places signaling device within reach
22. Performs hand hygiene

☐ TRANSFERS CLIENT FROM WHEELCHAIR TO BED (CHAPTER 16)

1. Performs hand hygiene
2. Explains procedure, speaking clearly, slowly, and directly, maintaining face-to-face contact whenever possible
3. Provides for privacy during procedure with curtain, screen, or door
4. Lowers bed
5. Raises head of bed to sitting position
6. Positions wheelchair close to bed so that person's strong side is next to the bed
7. Before transferring client, ensures client is wearing non-skid footwear
8. Folds up footplates
9. Before transferring the person, locks wheels on wheelchair and locks bed brakes
10. Removes and folds lap blanket
11. *With transfer (gait) belt:* Stands in front of client, positioning self to ensure safety of candidate and client during transfer (e.g., knees bent, feet apart, back straight), places belt around the person's waist, and grasps belt. Tightens belt so that fingers of candidate's hand can be slipped between transfer/gait belt and the person *Without transfer belt:* Stands in front of the person, positioning self to ensure safety of candidate and the person during transfer (e.g., knees bent, feet apart, back straight, arms around the person's torso under arms)
12. Provides instructions to enable the person to assist in transfer, including prearranged signal to alert the person to begin standing
13. Has the person hold on to armrests and lean forward
14. Grasps the transfer belt on each side if using it. Grasps underneath the belt
15. Braces the person's lower extremities with foot, knees, or leg to prevent sliding or falling
16. Counts to three (or says other prearranged signal) to alert the person to begin transfer
17. On signal, gradually assists the person to stand by pulling and straightening knees
18. Supports the person in standing position
19. Assists the person to pivot to edge of mattress. The legs touch mattress
20. Turns the person until the person can reach the mattress with both hands
21. Lowers the person onto bed as candidate bends hips and knees
22. Removes transfer belt, if used

23. Assists the person to remove non-skid footwear
24. Assists the person to move to center of bed
25. Provides for comfort and good body alignment
26. Places signaling device within reach
27. Performs hand hygiene

☐ WEIGHS AND MEASURES HEIGHT OF AN AMBULATORY CLIENT (CHAPTER 25)

1. Performs hand hygiene
2. Explains procedure, speaking clearly, slowly, and directly, maintaining face-to-face contact whenever possible
3. Asks the person to void
4. Starts with scale balanced at zero before weighing the person
5. Places paper towels on the scale platform
6. Has the person remove robe and footwear, assisting as needed
7. Assists the person to step up onto center of scale and place arms at sides
8. Determines the person's weight and height
9. Assists the person off scale before recording weight and height
10. Helps the person put on robe and footwear if client will be up
11. Places signaling device within reach
12. Records weight and height within required range
13. Discards paper towels
14. Perform hand hygiene

AFTER A PROCEDURE

- After you demonstrate a skill, complete a safety check of the room.
  - The person is wearing eyeglasses, hearing aids, and other devices as needed.
  - The signaling device is plugged in and within reach.
  - Bed rails are up or down according to the care plan.
  - The bed is in the lowest horizontal position.
  - The bed position is locked if needed.
  - Manual bed cranks are in the down position.
  - Bed wheels are locked.
  - Assistive devices are within reach. Walker, cane, and wheelchair are examples.
  - The overbed table, filled water pitcher and cup, tissues, phone, TV controls, and other needed items are within reach.
  - Unneeded equipment is unplugged or turned off.
  - Harmful substances are stored properly. Lotion, mouthwash, shampoo, after-shave, and other personal care products are examples.

AFTER THE TEST

Celebrate—you have completed the competency evaluation! The length of time for you to get your test results varies with each state. In the meantime, try to relax. Continue your daily routine and be the best nursing assistant you can be.

ANSWERS TO REVIEW QUESTIONS IN TEXTBOOK CHAPTERS REVIEW

Chapter 1
1. c
2. b
3. b

Chapter 2
1. d
2. a
3. b

Chapter 3
1. b
2. a
3. a
4. b
5. d
6. a
7. b
8. b

Chapter 4
1. c
2. c
3. b
4. a
5. d
6. b
7. c

Chapter 5
1. c
2. c
3. a
4. d
5. d
6. b

Chapter 6
1. a
2. c
3. d

Chapter 7
1. b
2. d
3. d
4. c
5. d
6. b
7. a
8. c
9. d
10. c
11. c
12. d
13. a
14. b

Chapter 8
1. b
2. d
3. c
4. b
5. d
6. a
7. b
8. a

Chapter 9
1. d
2. c
3. c
4. d
5. c
6. d
7. d
8. a

Chapter 10
1. b
2. d
3. a
4. d
5. c
6. c
7. b
8. b
9. c
10. b

Chapter 11
1. a
2. d
3. b
4. c
5. c
6. c

Chapter 12
1. a
2. c
3. a
4. a
5. b
6. b

Chapter 13
1. b
2. d
3. d
4. a
5. a
6. c

Chapter 14
1. c
2. b
3. c
4. c

Chapter 15
1. c
2. a
3. c

Chapter 16
1. b
2. a
3. d

Chapter 17
1. a
2. a
3. a
4. c
5. b
6. c
7. d
8. b
9. a
10. a
11. d
12. c
13. c
14. d
15. d

Chapter 18
1. c
2. d
3. b
4. d
5. c
6. b
7. a
8. c
9. a
10. a

Chapter 19
1. a
2. b
3. a
4. a
5. b
6. a
7. a
8. a
9. b
10. b
11. d

Chapter 20
1. b
2. d
3. c
4. c

Chapter 21
1. a
2. b
3. c

Chapter 22
1. b
2. d
3. d
4. a

Chapter 23
1. d
2. a
3. b
4. d
5. d

Chapter 24
1. c
2. a
3. a
4. b
5. a
6. c
7. c

Chapter 25
1. b
2. a
3. b
4. b
5. d
6. d

Chapter 26
1. d
2. a
3. a
4. b

Chapter 27
1. c
2. a
3. b
4. a

450

Chapter 28
1. d
2. c
3. d
4. b
5. d
6. c

Chapter 29
1. c
2. c
3. a
4. a

Chapter 30
1. c
2. b
3. a
4. c
5. d

Chapter 31
1. a
2. a
3. d
4. a
5. b

Chapter 32
1. c
2. b
3. a
4. a

Chapter 33
1. b
2. d
3. a
4. a
5. b
6. b
7. d
8. c
9. a
10. c
11. c
12. a
13. b
14. b
15. a
16. d
17. c
18. a

Chapter 34
1. a
2. a
3. a
4. c
5. d

Chapter 35
1. c
2. d
3. a
4. d

Chapter 36
1. c
2. a
3. b
4. c

Chapter 37
1. d
2. c
3. b
4. d
5. a

Chapter 38
1. a
2. d
3. b

1. **C** You never give drugs. You may politely refuse to do a task that you have not been trained to do. However, you need to tell the nurse. Do not ignore a request to do something. Page 27, Chapter 3.

2. **A** An ethical person does not judge others or cause harm to another person. Ethical behavior involves not being prejudiced or biased. Ethical behavior also involves not avoiding persons whose standards and values are different from your own. Page 31, Chapter 4.

3. **D** An ethical person is knowledgeable of what is right conduct and wrong conduct. Health care workers do not drink alcohol before coming to work and do not drink alcohol while working. Page 31, Chapter 4.

4. **A** Neglect is failure to provide a person with the goods or services needed to avoid physical harm, mental anguish, or mental illness. Page 36, Chapter 4.

5. **B** The person's information is confidential. Information about the patient or resident is shared only among health team members involved in his or her care. Page 46, Chapter 5.

6. **D** End-of-shift is a time for good teamwork. Continue to do your job. Your attitude is important. Page 45, Chapter 5.

7. **C** Write in ink, spell words correctly, and use only agency-approved abbreviations. Page 60, Chapter 6.

8. **B** Give a courteous greeting. End the conversation politely and say good-bye. Confidential information about a resident or employee is not given to any caller. Page 63, Chapter 6.

9. **C** Safety and security needs relate to feeling safe from harm, danger, and fear. Health care agencies are strange places with strange routines and equipment. People feel safer if they know what to expect. Be kind and understanding. Show the person the nursing center, listen to his or her concerns, and explain routines and procedures. Page 69, Chapter 7.

10. **B** When a person is angry or hostile, stay calm and professional. The person is usually not angry with you. He or she may be angry at another person or situation. Page 77, Chapter 7.

11. **D** Use words that are familiar to the person. Speak clearly, slowly, and distinctly. Also, ask one question at a time and wait for an answer. Page 11, Chapter 7.

12. **D** Follow the manufacturer's instructions. The excess strap should be tucked under the belt. The belt is applied over clothing and under the breasts. Page 128, Chapter 11.

13. **D** Listening requires that you care and have interest in the other person. Have good eye contact with the person. Focus on what the person is saying. Page 73, Chapter 7.

14. **C** Assume that a comatose person hears and understands you. Talk to the person and tell him or her what you are going to do. Page 75, Chapter 7.

15. **A** Protect a person's right to privacy when giving care. Politely ask visitors to leave the room. Do not expose the person's body in front of them. Show visitors where to wait. Page 76, Chapter 7.

16. **B** If a person wants to talk with a minister or spiritual leader, tell the nurse. Many people get comfort and strength from prayer and religious practices. Page 70, Chapter 7.

17. **A** Observe the person with a restraint at least every 15 minutes. Remove the restraint and reposition the person every 2 hours. Apply a restraint so that it is snug and firm but not tight. You could be negligent if the restraint is not applied properly. Page 137, Chapter 12.

18. **D** The skin becomes more dry, muscle strength decreases, reflexes are slower, and bladder muscles weaken. Pages 101–102, Chapter 9.

19. **B** Always act in a professional manner. Page 104, Chapter 9.

20. **C** Push the chair forward when transporting the person. Do not pull the chair backward unless going through a doorway. Page 205, Chapter 16.

21. **A** Tell the nurse at once. It is important to do the correct procedure on the right person. You have to be able to read the person's name on the ID bracelet or use the photo ID to identify the person. Page 109, Chapter 10.

22. **B** Clutching at the throat is the "universal sign of choking." Page 111, Chapter 10.

23. **D** When a person is on a diabetic diet, tell the nurse about changes in the person's eating habits. The person's meals and snacks need to be served on time. The person needs to eat at regular intervals to maintain a certain blood sugar. Always check the tray to see what was eaten. Page 338, Chapter 23.

24. **D** With mild airway obstruction, the person is conscious and can speak. Often forceful coughing can remove the object. Page 111, Chapter 10.

25. **A** Abdominal thrusts are used to relieve severe airway obstruction. Page 111, Chapter 10.

26. **B** Do not use faulty electrical equipment in nursing centers. Take the item to the nurse. Page 114, Chapter 10.

27. **C** If a warning label is removed or damaged, do not use the substance. Take the container to the nurse and explain the problem. Page 115, Chapter 10.

28. **C** An ethical person realizes a person's values and standards may be different from his or hers. Page 77, Chapter 7.

29. **D** Remind a person not to smoke inside the center. Page 116, Chapter 10.

30. **A** During a fire, remember the word RACE. Page 116, Chapter 10.

31. **C** If a person with Alzheimer's disease has sundowning (increased restlessness and confusion as daylight ends), provide a calm, quiet setting late in the day. Do not try to reason with the person because he or she cannot understand what you are saying. Do not ask the person to tell you what is bothering him or her. Communication is impaired. Complete treatments and activities early in the day. Page 513, Chapter 35.

32. **C** Make sure dentures fit properly. Cut food into small pieces and make sure the person can chew and swallow the food served. Report loose teeth or dentures to the nurse. Page 111, Chapter 10.

33. **A** Lock both wheels before you transfer a person to and from the wheelchair. The person's feet are on the footplates before moving the chair. Do not let the person stand on the footplates. Page 205, Chapter 16.

34. **B** Ease the person to the floor. Do not try to prevent the fall or yell at the person. The person should not get up before the nurse checks for injuries. Therefore the nurse needs to be told as soon as the fall occurs. Page 130, Chapter 11.

35. **B** Death from strangulation is the most serious risk factor when using a restraint. Restraints are not used for staff convenience or to punish a person. A written doctor's order is required before a restraint can be applied. Page 136, Chapter 12.

36. **C** Wash your hands before and after giving care to a person. Page 154, Chapter 13.

37. **D** Gloves need to be changed when they become contaminated with blood, body fluids, secretions, and excretions. Page 159, Chapter 13.

38. **D** When washing your hands, keep your hands and forearms lower than your elbows. Do not use hot water or let your uniform touch the sink. Push your watch up your arm so that you can wash past your wrist. Page 154, Chapter 13.

39. **C** Bend your knees and squat to lift a heavy object. Hold items close to your body when lifting a heavy object. For a wider base of support and more balance, stand with your feet apart. Do not bend from your waist when lifting objects. Page 174, Chapter 14.

40. **B** The head of the bed is raised between 45 and 60 degrees for Fowler's position. Page 224, Chapter 17.

41. **B** Negligence—an unintentional wrong in which a person did not act in a reasonable and careful manner and causes harm to a person or the person's property. Page 36, Chapter 4.

42. **A** Have the person's back and buttocks against the back of the chair. Feet are flat on the floor or on the wheelchair footplates. The backs of the person's knees and calves are slightly away from the edge of the seat. Page 182, Chapter 14.

43. **B** Help the person out of bed on his or her strong side. In transferring, the strong side moves first. It pulls the weaker side along. Page 206, Chapter 16.

44. **A** When a person tries to bite, scratch, pinch, or kick you, you need to protect the person, others, and yourself from harm. Page 77, Chapter 7.

45. **B** Protect the person's right to privacy at all times. Screen the person properly, and do not expose body parts. Page 189, Chapter 15.

46. **D** For comfort, adjust lighting to meet the person's changing needs. Nursing centers maintain a temperature range of 71°F to 81°F. Unpleasant odors may be offensive or embarrassing to people. Many older persons are sensitive to noise. Page 222, Chapter 17.

47. **A** Call lights are placed on the person's strong side and kept within the person's reach. Call lights are answered promptly. Page 228, Chapter 17.

48. **C** You must have the person's permission to open or search closets or drawers. Page 229, Chapter 17.

49. **C** When handling linens, do not take unneeded linen to a person's room. Once in the room, extra linen is considered contaminated. Because your uniform is considered dirty, always hold linen away from your body. To prevent the spread of microbes, never shake linen. Never put clean or dirty linens on the floor. Page 231, Chapter 17.

50. **C** To use a fire extinguisher, remember the word PASS. P—pull the safety pin, A—aim low, S—squeeze the lever, S—sweep back and forth. Page 117, Chapter 10.

51. **B** Mouth care is given at least every 2 hours for an unconscious person. To prevent aspiration, you position the person on one side with the head turned well to the side. Use a padded tongue blade to keep the person's mouth open. Wear gloves. Page 252, Chapter 18.

52. **B** A good attitude is needed at work. Be willing to help others. Be pleasant and respectful of others. Page 45, Chapter 5.

53. **B** During cleaning, firmly hold dentures over a basin of water lined with a towel. This prevents them from falling onto a hard surface and breaking. Clean and store dentures in cool water. Hot water causes dentures to lose their shape. To prevent losing dentures, label the denture cup with the person's name. Page 255, Chapter 18.

54. **C** Report and record the location and description of the rash. Page 257, Chapter 18.

55. **C** Gently wipe the eye from the inner aspect to the outer aspect of the eye. Clean the far eye first. Do not use soap. Page 259, Chapter 18.

56. **D** When giving a back massage, wear gloves if the person's skin has open areas. Warm the lotion before applying it to the person. Use firm strokes. Do not massage reddened bony areas. This can lead to more tissue damage. Page 242, Chapter 17.
57. **A** Separate the labia and clean downward from front to back. Wear gloves and use soap. Page 269, Chapter 18.
58. **C** Stay within hearing distance if the person can be left alone. Place the call light within the person's reach. Cold water is turned on first, then hot water. Direct water away from the person while adjusting the water temperature. Page 263, Chapter 18.
59. **B** Electric razors are used when a person is on an anticoagulant. An anticoagulant prevents or slows down blood clotting. Bleeding occurs easily. A nick or cut from a safety razor can cause bleeding. Page 279, Chapter 19.
60. **B** Remove clothing from the strong or "good" (unaffected) side first. Page 284, Chapter 19.
61. **C** Address a person with dignity and respect. Call the person by his or her title—Mr. or Mrs. or Miss. Address a person by his or her first name, or another name, if the person asks you to do so. Page 14, Chapter 2.
62. **D** Measure and record the amount of urine in the drainage bag. The catheter is secured to the person's thigh or abdomen. Do not disconnect the catheter from the drainage tubing. Do not let the person lie on the tubing. Page 311, Chapter 21.
63. **B** Carbohydrates provide energy and fiber for bowel elimination. Page 334, Chapter 23.
64. **D** When taking a rectal temperature, the thermometer is held in place so that it is not lost into the rectum or broken. Lubricate the bulb end of the thermometer for easy insertion and to prevent tissue damage. Provide for privacy. A glass thermometer remains in place for 2 minutes or as required by policy. Page 363, 367, Chapter 25.
65. **A** Report any systolic pressure below 90 mm Hg and any diastolic pressure below 60 mm Hg at once. Record the BP. It is your responsibility to tell the nurse. Page 373, Chapter 25.
66. **D** Oral temperatures are not taken on unconscious persons, persons receiving oxygen, or persons who breathe through their mouth. Page 361, Chapter 25.
67. **A** To assist with walking, offer the person your arm and have the person walk a half step behind you. When caring for a person who is blind or visually impaired, let the person do as much for himself or herself as possible. Use a normal voice tone. Do not shout at the person. Identify yourself when you enter the room. Do not touch the person until you have indicated your presence. Page 464, Chapter 32.
68. **D** The person with confusion and dementia has the right to personal choice. He or she also has the right to keep and use personal items. The family makes choices if the person cannot. Page 516, Chapter 35.
69. **D** Discuss your feelings with the nurse. No one can shout, scream, or hit the person. Nor can they call the person names. The person did not choose loss of function. Page 456, Chapter 31.
70. **C** Encourage the person to help as much as possible. Doors and windows are closed to reduce drafts. You wash from the cleanest areas to the dirtiest areas. Pat the skin dry to avoid irritating or breaking the skin. Page 257, Chapter 18.
71. **A** When a person is dying, always assume that the person can hear you. Reposition the person every 2 hours to promote comfort. Skin care, personal hygiene, back massages, oral hygiene, and good body alignment promote comfort. Page 536, Chapter 37.
72. **B** Foods that melt at room temperature (ice cream, sherbet, custard, pudding, gelatin, and Popsicles) are measured and recorded as intake. The nurse measures and records IV fluids and tube feedings. Page 350, Chapter 24.
73. **B** After bedrest, activity increases slowly and in steps. First the person dangles. Sitting in a chair follows. Next the person walks in the room and then in the hallway. Page 397, Chapter 27.
74. **B** Tell the nurse at once if you find or cause a skin tear. Page 412, Chapter 28.
75. **A** Treat the resident with respect and ensure privacy. The resident has a right not to have his or her private affairs exposed or made public without giving consent. Only staff involved in the resident's care should see, handle, or examine his or her body. Page 12, Chapter 2.

ANSWERS TO PRACTICE EXAMINATION 2

1. **C** You may politely refuse to do a task that is not in your job description. Page 27, Chapter 3.
2. **B** An ethical person realizes a person's values and standards may be different from his or hers. You may not agree with advance directives or resuscitation decisions. However, you must respect the person's wishes. Page 540, Chapter 37.
3. **C** Verbal abuse is using oral or written words or statements that speak badly of, sneer at, criticize, or condemn a person. Page 36–37, Chapter 4.
4. **C** Speak in a normal tone. Use words the person seems to understand and speak slowly and distinctly. Page 75, Chapter 7.
5. **C** Do not allow smoking in bed. Turn cold water on first, then hot water. Assist the person with drinking or eating hot food. Do not let the person sleep with a heating pad. Page 110, Chapter 10.
6. **B** Use three-pronged plugs on all electrical devices and follow the manufacturer's instructions on equipment. Wipe up spills right away. Do not use unfamiliar equipment. Ask for training if you are unfamiliar with something. Page 114, Chapter 10.
7. **D** Answer call lights promptly. Throw rugs, scatter rugs, and area rugs are not used. The person's bed should be in the lowest horizontal position, except when giving care. Grab bars should be used when the person showers. Page 124, Chapter 11.
8. **B** Decontaminate your hands after removing gloves. Page 154, Chapter 13.
9. **D** Sometimes multiple people or a mechanical lift is needed for moving and turning persons in bed. Page 189, Chapter 15.
10. **C** A person must not put his or her arms around your neck. He or she can pull you forward or cause you to lose your balance. Neck, back, and other injuries from falls are possible. Ask a co-worker to help you, and you should use a transfer or gait belt. Lock the wheels on the wheelchair. Page 208, Chapter 16.
11. **B** Wear gloves when removing linen. Linens may contain blood, body fluids, secretions, or excretions. Raise the bed for good body mechanics. The bed is flat when you place clean linens on it. Page 233, Chapter 17.
12. **B** Use a circular motion, start at the meatus, and work outward. Gloves are worn. Soap is used. Page 270, Chapter 18.
13. **C** Put clothing on the weak (affected) side first. Page 284, Chapter 19.
14. **D** The drainage bag hangs from the bed frame or chair. It must not touch the floor. The bag is always kept lower than the person's bladder. The drainage bag does not hang on the bed rail. Page 311, Chapter 21.
15. **A** Protein is needed for tissue repair and growth. Page 334, Chapter 23.
16. **C** Older persons may not feel thirsty (decreased sense of thirst). Offer water often. Page 350, Chapter 24.
17. **C** NPO means nothing by mouth. An NPO sign is posted above the bed. The water pitcher and glass are removed from the room. Oral hygiene is performed frequently. Page 350, Chapter 24.
18. **C** 1 oz equals 30 mL. 3 oz equals 90 mL. Page 350, Chapter 24.
19. **D** Allow time for chewing and swallowing. Fluids are offered during the meal. A teaspoon, rather than a fork, is used for feeding. Sit and talk with the person. Pages 343, Chapter 23.
20. **D** Support the part being exercised. Do not force a joint beyond its present ROM. Move the joint slowly, smoothly, and gently. Do not force the joint to the point of pain. Page 399, Chapter 27.
21. **B** A cane is held on the strong side of the body. If the left leg is weak, the cane is held in the right hand. Page 405, Chapter 27.
22. **B** Position the person in good alignment. Bed linens are kept tight and wrinkle free. Talk softly and gently. Avoid sudden and jarring movements of the bed or chair. Page 241, Chapter 17.
23. **C** Check behind the ears and under the nose for signs of irritation. Never remove an oxygen device. Do not adjust the oxygen flow rate. Do not fill the humidifier. Page 449, Chapter 30.
24. **A** Tell the nurse at once. Mercury is a hazardous substance. Do not touch the mercury. Follow special procedures for handling hazardous materials. Page 367, Chapter 25.
25. **C** Record and report at once a pulse rate less than 60 or more than 100 beats per minute. The radial pulse is used for routine vital signs. If the pulse is irregular, count it for 1 minute. Do not use your thumb to take a pulse. Page 369, Chapter 25.
26. **B** Count the respirations for 1 minute if an abnormal breathing pattern is noted. People change their breathing patterns when they know respirations are being counted. Therefore the person should not know that you are counting respirations. The healthy adult has 12 to 20 respirations per minute. Page 372, Chapter 25.
27. **A** Report at once any systolic pressure above 120 mm Hg and any diastolic pressure above 80 mm Hg. Record the BP. It is your responsibility to tell the nurse. Page 373, Chapter 25.

28. **C** Rectal temperatures are not taken if a person has diarrhea, is confused, or is agitated. Page 361, Chapter 25.

29. **C** Residents must be cared for in a manner that promotes dignity and self-esteem. Use the right tone of voice. Respect private space and property. Listen to the person with interest. Knock on the door and wait to be asked in before entering. Page 14, Chapter 2.

30. **B** Have the person void before being weighed. A full bladder adds weight. No footwear is worn. Footwear adds to the weight and height measurements. Weigh the person at the same time of day, usually before breakfast. Balance the scale before weighing the person. Page 379, Chapter 25.

31. **D** Keep the skin free of moisture from urine, stools, or perspiration. Reposition the person at least every 2 hours. Do not massage reddened areas. Keep the heels and ankles off the bed. Page 436, Chapter 29.

32. **C** Face the person when speaking. Reduce or eliminate background noise. Speak in a normal voice tone. Speak clearly, distinctly, and slowly. Page 460, Chapter 32.

33. **C** Explain the location of food and beverages. Keep furniture and equipment out of areas where the person walks. Provide lighting as the person prefers. Do not rearrange furniture and equipment. Page 464, Chapter 32.

34. **C** The person with confusion and dementia has the right to privacy and confidentiality. Information about the person's care and condition is shared only with those involved in providing the care. Protect the person from exposure. Page 517, Chapter 35.

35. **C** Ask clear, simple questions. Explain what you are going to do and why. Call the person by name every time you are in contact with him or her. Keep calendars and clocks in the person's room. Page 505, Chapter 35.

36. **D** Exercise the person as ordered. Adequate exercise often reduces wandering. Do not keep the person in his or her room. Involve the person in activities. Do not restrain the person or argue with the person who wants to leave. Page 513, Chapter 35.

37. **B** Restorative nursing programs promote self-care measures. They help maintain the person's highest level of function. The programs focus on the whole person. The care helps the person regain health, strength, and independence. Page 452, Chapter 31.

38. **C** Remind the person of his or her progress in the rehabilitation program. Focus on the person's abilities and strengths. Progress may be slow. Do not deny the disability. Page 455, Chapter 31.

39. **D** Respect the person's right to privacy. Do not expose the person's body unnecessarily. Only those involved in the person's care need to know the person's diagnosis. The final moments of death are kept confidential. So are family reactions. Page 530, Chapter 37.

40. **A** Remember the word RACE. Your first action is to Rescue the person in immediate danger. Then sound the Alarm, Confine the fire, and Extinguish the fire. Page 116, Chapter 10.

41. **B** Failure to provide a person with the goods or services needed to avoid physical harm or mental anguish is neglect. Page 36, Chapter 4.

42. **C** You have not been trained to give drugs or perform sterile procedures. Do not perform tasks that are not in your job description. Page 27, Chapter 3.

43. **C** Ask the nurse to observe urine that looks or smells abnormal. Then record your observation. Page 295, Chapter 20.

44. **D** A good attitude is needed at work. People rely on you to give good care. You are expected to be pleasant and respectful. Always be willing to help others. Page 45, Chapter 5.

45. **B** Unnecessary restraint is false imprisonment. Observe the person for complications every 15 minutes. The least restrictive type of restraint is ordered by the doctor. Restraints can increase confusion and agitation. Page 137, Chapter 12.

46. **C** The supine position is the back-lying position. For good alignment, the bed is flat and the head and shoulders are supported on a pillow. Place arms and hands at the sides. Page 180, Chapter 14.

47. **A** Hand washing is the most important way to prevent or avoid spreading infection. Page 153, Chapter 13.

48. **B** To gossip means to spread rumors or talk about the private matters of others. Gossiping is unprofessional and hurtful. If others are gossiping, you need to remove yourself from the group. Do not make or repeat any comment that can hurt another person. Page 46, Chapter 5.

49. **D** Ask a co-worker to help you. The head of the bed is lowered. The person flexes both knees. Friction and shearing cause skin tears and need to be prevented. Page 188, Chapter 15.

50. **A** On a sodium-controlled diet, high-sodium foods such as ham and canned vegetables are omitted. Salt is not added to food at the table. The amount of salt used in cooking is limited. Page 338, Chapter 23.

51. **B** Elastic stockings should not have wrinkles or creases after being applied. Wrinkles and creases can cause skin breakdown. Apply stockings before the person gets out of bed. Apply the correct size. Page 415, Chapter 28.

52. **C** When a person begins to fall, ease him or her to the floor. Also protect the person's head. Page 130, Chapter 11.

53. **A** Before bathing, allow the person to use the bathroom, bedpan, or urinal. Page 256, Chapter 18.

54. **A** Insert a glass thermometer 1 inch into the rectum. An electronic thermometer is inserted ½ inch into the rectum. Page 367, Chapter 25.

55. **A** Touch is a form of nonverbal communication. It conveys comfort and caring. Touch means different things to different people. Some people do not like to be touched. Page 71, Chapter 7.

56. **A** A person's information is confidential. The information is shared only among health team members involved in the person's care. Page 46, Chapter 5.

57. **A** Report and record complaints of urgency, burning, dysuria, or other urinary problems. Page 295, Chapter 20.

58. **C** Respect a person's culture and religion. Learn about his or her beliefs and practices. This helps you understand the person and give better care. Page 77, Chapter 7.

59. **C** Wear gloves when giving perineal care. Gloves are needed whenever contact with blood, body fluids, secretions, excretions, mucous membranes, and non-intact skin is likely. Pages 159, Chapter 13.

60. **D** Report any changes from normal or changes in the person's condition to the nurse at once. Then record your observation. Page 59, Chapter 6.

61. **A** If a person is standing, have him or her sit before fainting occurs. Page 528, Chapter 36.

62. **A** The person drinks an increased amount of fluid. Keep fluids within the person's reach. Offer fluids regularly. Page 350, Chapter 24.

63. **B** Communication fails when you talk too much and fail to listen. Page 75, Chapter 7.

64. **A** During bathing, a person has the right to privacy and the right to personal choice. Page 256, Chapter 18.

65. **C** People in late adulthood need to develop new friends and relationships. They need to adjust to retirement and reduced income, decreased strength, and loss of health. They need to cope with a partner's death and prepare for their own death. Page 99, Chapter 9.

66. **D** Blood pressure is not taken on an arm with an IV (intravenous) infusion. When taking a blood pressure, apply the cuff to the bare upper arm. Make sure the room is quiet. Talking, TV, radio, and sounds from the hallway can affect an accurate measurement. Place the diaphragm of the stethoscope over the brachial artery. Page 375, Chapter 25.

67. **C** Never put clean or dirty linen on the floor. The floor is dirty. You cannot use the linen. Page 245, Chapter 17.

68. **B** To prevent aspiration, position the unconscious person on one side when you do mouth care. Use a small amount of fluid to clean the mouth. Tell the person what you are doing. Dentures are not worn when the person is unconscious. Pages 252, Chapter 18.

69. **B** Encourage people to do their own hair care. Do not cut matted or tangled hair. The person chooses his or her hairstyle. Brushing and combing are done with morning care and whenever needed. Page 275, Chapter 19.

70. **D** Check between the toes for cracks and sores. These areas are often overlooked. If left untreated, a serious infection could occur. Fingernails are cut with nail clippers, not scissors. You do not trim or cut toenails if a person has diabetes or poor circulation. Page 282, Chapter 19.

71. **B** If an indwelling catheter becomes disconnected from the drainage system, you tell the nurse at once. Page 314, Chapter 21.

72. **B** Urinary drainage bags are emptied, and the contents measured at the end of each shift. Drainage bags must not touch the floor. The bag is always kept lower than the person's bladder. Page 311, Chapter 21.

73. **C** Use elastic tape to secure a condom catheter. Elastic tape expands when the penis changes size and adhesive tape does not. Do not apply a condom catheter if the penis is red and irritated. Always act in a professional manner. Page 316, Chapter 21.

74. **D** For comfort during bowel elimination, leave the person alone if possible. Provide for privacy. Help the person to the toilet or commode if possible. Page 322, Chapter 22.

75. **A** Help the person from the wheelchair to the bed on his or her strong side. In transferring, the strong side moves first. It pulls the weaker side along. Page 210, Chapter 16.